Addictions: Pathology and Physiology

Addictions: Pathology and Physiology

Edited by **Don Boles**

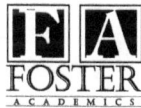

FA FOSTER
A C A D E M I C S

New Jersey

Published by Foster Academics,
61 Van Reypen Street,
Jersey City, NJ 07306, USA
www.fosteracademics.com

Addictions: Pathology and Physiology
Edited by Don Boles

International Standard Book Number: 978-1-63242-017-6 (Hardback)

Printed in the United States of America.

Contents

Preface

This book has been an outcome of determined endeavour from a group of educationists in the field. The primary objective was to involve a broad spectrum of professionals from diverse cultural background involved in the field for developing new researches. The book not only targets students but also scholars pursuing higher research for further enhancement of the theoretical and practical applications of the subject.

Addiction, increasingly discerned as a heterogeneous brain disorder, is one of the most distinct psychiatric pathologies in that its management includes often non-overlapping, resources from the biological, psychological, medical, economic, social, and legal realms. Despite various researches, till now there are no dependably effective treatments of addiction. This may result from a lack of acknowledgement of the etiology and pathophysiology of this disease and also from the lack of concern into the potential differences among patients in the way they interact compulsively with their drug. This book presents an outlook of general considerations and pathophysiology of addiction. The information available in this book would serve as a valuable guide for those involved in the field of addiction control.

It was an honour to edit such a profound book and also a challenging task to compile and examine all the relevant data for accuracy and originality. I wish to acknowledge the efforts of the contributors for submitting such brilliant and diverse chapters in the field and for endlessly working for the completion of the book. Last, but not the least; I thank my family for being a constant source of support in all my research endeavours.

Editor

General Considerations

Animal Models of Drug Addiction

Aude Belin-Rauscent and David Belin
INSERM U 1084, LNEC, Université de Poitiers,
INSERM AVENIR Team "Psychology of Compulsive Disorders", Poitiers,
France

1. Introduction

The study of drug addiction integrates a broad range of research fields including social sciences, psychology, psychiatry, behavioural neurosciences, pharmacology or genetics, each of which being represented in the different chapters of this book. Preclinical studies involving behaving animals have been pivotal for our increasing insights into the psychobiological substrates of addiction and so for about 100 years. Even today, our understanding and knowledge of addiction increase in parallel with the refinement of animal models of this pathology.

1.1 Necessity for animal models in drug addiction research

Whilst animal models can never reproduce the complex social and often personal reasons why people abuse drugs they nevertheless provide a rigorous means to precisely control environmental context, drug exposure as well as assessing behavioural and cognitive performance prior to drug administration. They also allow neural manipulations (e.g., using selective ligands) and so establish the causal influences of putative neural loci and, in turn, the cellular and molecular substrates, of drug addiction. Thus, to date, animal models provide a valuable means to investigate the different stages of the drug addiction cycle including especially the initiation of drug taking, the maintenance phase, which is often accompanied by binges and escalation of drug intake, and finally the switch to compulsive drug intake defined operationally by an increased motivation to take the drug, an inability to inhibit drug seeking and continued dug use despite negative or adverse consequences.

1.2 Definition and validity criteria of animal models

1.2.1 Definition of an animal model

An animal model is a preparation in one organism that allows for the study of one or several aspects of a human condition. Thus a model of drug addiction must provide insights into the neurobiological, psychological or etiological mechanisms of the pathology in humans, at least mimicking some aspects of the pathology.

Two strategies are generally used when designing animal models of drug addiction. Firstly, the model can address a specific symptom, a neurobiological or psychological feature or a behavioural / neurobiological construct associated with the pathology (figure 1).

DSM-IV diagnostic criteria for drug addiction	Psychobiological dimension	Monodimensional animal model	Polydimensional animal model
[1] Need for markedly increased amounts of a substance to achieve intoxication or desired effect, or markedly diminished effect with continued use of the same amount of the substance	Pharmacological tolerance		
[2] The presence of a characteristic withdrawal syndrome or use of a substance (or a closely related substance) to relieve or avoid withdrawal symptoms	Negative affect/mood depression, anhedonia, anxiety		
[3] Persistent desire to use drugs or one or more unsuccessful efforts to cut or control substance use	Impulsivity / compulsivity behavioural control failure	Reinstatement [1-4] Relapse [5]	3-criteria model of drug addiction: inability to refrain from drug-seeking [14-16]
[4] Substance used in larger amounts or over a longer period time than the person intented	Impulsivity / compulsivity behavioural control failure	Escalation of drug intake [6-7]	3-criteria model of drug addiction: escalation of drug intake during long access to cocaine [14-16]
[5] Important social, occupational, or recreational activities given up or reduced because of substance use	Impulsivity / compulsivity behavioural control failure	Resistance to punishment [8] Resistance to conditioned suppression [9]	
[6] A great deal of time spent in activities necessary to obtain, to use or to recover from the effects of substance used	Habit / compulsivity	Progressive ratio seeking-taking and second order schedule of reinforcement [10-13]	3-criteria model of drug addiction: increased break points in a progressive ratio schedule of reinforcement [14-16]
[7] Continued substance use despite knowledge of having a persistent or recurrent physical or psychological problem that is likely to be caused or exacerbated by continued use	Compulsivity	Resistance to punishment [8] Resistance to conditioned suppression [9]	3-criteria model of drug addiction: resistance to punishment or adverse consequences [14-16]

Fig. 1. Animal models of drug addiction in reference to the DSM IV diagnostic criteria for drug addiction (adapted from the DSM-IV [97]))

{1} Stewart J. & De Wit H. (1987). *Methods of assessing the reinforcing properties of abused drugs*, (M.A.Bozarth, Ed.). 211-227. Springer-Verlag, New-York.

{2} Shaham Y., Erb S. & Stewart J. (2000). *Brain research review*, 33: 13-33

{3} Grimm J.W., Hope B.T., Wise R.A. & Shaham Y. (2001). *Nature*, 412: 141-142

{4} Bossert J.M., Liu S.Y., Lu L. & shaham Y. (2004). *J. Neurosci.*, **24**(47): 10726-30

{5} Fuchs R.A., Branham R.K. & See R.E. (2006). *J. Neurosci.*, **26**(13): 3584-8

{6} Ahmed S.H. & Koob G.F. (1998). *Science*, **282**(5387): 298-300

{7} Ahmed S.H., Walker J.R. & Koob G.F. (2000). *Neuropsychopharmacology*, **22**(4):413-421

{8} Pelloux Y., Everitt B.J. & Dickinson A. (2007). *Psychopharmacology*, **194**(1): 127-137

{9} Vanderschuren L.J. & Everitt B.J. (2004). *Science*, **305**(5686): 1017-1019

{10} Goldberg S.R., Morse W.H. & Goldberg D.M. (1976). *J Pharmacol Exp Ther*, **199**(1): 278-286

{11} Arroyo M., Markou A., Robbins T.W. & Everitt B.J. (1998). *Psychopharmacology*, **140**(3): 331-344

{12} Everitt B.J. & Robbins T.W. (2000). *Psychopharmacology*, **153**(1): 17-30

{13} Olmstead M.C., Parkinson J.A., Miles F.J., Everitt B.J. & Dickinson A. (2000). *Psychopharmacology*, **152**(2): 123-131

{14} Deroche-Gamonet V., Belin D. & Piazza P.V. (2004). *Science*, **305**(5686): 1014-1017

{15} Belin D., Mar A.C., Dalley J.W., Robbins T.W. & Everitt B.J. (2008). *Science*, **320**(5881):1352-1355

{16} Belin D., Balado., Piazza P.V. & Deroche-Gamonet V. (2009). *Biological psychiatry* 65:863-868

{17} Amhed S.H. (2010). *Neurosci Biobehav Rev*, **35**(2): 172-84

These models have been widely developed the last 40 years and have provided substantial informations about the molecular targets of addictive drugs as well as the neurobiological and psychological adaptations resulting from either acute or chronic drug exposure. Indeed, models that focus on defined features of drug addiction provide a powerful heuristic framework for determining the brain mechanisms underlying the pathology. However, they rarely address other clinical dimensions of the disorder such as behavioural predictive factors or interactions between different symptoms of the pathology. Thus, the second type of models are those that try to incorporate several symptoms of the pathology in humans, thereby providing powerful tools for longitudinal studies or even testing pharmacological treatments, but are somewhat limited in the identification of underlying mechanisms. Indeed, the behavioural complexity of these models makes it difficult to implement causal investigative studies where the end-point is well defined. We discuss the general utility and application of both modelling approaches as complementary tools to investigate the neurobiological and psychological mechanisms of drug addiction and its vulnerability.

1.2.2 Validity criteria of animal models

The validation of animal models of addiction is based upon the same principles that have been established for models in general, namely fulfilling standard criteria amongst which reliability and predictive validity are the most important [1]. However, there are other criteria that have been used widely in validating animal models of drug addiction, including face validity and construct validity [1]. Briefly, reliability refers to the consistency and stability with which the independent and the dependent variables are measured. Thus a reliable model of drug addiction must allow for a precise and reproducible manipulation of the independent variable and an objective and reproducible measure of the dependent variable in standard conditions. A further key criterion for the validation of an animal model is its predictive validity. A valid animal model should predict either the therapeutical potential of a compound in humans (pharmacological isomorphism) or a variable that may influence both the dependent variable of the model and the process under investigation in humans.

Face validity refers to the similarities between the dependent variable of the model, i.e., behaviour in the case of drug addiction, and the human condition, i.e. the symptoms of the pathology. Thus face validity may be important in designing the model but is unlikely an objective criterion to actually assess its validity. Indeed, it is very difficult, if not impossible, to provide an objective criterion to evaluate the similarities between the behavioural output of a rat preparation and drug addiction in humans when the behavioural repertoire of the two species is so different.

Construct validity has been increasingly considered in animal models of drug addiction. It refers to the ability of a model to take into account psychological or neurobiological constructs that characterise the specific pathological processes in humans. Thus, incentive sensitisation, habit formation or top-down prefrontal executive control failure are examples of constructs which have been investigated in animal models.

2. Reinforcing effects of drugs of abuse, abuse liability

As previously mentioned all addictive substances show reinforcing properties in animals. Indeed, the abuse liability of a substance is often measured by its ability to support self-administration and a conditioned place preference [2]. In this section are reviewed the experimental designs that have been developed to investigate the reinforcing properties of addictive drugs. These procedures, combined with molecular biology and pharmacology, have been crucial in the identification and functional characterisation of the molecular targets of addictive drugs.

The seminal discovery by Olds and Milner of intra-cranial self-stimulation (ICSS) in 1954 marked a major turning point for research on the neural mechanisms of addiction [3]. The discovery that dopaminergic projections from the ventral tegmental area (VTA) to limbic cortico-striatal structures (nucleus accumbens, Acb), olfactory tubercle, amygdala, orbitofrontal cortex (OFC), medial prefrontal cortex (mPFC) were effective substrates for ICSS sparked considerable interest in the brain dopamine systems as neural substrates for the rewarding properties of both natural [food] and drug reinforcers. A few years later Weeks developed an operant procedure to deliver intravenous morphine infusions to relatively unrestrained rats [4], a method still widely used in many pre-clinical research laboratories today. That research continued on the opioid drugs morphine and heroin for some considerable time thereafter was no surprise given the strong emphasis at that time in the DSM-III on the symptomatology of opioid dependence and withdrawal [5].

Since then it has been established that addictive substances exert powerful effects on primary and secondary (i.e. conditioned) reinforcement mechanisms. As instrumental reinforcers they strongly encourage behaviours that lead to the availability of a drug, a process subserved by stimulus-response associative mechanisms (instrumental conditioning). Abused drugs also facilitate Pavlovian conditioning whereby previously neutral stimuli in the environment become conditioned to the drug, and can predict it, or even act as conditioned reinforcers.

In operational terms, a reinforcer is a stimulus that increases the probability of a response consequent upon its presentation. Thus, all addictive drugs are reinforcers since they are self-administered by animals and humans and support conditioned place preference (a form of contextual Pavlovian conditioning). Pavlovian conditioned stimuli can act as conditioned reinforcers when presented contingently. Then they can have powerful motivational effects and support long sequences of instrumental drug-seeking behaviour by bridging delays to future drug reinforcement [6-8].

2.1 Conditioned place preference

Conditioned place preference (CPP), has been used extensively to probe the psychological [9] and neurobiological [10-11] mechanisms underlying the rewarding properties of addictive drugs [10;12], as well as negative emotional states associated with drug withdrawal [13-15]. Indeed, through Pavlovian conditioning, the negative affective state caused by drug withdrawal can induce a reliable conditioned place aversion [13-15].

The first study based on the modern paradigm of CPP was reported by Rossi and Reid in 1976 [16] although earlier demonstration of preference for a drug paired environment was published as early as the 1940's [10]. In this procedure two different unconditioned stimuli (US) are paired with two distinct environments. These contextual cues differ in their spatial configuration, colour, flooring, and sometimes even olfactory cues. Briefly, the CPP procedure involves injecting animals with either the drug in question or a control solution, each being administered in a different environment often over successive days. The conditioning phase may combine several pairings, ideally according to a Latin square and unbiased design such that every pairing does not predict subsequent pairings, and that any spontaneous bias or preference for a compartment is initially controlled for. CPP is then tested during a drug-free choice phase where subjects are given access to both compartments. Preference for the drug-paired environment is indicative of the rewarding properties of the drug. CPP can be established not only for addictive drugs but also for natural rewards such as food, water, sexual partner and novelty [10]. Based on a plethora of studies, it is widely accepted that increased dopamine transmission is necessary for the establishment of CPP [17]. Although some authors suggest that CPP is a model of drug seeking behaviour [or drug craving], being essentially dependent upon Pavlovian associations, CPP alone cannot account for the instrumental nature of drug seeking and drug taking behaviour, which is perhaps better modelled by drug self-administration procedures.

2.2 Drug self-administration models

Drug self-administration procedures lie at the core of the most sophisticated preclinical models of drug addiction that have been developed over the last twenty years, ranging from relapse to drug taking [18-20], to loss of control over intake [21-22], compulsive drug taking [23-25] and addiction-like behaviour [8;26-28].

Addictive drugs act as reinforcers, in that they increase the probability of a behavioural response that leads to their presentation, through instrumental conditioning. Thus, animals can readily detect the contingency between an instrumental response and the delivery of a particular drug (e.g., an intravenous infusion of heroin, cocaine, nicotine or THC, or a small volume of alcohol in a magazine) and respond in an instrumental manner to obtain such drugs. The acquisition of drug self-administration is a behavioural marker of its reinforcing properties and abuse liability [2]. Indeed, apart from LSD, all drugs abused by human are self-administered by animals.

Drugs of abuse can be self-administered by a variety of routes across preclinical models, including intramuscular, intranasal, oral, and intravenous [29].

Drug self-administration was initially developed in non human primates, however since the pioneering work of Weeks (1962), rats have extensively been used to investigate the psychological, neural and cellular mechanisms underlying drug self-administration.

Self-administration procedures can be arranged according to different schedules of reinforcement [29]. In fixed ratio schedules, the drug is delivered after the completion of a fixed number of responses by the animal, thereby providing a direct relationship between the actual response and drug delivery. By contrast, in fixed interval schedules, the animal is trained to seek the drug for prolonged periods of time.

Different schedules allow for the investigation of different processes of drug taking or drug seeking behaviour which are beyond the scope of this chapter. However, insightful descriptions of, and discussions about, these schedules can be found in [6;29-32].

The acquisition of drug self-administration is widely considered to depend on the functional integrity of the olfactory tubercle and the shell of the nucleus accumbens (AcbS) [7]. An important role for mesolimbic dopamine in this process was inferred by findings in freely moving rats that dopamine concentration is greatly increased in the striatum, and especially the Acb, following the self-administration of drugs commonly abused by humans [33]. This important study supported the influential hypothesis at that time that addictive drugs exert their primary reinforcing effects and addictive properties through activation of the mesolimbic dopamine system [34-37]. Although it is now clear that increased dopamine release in the Acb does not provide a sufficient account for the addictive properties of drugs such as cocaine, alcohol and heroin, dopamine still remains one of the most important neurotransmitters in the aetiology and pathophysiology of drug addiction, a role underscored by its proposed involvement in salience detection and learning [7;38-52].

In its classic form, the drug self-administration paradigm has provided valuable insights into the brain substrates mediating drug taking behaviour, which differ somewhat according to the particular drug under investigation [53-56]. Addictive drugs not only influence the function of the mesolimbic dopamine system [33] they also trigger a variety of between-systems anatomical [57-62] and functional neuroadaptations [63-66] as well as changes in gene transcription and function in a number of brain systems including the hypothalamus [67], the VTA [68], the amygdala [69-74], Acb [75-79], dorsal striatum [80], orbital [81-82] and prefrontal cortices [83-85], with important effects on stress responsivity [86-88] and epigenetic processes in the limbic system [77;89-92].

However, even though these data have increased our knowledge about the neurobiological substrates of the reinforcing effects of addictive drugs and the neurobiological adaptations to drug self-administration, they provide only limited insights into the neurobiology of drug addiction. As very well brought to remembrance by Serge Ahmed [93], intravenous (intrajugular) self-administration of saline had been demonstrated in water-deprived monkeys [94] a year before the pioneer morphine self-administration work in rats of Weeks (1962), thereby demonstrating that drug self-administration is a measure of instrumental conditioning, but not really a model of drug addiction.

Thus, when one considers working on drug addiction one has to keep in mind that studying drug taking behaviour is not a way of studying drug addiction. This was already stated long ago by Wise and Bozart [95] and quoted by Robinson & Berridge [96]: "To assert that all addictive drugs are reinforcers is to do little more than redefine the phenomenon of addiction."..."To identify a drug as reinforcing goes no further than to identify the drug as addicting"; indeed, there is an obvious gulf between taking a drug on a social basis, as most of us often do, at least when one considers a glass of wine, and compulsively taking drugs. Nevertheless, even after the publication of the DSM-IV in 1994 [97] and the new diagnostic criteria for compulsive drug use that now form the hallmark of the clinical features of drug addiction many, if not all, of the early animal models focused on the "rewarding" properties of addictive drugs and their acute and chronic neurobiological effects.

Thus, during the last ten years pre-clinical research in drug addiction has attempted to better integrate one or more clinical features of the pathology according to the DSM-IV diagnostic criteria. New phenotypes have been identified based on craving or either reinstatement [20;98-99] or relapse to drug seeking [100], a loss of control over drug taking [21-22], habitual / compulsive cocaine seeking and taking [6;23-25;101] and inter-individual vulnerability to addiction-like behaviour [8;26-28].

3. Monodimensional animal models of addiction

3.1 Craving and relapse

Drug addicts show a high propensity to relapse, even after protracted abstinence [102]. This hallmark feature of addiction can be modelled in animals using two main procedures: extinction-reinstatement, initially developed by Stewart and colleagues [18-19] and abstinence-relapse [103]. Reinstatement of responding for drug can be induced by stress, low doses of the drug itself and by the presentation of drug-associated cues [20;104-112]. In the extinction-reinstatement procedure [18-19], animals experience a series of extinction sessions following a short period of drug self-administration, leading to a progressive decline in responding. Following extinction, responding for drug is reinstated by a stressful stimulus, a priming injection of drug, a presentation of a conditioned stimulus (CS) or by placing the animal in a drug-associated environment.

Reinstatement of drug seeking depends upon a broad neurobiological network which subsets are recruited based on the nature of the trigger of reinstatement, be it stress, the drug or drug associated cues and context [105]. Overall, reinstatement to drug seeking depends upon the extended amygdala, prefrontal cortex and dopaminergic neurons [105;113-114]. A large impetus has recently been put on the prominent role of glutamate homeostasis in reinstatement to drug seeking, especially focusing on prefrontal – accumbens pathways [111;115-116].

Interestingly, it has been shown that levels of reinstatement induced by contingent presentations of drug-associated cues increase with prolonged time of withdrawal. This observation suggests that drug craving increases with withdrawal duration [117-118], an adaptation that was specifically related to increase dopamine transporter (DAT) and N-Methyl-D-Aspartate receptor 1 (NMDA R1) protein levels in respectively the prefrontal cortex and the mesolimbic system [118]. However, incubation process has also been reported for food and fear, thereby suggesting that it is a common neurobehavioural adaptation to cessation of stimulation, whatever the nature of the unconditioned stimulus, rather than a specific neurobiological substrate of drug addiction.

In the abstinence-relapse procedure [103], animals are given a forced abstinence period after a brief period of drug self-administration. They are then maintained in their home cage until they are exposed again to the self-administration chamber where they are tested under extinction.

Whereas the reinstatement procedure clearly involves the Acb and both its dopaminergic and glutamatergic inputs, relapse to drug seeking depends upon the dorsolateral striatum [100;103]. Thereby, this neurobiological dissociation suggests that parallel, not necessarily mutually exclusive, neurobiological systems are involved in relapse to drug seeking. However, their respective contribution to the human craving and relapse situation remains unclear, especially the one of reinstatement since the situation in which human addicts go through extinction before responding to drug-associated stimuli or stress is very unfrequent.

3.2 Escalation of drug taking

The first well-established animal model of loss of control over drug intake, namely escalation of drug self-administration, is based on the fourth diagnostic criterion of drug addiction and was developed by Serge Ahmed and George Koob in 1998 for cocaine [21] and 2000 for heroin [22]. Short access ("ShA") to addictive drugs generally results in stable levels of self-administration such that plasma drug levels are controlled within an optimal level of reinforcement [119]. As mentioned previously, this pattern of self-administration does not account for the clinical features of drug addiction in humans. Ahmed and Koob thus gave extended access to cocaine to a group of animals ("LgA", or long access) following a period of moderate exposure (ShA, fixed ratio 1, one hour a day). A second group of rats received short access to cocaine throughout the experiment.

Introduction of the long access was immediately associated with higher drug intake, as compared to ShA rats. In other words, the LgA rats escalated their rate of cocaine self-administration compared with ShA rats, which maintained a constant level of cocaine intake. LgA rats also exhibited higher rates of cocaine self-administration during the first hour of each session. Escalation of cocaine intake has been associated with an upward shift in the intracranial self-administration threshold (ICSS), indicative of reward dysfunction [21] that has been postulated by the hedonic allostasis theory [2;86-88]. However, escalation of cocaine self-administration is not associated with psychomotor sensitisation but, instead, with a sensitization of the incentive motivational properties of cocaine [120], thereby suggesting a dissociation between loss of control over drug intake and behavioural sensitisation.

Escalation of drug intake has also been associated with higher resistance to shock-induced suppression of drug self-administration and conditioned suppression [24;121], and therefore might contribute to the instantiation of addiction.

However, all rats subjected to extended access to heroin do not necessarily escalate their intake [122]. Thus, when the upper and lower quartile of a population of Lister-Hooded rats are selected on the basis of the escalation slope (a direct measure of the magnitude of escalation of drug intake over time), marked differences can be observed [122]. Whereas low escalation (LE) rats show a marked increase in their intake when extended access is introduced and then reach a plateau in their daily drug intake, high escalation (HE) rats tend to show a slower adaptation to extended access, in that they do not increase their intake as quickly as LE rats, but progressively lose control over heroin self-administration (figure 2). This first formal description of inter-individual differences in the propensity to escalate heroin intake lead to the investigation of the behavioural markers of loss of control over heroin and cocaine intake (see "Vulnerabilities to drug addiction" section). This observation may resonate well with the demonstration that escalation of drug intake does not necessarily render rats insensitive to alternative reinforcers, i.e., despite escalation of cocaine self-administration rats have been reported to prefer a saccharine solution when given the choice between this reinforcer and the drug [123]. This suggests that schedule-induced escalation of drug intake, when considered without the individual dimension, does capture one criterion of drug addiction, namely, drug is used in larger amounts, but not necessarily extends to other criteria. However, inter-individual differences can also be observed in the resistance to alternative reinforcers after extended access to cocaine [93].

3.3 Animal models of drug seeking: The distinction between drug seeking and drug taking behaviour: Second-order and two-link heterogeneous chained schedules of reinforcement

Drug addiction does not involve only taking drugs, drug addicts spend most of their time foraging for the drug. It is therefore vital to dissociate drug taking from drug seeking. In trying to separate drug seeking from drug taking, schedules of reinforcement must be implemented in which operant responding for the drug during the drug seeking phase is not affected by the drug itself, i.e., so that drug seeking behaviour can be measured without interference by stimulant or sedative actions of the self-administered drug.

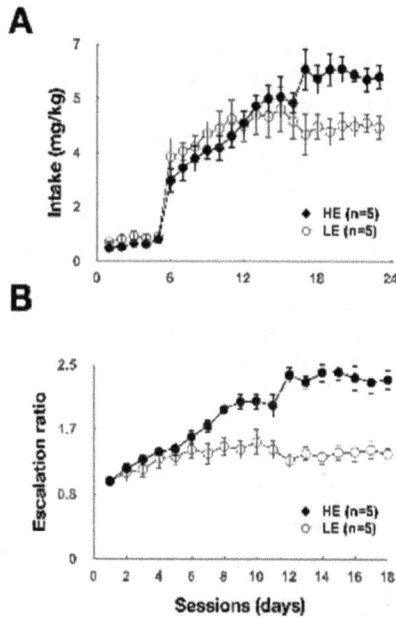

Fig. 2. Inter-individual propensity to lose control over heroin intake, after (122)
Marked inter-individual differences were revealed when the upper (high-escalation rats, HE, n=5) and lower quartile (low-escalation rats, LE, n=5) of a population of lister hooded rats were selected based on the slope of drug intake over all 18 days of the LgA phase [group: $F_{1,8}$ = 59.44, P < 0.001]. Thus, HE and LE rats displayed a different profile both in terms of heroin intake (A) and escalation ratio (B) [group x session interaction: $F_{22,176}$ = 8.26, P < 0.001 and $F_{16,128}$ = 10.20, P < 0.001, respectively]. Post-hoc analysis confirmed that HE rats displayed a daily increase in both intake and escalation ratio from the 4th and 6th day of extended access, respectively (vs. LgA d1, all Ps < 0.05), whereas LE rats showed no escalation at all.

Two-link heterogeneous chained schedules of reinforcement aim to dissociate spatially, temporally, and instrumentally drug seeking from drug taking behaviour. Second-order schedules of reinforcement allow the investigation of cue-controlled drug seeking over prolonged periods of time.

3.3.1 Two-link heterogeneous chain schedules of reinforcement

In this procedure completion of the first link of the chain, designated as the seeking link, results in access to the second link, or taking link, which permits, once performed, the delivery of the reinforcer. Acquisition of the chain schedule is achieved through successive steps of increasing complexity which start with introduction of the taking lever. A lever press is then reinforced under a fixed ratio (FR) 1 schedule so that each lever press produces drug reinforcement accompanied by the withdrawal of the taking lever. After several sessions of stable responding, the seeking lever is introduced while the taking lever is retracted. The first press on the seeking lever initiates a random interval (RI) schedule with the first seeking lever press occurring after the RI has elapsed terminating the first link of the chain; this results in retraction of the seeking lever and insertion of the taking lever to initiate the second link. One press on the taking lever results in the presentation of the reinforcer followed by a time-out period. Thereafter, the seeking lever is reinserted to start the next cycle of the schedule. The effects of experimental manipulation can thus be assessed through measures of seeking responding (latency, number or response rate) as well as taking responding (latency). The interest in dissociating seeking and taking behaviour is obvious when considering that the two instrumental components are influenced by dissociable processes since they are differentially sensitive to devaluation, incentive learning or Pavlovian manipulations [124]. In addition, cocaine seeking performance is monotonically related to the dose of drug with a relatively long time out [125]. Whereas early cocaine seeking performance is profoundly affected by extinction of the taking link [126-127] but not by inactivation of the dorsolateral striatum [127], after extended training it becomes automatic, i.e., insensitive to extinction of the taking lever and sensitive to inactivation of the dorsolateral striatum [127], thereby suggesting a shift in both the psychological and neurobiological mechanisms governing drug seeking when it becomes well established [128].

3.3.2 Second-order schedule of cocaine reinforcement

In the street, drug seeking behaviour is stimulus-bond in that drug addicts forage for their drug under the control of stimuli in the environment, acting as conditioned reinforcers, that support long sequences of behaviour in the absence of the outcome. More formally, conditioned reinforcers are stimuli that have themselves acquired rewarding properties after repeated associations with unconditioned rewards. Conditioned reinforcers bridge delays between seeking and obtaining the drug. Psychostimulants, opiates, speedball, cannabis, or nicotine-associated CSs act as powerful conditioned reinforcers since they greatly enhance drug seeking behaviour when presented contingently, but not non-contingently, upon instrumental responding during, usually, interval schedules of reinforcement [6;30;32;129-130]. Conditioned reinforcers can also support the acquisition of a new instrumental response [131-132]. Such properties are clearly demonstrated in procedures where animals work to obtain presentation of a conditioned stimulus, often in the absence of the unconditioned reward.

In second-order schedules of reinforcement, the CS is presented response-contingently usually under a fixed ratio schedule, during an overall fixed interval or fixed ratio schedule for the primary reinforcer, and markedly enhances and maintains responding for long periods of time (figure 3). Thus, under a second-order schedule of reinforcement, a strong contingency exists between the instrumental response and the presentation of the CS (under a fixed ratio) as well as the relatively weaker contingency that is arranged between instrumental performance and the outcome (the drug) that is reinforced only after completion of the first ratio after each interval has elapsed. Such schedules therefore facilitate the development of stimulus-response (S-R) control over instrumental responding. In addition, it has been shown that omission of CS presentation in second-order schedules of reinforcement disrupts cocaine seeking more than food seeking behaviour [130], suggesting that prolonged psychostimulant seeking is particularly dependent upon conditioned reinforcement.

Thus, instrumental responding during the first interval of a second-order schedule of reinforcement shows face and construct validity with regards to the behavioural features of drug seeking in humans: stimulus-bound, somewhat dissociated from the unconditioned effects of the drug and long lasting.

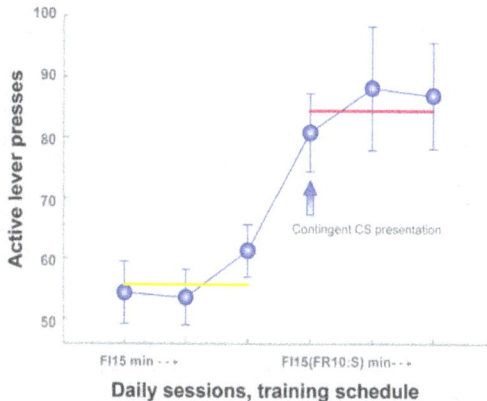

Fig. 3. Acquisition of cocaine seeking under a second-order schedule of reinforcement. Instrumental performance of a population of 24 Lister Hooded rats during the first interval of a FI15 and FI15(FR10:S) schedule of reinforcement (see text for explanation). Once animals have acquired self-administration under continuous reinforcement, the reinforcement schedule is switched to fixed intervals, with daily increments: FI1 min, FI2 min, FI4 min, FI8 min, FI10 min, and FI15 min. After 3 days of training under the FI15 schedule (*left part of the figure*), contingent presentations of the CS are introduced under a FR10 schedule such that rats are now trained under a FI15(FR10:S) second-order schedule of reinforcement. This acquisition procedure provides a direct measure of the potentiation of responding during interval schedules by the contingent presentation of the CS since they are introduced only once responding under fixed interval has stabilized. Thus, although the average response rate is 50 during the first interval of a FI15 schedule, it reaches 90-100 when the CS is contingently presented (Belin-Rauscent & Belin, unpublished).

Second-order schedules of cocaine and heroin self-administration were initially developed by Goldberg and colleagues in non human primates to assess the influence of environmental stimuli upon drug self-administration [30;129-130]. Everitt and colleagues have also established second-order schedules of drug reinforcement in rats [133]. In the study by Arroyo and colleagues (1998), rats were initially required to learn cocaine to self-administer under continuous reinforcement, i.e., FR1. After stabilisation of responding, (5 to 7 daily 2 hours sessions), a second-order schedule with fixed ratio components of the type FRx(Fry:S) was introduced, with initial values of x and y set to 1, so that each active lever press resulted in the presentation of the CS and and the delivery of 0.25 mg of cocaine. Then x and y values were progressively increased with increments in response requirements starting with x i.e., FR5(FR1:S) and FR10(FR1:S), then y, i.e., FR10(FR2:S), FR10(FR4:S), FR10(FR7:S) and FR10(FR10:S). After stabilisation of responding under this FR10(FR10:S) schedule of reinforcement which therefore requires 100 active lever presses and 10 one second presentations of the CS to obtain a cocaine infusion, a final fixed interval schedule FI15(FR10:S) was introduced such that a cocaine infusion was delivered only following the tenth active lever press that occurred when the 15 min interval had elapsed. Finally rats were allowed to perform cocaine seeking behaviour under this schedule for ten days. This acquisition procedure produces robust and stable CS-dependent rates of responding [133] and has been used extensively to probe the neural mechanisms involved in the acquisition, and the performance of, cue-controlled cocaine-seeking [101;134-135].

It is also possible to decrease the acquisition period to 11 days [101;136] (figure 3). In this case the training phase consists of three days of FR1 training, 2 hour daily sessions, 30 infusions (0.25 mg cocaine / infusion) followed by the introduction of interval schedules, with daily increments: FI1 min, FI2 min, FI4 min, FI 8 min, FI10 min, FI15 min. After three days of training under the FI15 schedule, contingent presentations of the CS are introduced under a FR10 schedule such that rats are now trained under a FI15(FR10:S) second-order schedule of reinforcement. This acquisition procedure provides a direct measure of the potentiation of responding during interval schedules by the contingent presentation of the CS since they are introduced only once responding under fixed interval has stabilised.

Thus, although the average response rate is 50-70 during the first interval of a FI15 schedule, it reaches 100-150 when the CS is contingently presented (figure 3), as described in several studies from Everitt's laboratory [101;137-138]. Indeed, short and long-term training under second-order schedules of reinforcement for cocaine have been very useful for investigating the neural mechanisms involved in the transition from newly acquired to well established or habitual cue-controlled cocaine seeking. Thus, acquisition of cue-controlled cocaine seeking depends upon the core of the Acb (AcbC) and its functional relationships with the basolateral amygdala [139] as well as dopamine transmission into the posterior dorsolateral striatum [137]. However, when it is well established, or habitual, cue-controlled cocaine seeking rather depends upon dopamine transmission into the dorsolateral striatum and its functional relationship with the AcbC, as demonstrated by functional disconnections between these two structures [101].

A dorsomedial to dorsolateral striatal shift in the control over drug seeking has recently been demonstrated to occur in alcohol self-administration after eight weeks of training [140a] and cocaine seeking after two weeks of training under an FI15(FR10:S) schedule of reinfocement [140b], a stage at which alcohol seeking was shown to be impervious to devaluation, i.e., was habitual. Thus addiction to both stimulants and alcohol may be dependent upon a shift from goal-directedness to habits that parallels, at the neural systems level, a progressive recruitment of the dorsolateral striatum. These data obtained in preclinical models resonate well with the recent demonstration of dorsal striatum implication cue-induced in alcohol [141] or cocaine [142] craving in humans.

3.4 Animal models of compulsive drug seeking and drug taking

As emphasised previously, addicted individuals not only consume large amounts of drugs but are also unable to repress their drug use regardless its consequences. Thus addiction shares common features with other compulsive disorders which are characterised as the uncontrollable and irresistible urge to performance an act, often to relieve anxiety or stress, but regardless of the rationality of the motivation.

The compulsive aspect of drug use in addicted subjects is even more obvious when similarities between addiction and obsessive compulsive disorder (OCD) are considered. Indeed, compulsive behaviour in the 4th version of the DSM [97] as a criterion for OCD is defined by the repetitive behaviours or mental acts that the person feels driven to perform in response to an obsession, or according to rules that must be applied rigidly aiming at preventing or reducing distress or some dreaded event or situation; but are either not connected to the issue or are excessive. Similarities between addiction and OCD have led, based on a modified version of the Yale–Brown Obsessive Compulsive Scale (Y-BOCS-hd) [143-144], to the development of the Obsessive Compulsive Drinking Scale (OCDS), a self-rated questionnaire which is able accurately to discriminate between alcoholic out-patients and social drinkers with high sensitivity and specificity [145], suggesting that obsessionality and compulsivity are key features of the heavily addicted individual [145].

Clinical data on abstinence from cocaine use suggest that the negative consequences directly related to use are a major reason for cessation [146]. Indeed, drug use is a high risk behaviour as it often compromised health, work and social relationships [147-148].

Preclinical models of drug addiction might therefore attempt to resemble in several respects the human conditions of compulsivity and fulfil some important features of the pathology in order to meet the necessary requirements of construct, face and predictive validity essential for the clinical application of data obtained from animal studies [1]. Of course, in animals it is extremely difficult to exactly reproduce compulsive drug seeking and taking as seen in human drug addicts because of obvious limitations including the absence of direct personal costs such as family or society problems associated with drug abuse, or limited alternative reinforcement choices.

However, despite such limitations, compulsivity in preclinical models of drug addiction should and must be defined as an inability to cease drug seeking and taking under conditions in which the drug is constantly available but its obtainment is associated with adverse consequences.

In recent years, progress has been made in an attempt to mimic human conditions of compulsive drug use.

3.4.1 Maintained drug use despite adverse consequences

1.   Resistance to devaluation / adulteration

In addition to their reinforcing properties, most addictive drugs have toxic effects, which after repeated use can lead to severe health complications. Such aversive properties would normally progressively devalue any reinforcer, and facilitate the engagement of the subject in alternative responses, incompatible with the pursuit of the initial reinforcer. However, despite often acknowledging the deleterious outcome of drug use, addicts rarely achieve spontaneous voluntary abstinence, and when they manage to do so, often relapse to compulsive drug use.

Similarly, rats differentially respond to devaluation of drugs of abuse and natural reinforcers. Performance for food is markedly affected by pairing its ingestion with illness produced by injection of lithium chloride. In contrast, devaluation of orally administered alcohol and cocaine does not greatly decrease drug seeking performance [140;149-150].

Similarly, extended access to free choice between drug solutions and water interrupted by periods of withdrawal in rats results in high levels of drug intake even when solutions are adulterated with bitter tasting quinine, evidencing the compulsive pattern of alcohol drinking after protracted exposure to the drug [151-153].

2.   Conditioned suppression

Until drug users explicitly experience the aversive consequences of drug use, drug taking is mainly moderated through warnings rather than actual punishment. Once experienced, aversive stimuli temporally distant from drug intake can appear, thereby rendering aversive contingencies less distinguishable. Moreover, the aversive consequences of drug use are counter-conditioned by previously extended drug presentation, which has been described as retarding the development of the conditioned emotional response [154]. All these processes may facilitate the attribution of aversive consequences to irrelevant stimuli. Adding a stimulus previously associated with an aversive outcome to the training context should normally reduce the frequency of a conditioned response. Indeed, although the aversive stimuli are not directly associated with drug use itself, a conditioned suppressor may be viewed as 'devaluing' the drug reinforcer since subjects would be required to respond for the drug in a state of conditioned fear [121].

However, Vanderschuren and Everitt (2004) found that the presentation of a Pavlovian conditioned fear stimulus after an extended self-administration training history failed to suppress cocaine self–administration, whereas after a brief cocaine taking history it did. These data support the view that while instrumental behaviour directed at obtaining drugs is initially a flexible, goal-directed form of behaviour, following prolonged drug exposure, drug seeking becomes insensitive to signals of punishment, thereby indicating its compulsive nature. However, it remains unclear whether in the multi-operant environment that drug addicts are normally exposed to, presentation of aversive conditioned stimuli may favour avoidance rather than abstinence.

4. Punishment

Aversive stimuli might eventually be perceived as directly associated with drug use. Punishment has often been debated as a treatment procedure, both in terms of its ethical acceptability and its efficacy. Nevertheless, it remains an undoubtedly important component of the every day life of drug addicts.

In animals, even though differing in many procedural parameters such as the locus or intensity of punishment, foot shock-induced punishment has been used in several recent models of compulsive drug seeking and drug taking behaviour. Thus we will focus here on this punisher, although foot shock-induced suppression may not easily be generalised to the human condition.

In most of the studies on drug taking despite adverse consequences, mild foot shocks, set at a constant intensity, are applied contingently upon a response reinforced by a constant dose of drug. In this case resistance to punishment is assessed through the persistence of the instrumental response despite contingent delivery of the punisher. Alternatively, the degree of response suppression is both dependent upon the magnitude of the reinforcer, the intensity of the punishment event, the schedule of their respective presentation and the delay between the instrumental responses and their consequences [155].

Consequently, Cooper et al. [156] increased daily by 0.04 mA the intensity of a shock that was initially set to 0.25 mA until rats stopped responding (lever pressing) during the 30 min daily sessions for three consecutive days. Whereas such a procedure has the advantage of assigning for each rat the final shock intensity that led to self-imposed abstinence, it constrains the opportunity for repeated testing when required.

The punishment contingency has been used at different loci of the instrumental drug taking action. Thus taking [157] or seeking behaviour [24] have been specifically punished. Since preparatory and consummatory responses have been shown to be under the influence of dissociable processes [158], it is conceivable they are differentially sensitive to punishment. In order to assess the sensitivity of seeking and taking responses to punishment Pelloux et al. used punishment in the seeking taking task that spatially and temporally dissociates the "preparatory" and "consummatory" behaviours [125]. Pelloux et al. conducted a study where either 50% of the seeking sequences where associated with the delivery of a shock instead of the activation of the taking lever or 50% of the instrumental responses on the taking lever were punished. With this probabilistic schedule of punishment both types of punishment induced a progressive suppression in performance but punishment of the taking response resulted in less suppression than punishment of the seeking response.

Finally, the efficacy of the punishment of drug seeking or taking seems to greatly depend on drug history. After short exposure to amphetamine or an opiate (remifentanil) punishment produces robust suppression of self-administration that resumed for the opiate in all subjects approximately 5 days after punishment was discontinued [159]. However, the punishment effect obtained for amphetamine lasted much longer [157]. After extended access to cocaine, punishment produced suppression of a seeking response except in a subgroup of animals (about 25%). Thus, compulsive drug seeking appears, as in humans, only after extended exposure to the drug in a small proportion of subjects conferring on these models good predictive validity.

5. Multidimensional animal model of drug addiction: addiction-like behaviour

As previously presented, there are two main strategies when developing preclinical models of drug addiction. The first category refers to models developed to understand the psychobiological, neurological, cellular and molecular processes involved in a particular aspect of the pathology. Therefore, these models specifically address one aspect of the pathology, whether a diagnostic criterion, such as escalation of intake, resistance to punishment, high motivation for the drug, habitual instrumental performance, vulnerability to relapse, or impaired cognitive flexibility. They may also be relevant to influential theories such as behavioural sensitisation [44;96;160-161] and hedonic allostasis [2;86-88]. Such models generally assume that drug exposure triggers rather similar behavioural, neural or molecular effects in all the subjects tested.

However, these models cannot address other crucial aspects of drug addiction, such as inter-individual differences in the vulnerability to develop the pathology and their behavioural and biological correlates. They also fail to capture the multi-symptomatic nature of drug addiction. Thus, the second category of animal models of drug addiction takes into accounts both inter-individual differences and the complementary strategy of meeting diagnostic criteria of the pathology in humans according to the DSM-IV. Thus, to be diagnosed as 'addicted' an individual must fulfil three out of seven diagnostic criteria of drug addiction over the last 12 months. This approach forms the basis of a new pre-clinical animal model based on vulnerability to addiction-like behaviour in the rat [26].

In this model, three diagnostic criteria, namely [i] an inability to refrain from drug seeking, [ii] high motivation for the drug, and [iii] maintained drug use despite negative consequences, have been operationalised by, respectively, [i] drug seeking during periods when the drug is not available and signalled as so, [ii] break points during progressive ratio schedules of reinforcement, and [iii] persistence of self-administration despite punishment by contingent electric foot-shocks.

When the population is large enough, as it has been the case in several of our studies [26;28], a systematic analysis of the distributions of each of the three addiction-like behaviours revealed that the distribution of the motivation for the drug and the persistence of drug seeking (n=40) were best fitted by a log-normal regression (Khi^2 and K-S: p>0.05, R^2 = 0.96 and 0.99, respectively) (figure 4, left and middle panel). In contrast the distribution of resistance to punishment was bimodal, composed of a first log-normal distribution (n=27 or 67.5% of the total population, K-S: d = 0.22451, p>0.1), and a second normal sub-distribution (n=13 or 32.5% of the total population, K-S: d = 0.15604 p>0.1) (figure 4, right panel) which general regression fit can be described as a 3 order polynomial equation y=3.24x^3 + 37.33x^2 +130.86x +146.67 [28].

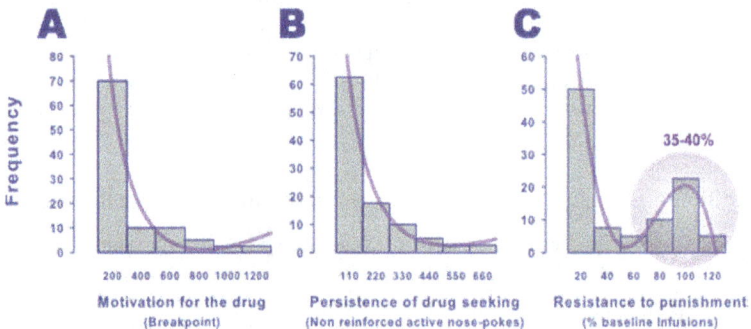

Fig. 4. Distribution of each of the addiction-like criteria, after (28)
The distribution of motivation for the drug and persistence of drug seeking (left and middle panel, respectively) (n=40) were best fitted by a log-normal regression (Khi2 and K-S: P>0.05). In contrast the distribution of resistance to punishment was bimodal, composed of a first log-normal distribution (n=27 or 67.5% of the total population, K-S: d=0.22451, p> 0.1) , and a second normal sub-distribution (n=13 or 32.5% of the total population, K-S: d=0.15604, p>0.1) (right panel) which general regression fit can be described as a 3 order polynomial equation: y=3.24x3+37.33x2+130.86x+146.67

The bimodal nature of the distribution of resistance to punishment we demonstrated in this study is in agreement with the observation of Pelloux et al. [24]. Bimodal distributions are very common in life science literature, especially during speciation process [162] whereby one whole population is somehow giving birth to two independent populations [163]. Rare in behavioural neuroscience, bimodal distributions have however been observed for drug-induced behaviours [164], suggesting that the neurobiological substrates of behavioural inter-individual differences need in some cases to be challenged in order to reveal bimodal distribution. Our results suggest that a specific subpopulation in the rat has diverged so that it has become specifically more vulnerable to maintain drug use despite averse consequences, as measured as resistance to punishment, when chronically exposed to the drug. This hypothesis, although speculative, when transferred to the human situation may actually resonate well with the Nesse and Berridge's suggestion that the vulnerability to drug addiction is a matter of evolution [165].

In practical terms, this bimodal distribution is particularly handy because it provides us with an objective criterion to determine a threshold in the population in order to carry out a dichotomous, categorial, strategy to identify animals that show addiction-like behaviour, i.e., 30-40% highest part of the population, depending on the study. Thus, for each of these three addiction-like criteria animals are ranked according to their score. If a rat's score is included in the 30-40% highest percentile of the distribution, this rat is considered positive for that addiction-like criterion and is given an arbitrary criterion score of 1. Then the arbitrary criteria scores for each of the three addiction-like criteria are added, and consequently four distinct groups are identified according to the number of positive scores: 0 criteria, 1 criterion, 2 criteria and 3 criteria rats (figure 5).

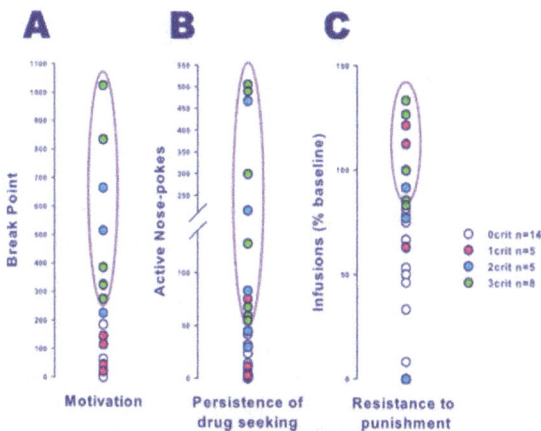

Fig. 5. Selection strategy of rats addicted (3crit rats) and rats resistant (0crit rats) to cocaine
Data analysed from (11). For each of these three addiction-like criteria animals are ranked according to their score. If a rat's score is included in the 30-40% highest percentile of the distribution, this rat is considered positive for that addiction-like criterion and is given an arbitrary criterion score of 1. Then the arbitrary criteria scores for each of the three addiction-like criteria are added, and consequently four distinct groups are identified according to the number of positive scores: 0 criteria, 1 criterion, 2 criteria and 3 criteria rats

Behaviourally, the categorial selection is associated with a criteria-dependent magnitude in each of the addiction-like criteria (figure 6). Our model is based on the comparison of three criteria (3crit) and 0 criteria (0crit) rats. 3crit rats show high scores for each of the three addiction-like criteria and are therefore considered "addicted", whereas 0crit rats are considered resistant to addiction. 3crit rats represent approximately 20% of the population exposed to cocaine, an incidence observed in several independent studies with Lister-

Hooded or Sprague-Dawley rats as well as either nose-poke or lever press as instrumental response [26;28;101;166], that is remarkably similar to that reported in humans [167].

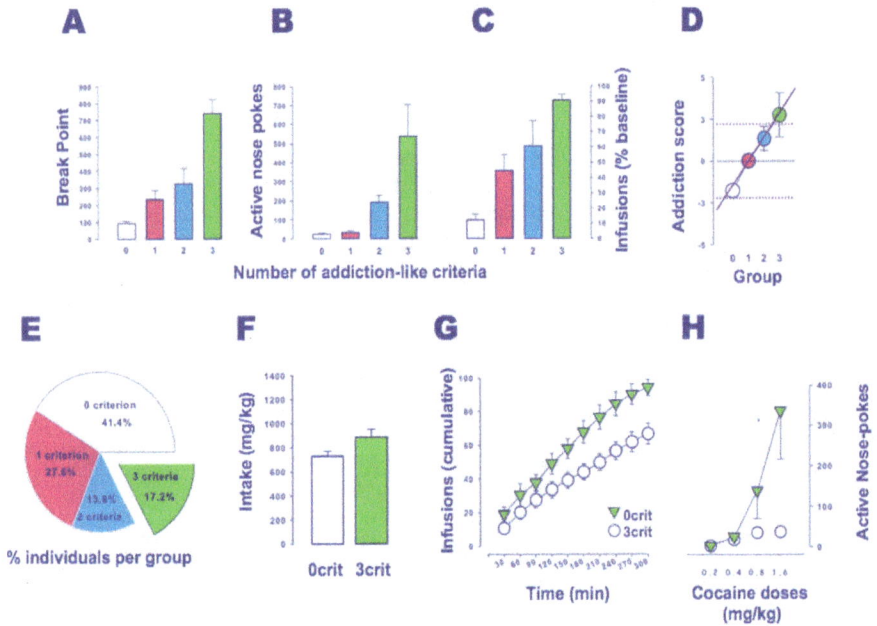

Fig. 6. Behavioural characterisation of addiction-like behaviour in the rat
A dichotomous approach to the diagnosis of addiction-like behaviour can be implemented in preclinical models of addiction on the understanding that some, but not all, animals chronically exposed to drug self-administration eventually develop one or more behavioural features resembling a clinical criterion for drug addiction as defined in the DSM-IV (see table 13.1). Thus we have operationally defined three addiction-like criteria, namely, (i) an inability to refrain from drug seeking (A), (ii) maintained drug use despite aversive consequences (B) and (iii) increased motivation to take the drug (C). Rats positive for none of the three criteria (0 criteria rats) are resistant to addiction, whereas rats that have three addiction-like criteria (3 criteria rats) are considered "addicted," and represent 15 to 20% of the population initially exposed to cocaine (D). Importantly these behavioural differences are not attributable to differential levels of cocaine intake, since throughout protracted exposure 3 criteria and 0 criteria rats do not differ in this measure (E). Although selected on three addiction-like criteria, 3criteria rats display complementary features of drug addiction, such as inability to limit drug intake when offered extended access to cocaine (F) and high vulnerability to relapse, as measured by reinstatement of cocaine seeking behaviour by increasing doses of non contingent cocaine infusions (G). A-E: after (11), F: after (8)

Although 3crit rats do not differ significantly from 0crit rats in terms of cocaine self-administration [26;28;166], 3crit rats eventually develop higher motivation for the drug, an inability to refrain from drug-seeking, and resistance to punishment [8;26;28;101;166].

More importantly, although selected on three addiction-like behaviours, 3crit rats also display enhanced escalation of cocaine self-administration as compared to 0crit rats (figure

6F). 3crit rats therefore fulfil a fourth criterion of addiction, namely an inability to control drug intake [26] classically established after extended access to the drug [21]. This results demonstrate that loss of control over drug intake does not necessarily follow extended access to the drug, but instead develops in some vulnerable subjects exposed to cocaine self-administration for prolonged periods of time.

The predictive validity of the model is further supported by de demonstration that 3crit rats also show a high vulnerability to relapse in response to non-contingent infusions of cocaine (figure 6G) [8] or contingent presentations of a drug-associated stimulus [26]. Thus, even though selected on three addiction-like criteria, after chronic exposure to cocaine, 3crit rats display important features of clinical addiction as defined in the DSM-IV. These observations provide the model with both construct and predictive validities.

Moreover, since addiction-like behaviour emerges in three criteria rats only after extended exposure to the drug, i.e., after at least 50 daily self-administration sessions, these results highlight the importance of the interaction between a vulnerable phenotype and chronic drug exposure in the development of compulsive drug self-administration.

6. Vulnerabilities to drug addictions

Like many other psychiatric disorders, we are not all equally vulnerable to develop drug addiction. Epidemiological studies have revealed that between 15 to 35% of the population exposed to addictive drugs will develop compulsive drug use [167]. The results described in the previous section illustrate very well that inter-individual differences in vulnerability to develop compulsive cocaine self-administration can also be observed in rats. Thus, in any given population of rats exposed to cocaine only some develop addiction-like behaviour, thereby demonstrating that animal models provide a realistic estimate of risk for addiction in humans [41;166;169].

As already discussed, the underlying aetiology of the different pathways to addiction are likely to involve interactions between a vulnerable phenotype, environmental influences and drug exposure itself [170-171]. It is therefore important to identify the psychobiological substrates of vulnerability to develop compulsive drug use both in drug naive subjects and drug experienced individuals, thereby being able to develop preventive and therapeutic strategies at different stages of drug use history.

6.1 Psychobiological factors of vulnerability to drug addiction: contribution of behavioural traits

Epidemiological studies in human populations have revealed striking associations between drug use [172-173b], and certain behavioural traits [174-189] such as anxiety [190-193], impulsivity [187;194-195] and sensation-seeking [176;183;196-199]. The relevance of these traits for animal models of addiction is discussed below.

6.1.1 Anxiety

Anxiety can be assessed in preclinical models using various procedures which include the elevated plus maze (EPM) [200-201]. During the classic 5-min test session on the EPM a variety of behaviours are measured including the ratio of open and closed arms entries, time spent in the open and closed arms, as well as self-grooming which are all indices of anxiety. High levels of anxiety including high grooming behaviour and a low percentage of time spent in the open arms of the EPM have been associated with an enhanced propensity to acquire cocaine CPP [202] as well as an increased motivation to self-administer cocaine [203], but see [204]. Trait anxiety has also been associated with an enhanced preference for alcohol [205-206], consistent with the notion that alcohol use may self-medicate underlying mood disorders related to anxiety and stress [207-208].

We have recently established that high anxiety in the EPM predicts escalation of cocaine, but not heroin self-administration in the rat (figure 7) [209].

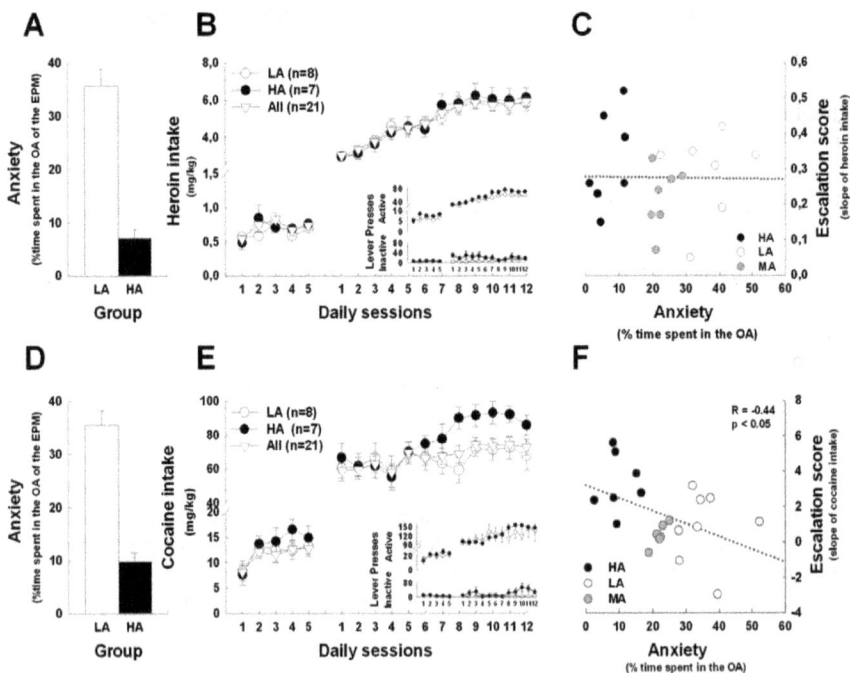

Fig. 7. High anxiety trait predicts loss of control over cocaine, but not heroin, self-administration in the rat, after (122)
High anxious (HA) and low anxious (LA) rats were selected in the upper and lower 33% of a Lister Hooded population (A & D). Whereas HA did not differ from either LA and the overall population in their escalation of heroin intake throughout 12 sessions of 6 h extended access to the drug (B) HA rats showed a marked increase in their cocaine intake as compared to LA or the overall population (E). Thus, high anxiety is related to the magnitude of cocaine escalation (F) whereas it is not related to the slope of escalation of heroin intake (C).

These data suggest that if high anxiety trait may contribute to the choice of the drug used, i.e., preference for alcohol or opiates [210], it does not necessarily contribute to the development of compulsive use when the drug is initially used as a self-medication [211]. However, the striking relationship between high anxiety levels in the EPM and subsequent vulnerability to escalate cocaine intake suggest that high anxiety may facilitate a tolerance to anxiogenic properties of cocaine [212] perhaps because of a ceiling effect, or, instead enhance the potential anxiolytic properties of cocaine that have been suggested for low doses of the drug [213].

6.1.2 Sensation seeking / Novelty-seeking

Sensation- and novelty-seeking traits have been the focus of a large number of pre-clinical studies on addiction vulnerability (for review, see [12]).

In preclinical studies, sensation/novelty seeking trait has been suggested to be modelled both by high locomotor reactivity to a new inescapable environment (high responder phenotype, HR) [214-215], and high propensity to visit a new environment in a free-choice, novelty-induced CPP, paradigm (high novelty preferring phenotype, HNP) [12;216].

Piazza and colleagues were the first to investigate the role of sensation-seeking in this context by measuring the locomotor response of rats to an inescapable novel environment [217]. In this model, rats are placed for two hours in a new environment and their horizontal activity is monitored. Based on inter-individual differences in locomotor response animals are either selected as high (HR) or low responders (LR) according to a median division [217]. HR rats show a greater propensity to acquire psychostimulant self-administration [217] since they more readily self-administer low doses of amphetamine than LR rats [2;217]. Moreover, HR rats show a greater propensity for drug-induced neural plasticity [218-219] and increased stress-evoked dopamine release in the Acb than LR rats [220].

However, sensation seeking does not predict the acquisition of CPP for addictive drugs, which instead is predicted by novelty-seeking [12;216;221-223], the latter being a behavioural trait dissociable from the former [9;28;224].

Novelty-seeking is normally assessed by measuring the preference of rats for a novel versus familiar compartment using a procedure quite similar to CPP [225], although broad methodological differences are observed in the literature that can impact onto the nature of the behavioural construct one is investigating. Indeed, depending on the study, novelty preference has been measured as (1) the number and time duration of visits of a new arm in a Y-maze during the first 2 or 5 min, respectively, of a test session taking place 30 min after the habituation to the other two arms of the set-up [226], (2), novelty-induced place preference tested for 15 min on the third day of a protocol during which animal were exposed 30 min daily to one compartment of a CPP box [223-224] whereas locomotor reactivity to novelty has been measured in (1) circular corridors [226-227], playground maze [228] or (2) activity chambers [216;229], each environment differing from one other in terms of light intensity, openness and area.

Overall, animals selected as novelty-seekers, or novelty-preferring (HNP), are those that fall in the upper quartile range. Unlike animals selected from the lower quartile of the population, high novelty seekers readily develop a conditioned place preference to amphetamine [224;228] and self-administration of cocaine under an autoshaping procedure [230].

Thus, although both traits are dependent upon the dopaminergic system [12], they are mutually exclusive [12;216], but see [231] and therefore may predict different dimensions of vulnerability to drug addiction [12].

We have investigated the respective role of HR and HNP phenotypes in inter-individual vulnerability to switch from controlled to compulsive cocaine SA. A cohort of rats were tested for their locomotor response to inescapable novelty and, subsequently for their preference propensity to express novelty-induced CPP.

After extended cocaine self-administration these rats were tested for each of the three addiction-like criteria. Whereas LR and HR rats were highly represented in the 0 and 1crit populations, 60% of the LNP rats were included in the 0crit population as opposed to 70% of the HNP rats that showed 2 or 3 addiction-like criteria, none belonging to the 0crit population (figure 8A). This asymmetric distribution specific to LNP and HNP rats was further investigated, as illustrated in figure 8B-D which depict the representativity of LR, HR, LNP and HNP rats within the distributions for each of the addiction-like criteria. Importantly, HNP rats, as opposed to LNP rats, represented the great majority of the subpopulation resistant to punishment (figure 8D).

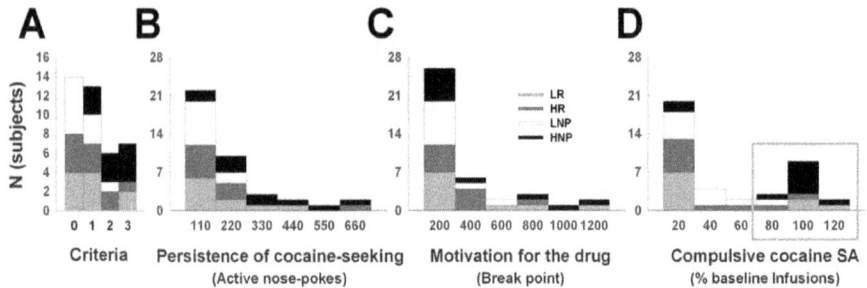

Fig. 8. High novelty preference (HNP) and sensation seekers (HR) rats are not equally distributed within the different addiction-like criteria.
A. Addiction score.The great majority of HNP rats are represented in the 2 and 3crit subgroups of the population whereas HR rats are equally distributed throughout the different groups. B-C. HNP and LNP rats are distributed asymmetrically within the population relative to persistence of drug seeking (B) and motivation for the drug (C). LNP rats are clustered on the right side of the distribution whereas HNP rats are also represented in the right part of the distribution. Such asymmetry is not observed for LR and HR rats which are equally distributed throughout the overall population for these two criteria. D. Distribution of LNP, HNP, LR and HR rats for compulsive cocaine self-administration. Whereas LR and HR rats did not show any difference in their distribution throughout the population, HNP rats were highly clustered in the compulsive subpopulation as emphasised by the encircling square. Thus HNP rats may be highly vulnerable to compulsive cocaine self-administration. Analysis of data from (28)

Thus although no differences were observed between HR and LR rats for their scores in each of their addiction-like criteria, HNP rats displayed higher scores than LNP rats in each of the addiciton-like criteria, namely resistance to punishment, inability to refrain from cocaine-seeking even if the drug is not available since they persisted, responded, more on the active nose-poke than LNP rats during "no-drug" periods and motivation for cocaine (figure 9D).

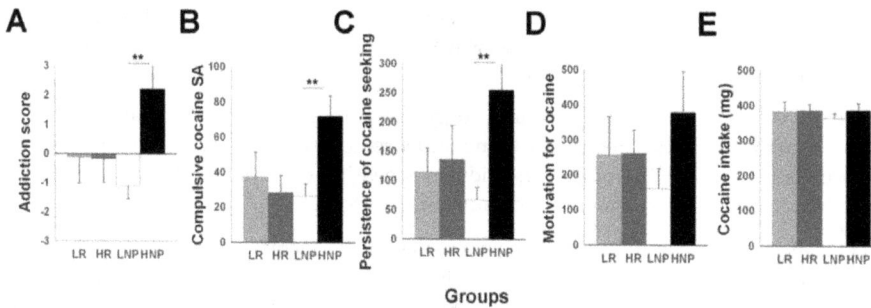

Fig. 9. Novelty Preference, but not locomotor reactivity to novelty predicts the switch to compulsive cocaine self-administration.

ANOVAs with HNP/LNP groups as between-subject factors revealed that HNP rats showed higher addiction score than LNP rats [$F_{1,18}$=10.59, p<0.01] (A). Compared to LNP rats, HNP rats developed compulsive cocaine SA as measured by high level of resistance to punishment [$F_{1,18}$=11.16, p<0.01] (B) and were unable to stop seeking cocaine when it was not available and signaled as so [$F_{1,18}$=9.03, p<0.01] (C). HNP rats tend to show higher motivation for cocaine than LNP though this difference did not reach statistical significance (D). These behavioral differences between HNP and LNP rats could not be attributable to differential cocaine intake since the two groups have been exposed to the same amount of cocaine throughout the experiment [$F_{1,18}$<1] (E). When compared to LR rats, HR rats showed no difference in the addiction-like behavioral measures. These two groups had behavioral scores similar to those of LNP rats, thereby illustrating that locomotor reactivity to novelty, as opposed to novelty preference, doesn't predict addiction-like behavior for cocaine.

The relationship between high novelty preference trait and vulnerability to switch to compulsive cocaine SA was further supported by a clear relationship assessed with a non parametric Spearman correlation analysis R=0.32, p<0.05, with the percentage of time spent in the new environment of the novelty-induced place preference procedure and the percentage of infusions compared to baseline when punished contingently by electric foot shocks as variables. However, no relationship was observed between locomotor reactivity to novelty and resistance to punishment (Spearman R=-0.15, p=0.36). Importantly, the behavioural differences observed between HNP and LNP rats cannot be attributed to a difference in the total amount of cocaine intake since the two groups did not differ for their total cocaine intake during the 60 days preceding the assessment of the addiction-like criteria [$F_{1,18}$<1] (figure 9E).

Since a great majority of the HNP, and none of the LNP, rats was clustered in the compulsive subpopulation, HNP rats, even though identified from a normally distributed population, may represent a specific sub-population vulnerable to compulsive cocaine intake after protracted exposure to the drug. Thereby the high novelty preference trait in the rat, as identified as the upper quartile of the population tested with the present paradigm is a promising behavioural tool for the study of the neurobiological substrates of vulnerability to compulsive cocaine intake.

While providing the first evidence for a causal relationship between novelty preference and compulsive cocaine use, this study confirms that locomotor reactivity to novelty does not predict the vulnerability to develop cocaine addiction, but does rather predict the propensity to self-administer drugs [27;217]. Altogether, these data suggest that the HR phenotype and its underlying neurobiological mechanisms may be involved in facilitating cocaine use, but not in the transition to switch from controlled to compulsive cocaine use, the hallmark of cocaine addiction [97].

Thus two different behavioural measures suggested to reveal a putative sensation/novelty seeking trait in rats [12], namely novelty-induced locomotor activity and novelty preference, are differentially predictive of inter individual propensity to self-administer cocaine and to switch from controlled to compulsive cocaine use, respectively.

These preclinical data suggest that the correlates of the increased propensity shown by human sensation seekers to use addictive drugs [175] should be dissociated from those associated with the transition from controlled to compulsive drug use. Indeed, not only is sensation seeking a heterogeneous, multifaceted, construct [232] but it is quantified according to different, not necessarily overlapping [233], personality scales including the Zuckerman, Eysenck, Arnett and Cloninger's scales. A factorial analysis of the different items of the sensation seeking scale developed by Zuckerman [197] revealed four dimensions [234] namely Thrill and Adventure Seeking [TAS], Experience Seeking [ES], Disinhibition [Dis], and Boredom Susceptibility [BS], of which the TAS and DIS sub-scales have been suggested to refer to sensation seeking whereas the ES and BS sub-scales would refer to novelty seeking [234-235]. Further research is needed to investigate which of these sub-scales is the most predictive of the vulnerability to switch to compulsive cocaine use, thereby clearly refining the relationships between sensation seeking trait and vulnerability to cocaine addiction.

6.1.3 Impulsivity

A popular paradigm used to assess impulsivity in rodents is the 5-choice serial reaction time task (5-CSRTT), which was developed originally as an analogue of the human continuous performance task of sustained attention [236]. The 5-CSRTT requires animals to detect brief flashes of light presented pseudo-randomly in one of five holes and to make a nose-poke response in the correct spatial location in order to receive a food reward. The rat is thus required to monitor a horizontal array of apertures and to withhold from responding until the onset of the stimulus. Generally, the accuracy of stimulus discrimination provides an index of attentional capacity, while premature responses – made before the presentation of the stimulus – are regarded as a form of impulsive behaviour and hence a failure in impulse control [237-238]. The neural and neurochemical basis of impulsivity on the 5-CSRTT has been extensively investigated, involving important contributions from the anterior cingulate cortex (ACC), infralimbic cortex, Acb, medial striatum and by the ascending monoaminergic systems [239-240].

More recently, the 5-CSRTT has been used to screen for spontaneously high levels of impulsivity in rats, a phenotype associated with increased cocaine, sucrose and nicotine self-administration [241-243]. Interestingly, Dalley and colleagues have recently shown using microPET brain imaging that high impulsive rats have lower dopamine D2/3-binding levels in the ventral striatum as compared to low impulsive littermates [241], thereby suggesting that alteration of dopamine D2/3-receptors in the Acb may contribute to high impulsivity and vulnerability to drug addiction.

We have used the animal model of addiction-like behaviour for cocaine described in previous sections to investigate whether high impulsivity trait predicts the switch to compulsive cocaine SA.

A cohort of 40 Lister Hooded rats was screened in the 5-CSRTT for their impulse control. These rats were then tested for their locomotor response to a new, inescapable environment. Thus, prior to cocaine exposure, rats were identified as high (HI) and low (LI) impulsive or HR and LR (figure 10).

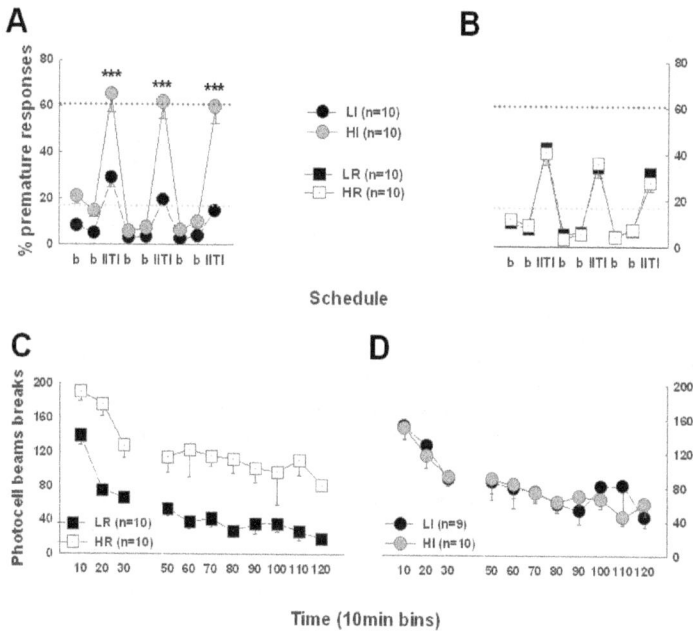

Fig. 10. Impulsivity and novelty-induced locomotor activity: two distinct phenotypes. After (27)

On two baseline days (B), premature responses in the 5_CSRTT were measured. (A and B) During long intertrail intervals (LITIS), HI rats showed more premature responses than LI rats (Group: $F_{3,36} = 14.4$, $p < 0.01$; scedule: $F_{8,288} = 130.22$, $p < 0.01$; Schedule x Group: $F_{24,288} = 7.01$, $p < 0.01$) (***$p < 0,001$) (A) and HR ($p < 0.01$) or LR rats ($p < 0.05$) (B). HR rats did not differ from LR rats or from LI subjects (B). (C and D) HR rats were more reactive to novelty tha LR rats ($F_{3,35} = 17.63$, $p < 0.01$). HI and LI subjects never differed from each other. *Comparison with HR: *$p < 0.05$, **$p < 0.01$, ***$p < 0.001$. (D) Pink and blue dotted lines represent the average premature responses during the last two intertrial intervals for HI and LI rats, respectively.

High impulsivity trait and locomotor response to novelty were demonstrated to be independent behavioural traits. We then tested whether high locomotor response to novelty and high impulsivity traits predicted higher propensity to acquire cocaine self-administration. We allowed animals to acquire cocaine SA with daily increasing doses of the drug. We demonstrated that HR rats acquire cocaine self-administration at doses at which

LR rats do not, thereby confirming that HR rats are more prone to acquire stimulants self-administration than LR animals [217]. However, HI rats did not differ from LI in their propensity to acquire cocaine SA (figure 11).

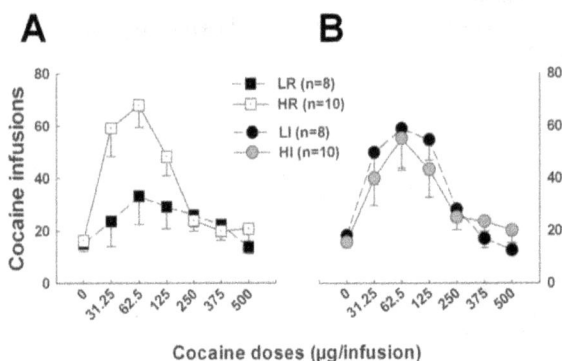

Fig. 11. Novelty-induced locomotor activity predicts the propensity to acquire cocaine self-administration, after (27)

(A) HR rats showed an upward shift of the cocaine dose-response curve compared with LR littermates (Group: $F_{1,16}$ = 4.9, p<0.05; Dose: $F_{6,96}$ = 11.73, p<0.01; Group x Dose: $F_{6,96}$ = 4.39, p<0.01). HR rats infused more cocaine at the lowest three doses than vehicle (p<0.01). (B) HI and LI subjects did not differ in the number of self-administered cocaine infusions (Group: $F_{1,16}$<1; Dose: $F_{6,96}$ =10.79, p<0.01; Group x Dose: $F_{6,96}$<1)

When subsequently exposed to protracted cocaine self-administration and tested for their addiction-like behaviour, rats were identified as 0, 1, 2 and 3crit rats and each animal was given an addiction score (figure 12). We then retrospectively compared HI vs LI and HR vs LR rats for their addiction score and revealed that HI rats had higher addiction score than LI whereas HR did not differ from LR rats.

This increased addiction score observed in HI rats was specifically attributed to the development of compulsive cocaine SA in these rats since they maintained cocaine SA despite punishment to the same extent as 3crit rats did. However, HR and LR rats did not differ in this behavioural criterion. The specific relationship between high impulsivity and compulsivity was further demonstrated by a correlational analysis between the percentage of premature responses in the 5-CSRTT and resistance to punishment, as assessed by a non parametric correlation analysis (figure 12).

This evidence suggests that the predisposition to initiate drug use is independent of the vulnerability to shift from controlled to compulsive drug taking, and therefore provides new insights into the various behavioural and psychological factors that influence the pathways to addiction. In particular, the demonstration that the high impulsive trait predicts the shift to compulsive drug taking behaviour is of major interest since a shift from impulse control failure to compulsivity has been suggested to play a major role in the development of drug addiction in humans [87;244] (figure 13).

Together with the demonstration that novelty preference predicts addiction-like behaviour for cocaine [28] the present data suggest that further investigations should focus on the additive or interactive contribution of high impulsivity and novelty seeking traits to the vulnerability to switch to compulsive cocaine SA.

This suggestion is timely since we [245] have recently demonstrated that high impulsive rats, as identified in the 5-CSRTT, prefer a novel compartment in a novelty-induced CPP procedure [245] (figure 14).

Thus both novelty preference and impulsivity, but not locomotor response to novelty, contribute to inter-individual propensity to switch from controlled to compulsive cocaine SA.

However, this conclusion may be taken with caution since it might be true only for stimulants. Indeed, we [122] have recently demonstrated that high impulsivity trait does not predict inter-individual differences in escalation of heroin self-administration (figure 15). This propensity was instead predicted by pharmacological flexibility in response to extended access to heroin, i.e., increased titration in response to increased availability of the drug.

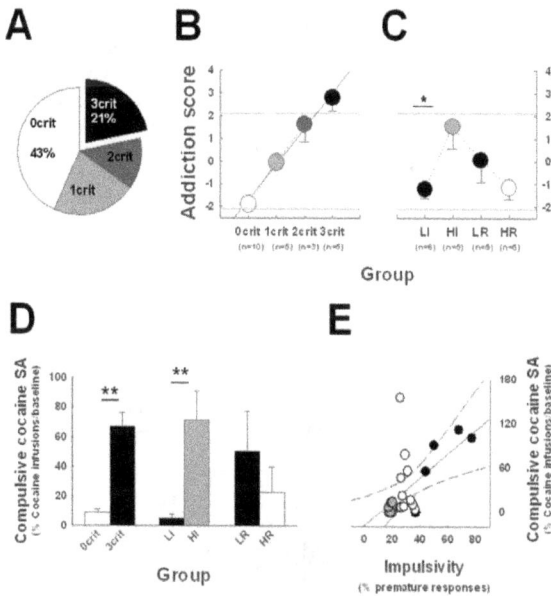

Fig. 12. Impulsivity predicts the transition to compulsivity

After extended exposure to cocaine SA 0, 1, 2 and 3crit rats were identified and were distributed similarly to previously described (A) in that 3 crit rats represented 20% of the overall population. When ranked on a linear addiction scale ($R^2 = 0.99$, Group: $F_{3,19}=34.43$, p<0.01), three-criteria rats had addiction scores (2.8 ± 0.6) above the standard deviation (2.1), and higher than all the other groups (B). (C) HI rats displayed higher addiction score than LI rats ($F_{1,9} = 7.55$, *p<0.05), whereas HR rats did not differ from LR rats. (D) HI rats (n=5) displayed higher resistance to punishment than LI rats (n=6) ($F_{1,9} = 12.79$, p<0.01), whereas HR (n=5) rats did not differ from LR rats (n=5). (E) Impulsivity predicts compulsive cocaine self-administration (R= 0.42, p<0.05). Gray and black shadings represent LI and HI rats, respectively.

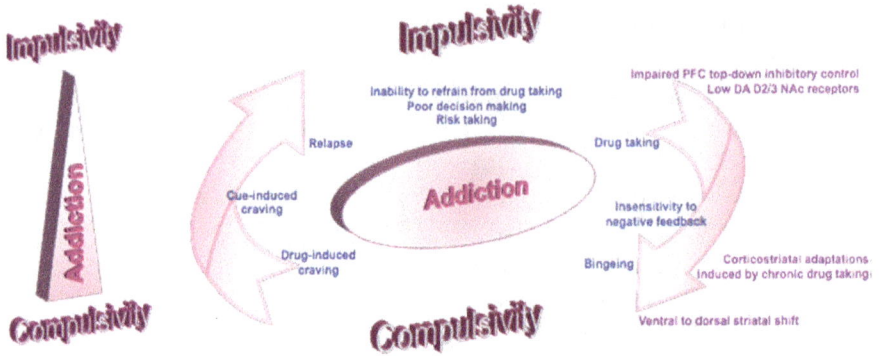

Fig. 13. Impulsivity and compulsivity in drug addiction.
It has been suggested that a shift occurs from impulsivity to compulsivity in the control over drug seeking during the development of drug addiction (left). According to this theoretical framework, drug use is initially controlled by the positive reinforcing properties of drugs. However, when addiction develops drug taking is no longer controlled by positive reinforcement but, instead, is controlled by negative reinforcement and the need to avoid the negative consequences of withdrawal. Other theoretical frameworks suggest a contribution of both impulsivity and compulsivity to different stages of the addiction cycle (right). Impulsivity might then be associated with drug taking and relapse, whereas compulsivity might be associated with craving, bingeing and insensitivity to negative feedback.

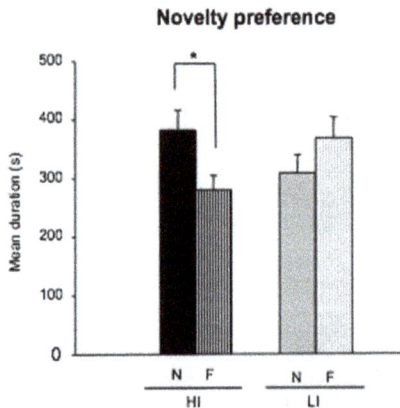

Fig. 14. High impulsive rats seek novelty
HI rats explored the novel compartment of the CPP apparatus for significantly longer period of time compared with the familiar compartment, a preference that was not observed in LI rats (group x compartment interraction: $F_{1,24} = 6.53$, p=0,017; post hoc t-test p=0.031). Howerver, there was no significant difference between HI and LI rat in the total time spent in the novel compartment. LI rats showed a trend increase in time spent in the familiar compartment compared with HI rats (p=0.059).

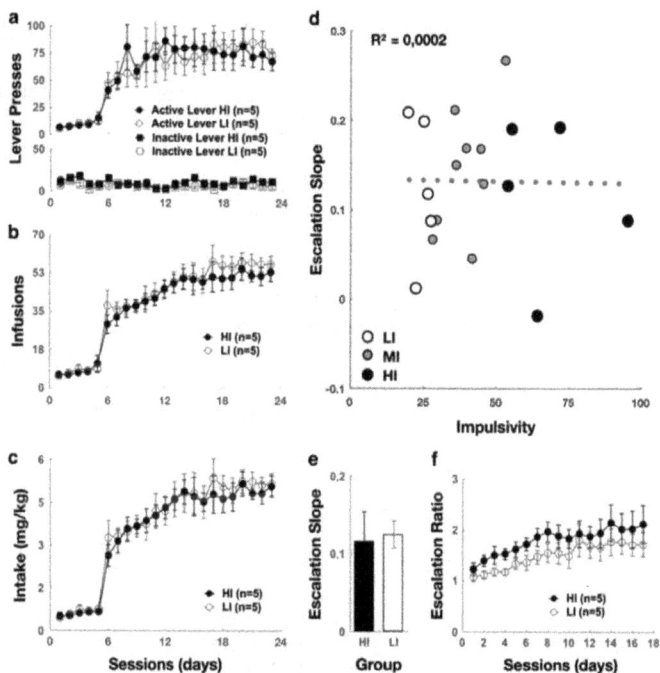

Fig. 15. High impulsivity trait does not predict a greater propensity to escalate heroin SA. After (122)

Extended access to heroin resulted in escalation of heroin SA over time in both HI and LI rats (a-d). After 5 days of 1-hour access to heroin, an 18-day 6-hour daily self-administration period was introduced. Following initiation of the LgA sessions, HI rats (n=5) and LI rats (n=5) did not differ in their time-dependent increase in active lever presses (a), heroin infusion (b), and intake (calculated as the amount of heroin self-administered by each rat in milligrammes per kilogramme bidy weight) (c). A dimentional analysis based on the overall population tested (n=19) did not reveal any correlation between the individual level of impulsivity (percentage of premature responses during the last two 7 s-LITI sessions) and the propensity to escalated heroin SA (escalation score; calculated as the slope of intake over 18 days od LgA for each subject) (d). Consequently, HI and LI rats differed neither in their escalation slope (e) not in the increase of their ER (intake for each LgA day divided by intake for day 1) over the 18 LgA sessions (f).

This observation is of interest since it suggests that pharmacological flexibility in response to changes in drug availability and individual propensity to titrate drug intake according to drug availability may protect against loss of control over heroin SA. Nevertheless, the marked dissociation between high impulsivity trait and individual propensity to lose control over heroin intake is in marked contrast with the demonstration that high impulsivity predicts increased vulnerability to lose control over cocaine SA [241]. Such dissociation suggests that heroin and cocaine addiction may not necessarily share common etiological factors, or, since impulsivity is a multifaceted construct [246], that other forms of impulsivity predict vulnerability to opiates addiction.

7. Conclusions

Major advances in the understanding of the neurobiological substrates of addictive drugs and their short and long-term consequences on the brain have been provided by CPP or self-administration models. Refined preclinical models, that go beyond drug reinforcement or neurobiological adaptations to repeated exposure to addictive drugs, hence with heuristic value with regards to the compulsive nature of drug seeking in drug addicts, have provided new insights into the aetiology and pathophysiology of drug addiction. Nevertheless, to date several critical behavioural aspects of drug addiction remain under-investigated, including the influence of alternative reinforcers during self-administration sessions and the role of environmental conditions, and especially environmental enrichment in inter-individual vulnerability to switch to compulsive drug use. Additionally, the recent data we have acquired on inter-individual differences in loss of control over heroin intake and the marked dissociation between high impulsivity trait and escalation of heroin SA reveal the necessity to develop preclinical models of addiction-like behaviour for other classes of drugs than stimulants. Only then will we be able to determine whether drug addiction is one pathology characterised by common etiological and pathophysiological factors or whether it should instead be considered as multifaceted, with different etiological and pathophysiological pathways, depending, at least, on the drug [56].

8. Acknowledgements

This work was supported by the INSERM AVENIR program, the IREB, the Fondation pour la recherche Médicale (FRM) and the University of Poitiers. Aude Belin-Rauscent was supported by the AXA research fund and an INSERM post-doctoral fellowship. The authors would like to thank Drs Yann Pelloux, Daina Economidou and Pr Barry Everitt for previous work on contents of this chapter.

9. References

[1] Geyer MA, Markou A, Bloom FE, Kupfer DJ. Animal models in psychatric disorders. 1995. p. 787-798.

[2] Koob G, Le Moal M. Plasticity of reward neurocircuitry and the 'dark side' of drug addiction. Nat Neurosci. 2005; 8: 1442-1444.

[3] Olds J, Milner P. Positive reinforcement produced by electrical stimulation of septal area and other regions of rat brain. Jcomp Physiol Psychol. 1954; 47: 419-427.

[4] Weeks JR. Experimental Morphine Addiction: Method for Automatic Intravenous Injections in Unrestrained Rats. Science. 1962; 138: 143-144.

[5] DSMIII. Diagnostic and Statistical Manual of Mental Disorders [Third Edition]. American Psychiatric Association.; 1985

[6] Everitt BJ, Robbins TW. Second-order schedules of drug reinforcement in rats and monkeys: measurement of reinforcing efficacy and drug-seeking behaviour. Psychopharmacology. 2000; 153: 17-30.

[7] Everitt BJ, Robbins TW. Neural systems of reinforcement for drug addiction: from actions to habits to compulsion. Nat Neurosci. 2005; 8: 1481-1489.

[8] Belin D, Balado E, Piazza PV, Deroche-Gamonet V. Pattern of intake and drug craving predict the development of cocaine addiction-like behavior in rats. Biol Psychiatry. 2009; 65: 863-868.

[9] Pelloux Y, Costentin J, Duterte-Boucher D. Differential effects of novelty exposure on place preference conditioning to amphetamine and its oral consumption. Psychopharmacology. 2004; 171: 277-285.

[10] Bardo M, Bevins RA. Conditioned place preference: what does it add to our preclinical understanding of drug reward? Psychopharmacology [Berl]. 2000; 153: 31-43.

[11] Kusayama T, Watanabe S. Reinforcing effects of methamphetamine in planarians. Neuroreport. 2000; 11: 2511-2513.

[12] Bardo M, Donohew RL, Harrington NG. Psychobiology of novelty seeking and drug seeking behavior. Behavioural Brain Research. 1996; 77: 23-43.

[13] Frenois F, Cador M, Caille S, Stinus L, Le Moine C. Neural correlates of the motivational and somatic components of naloxone-precipitated morphine withdrawal. Eur J Neurosci. 2002; 16: 1377-1389.

[14] Frenois F, Le Moine C, Cador M. The motivational component of withdrawal in opiate addiction: rôle of associative learning and aversive memory in opiate addiction from a behavioral, anatomical and functional perspective. Rev Neurosci. 2005; 16: 255-276.

[15] Frenois F, Stinus L, Di Blasi F, Cador M, Le Moine C. A specific limbic circuit underlies opiate withdrawal memories. J Neurosci. 2005; 25: 1366-1374.

[16] Rossi NA, Reid LD. Affective states associated with morphine injections [dissertation]. Bradley University.; 1976.

[17] Tzschentke T. Behavioral pharmacology of buprenorphine, with a focus on preclinical models of reward and addiction. Psychopharmacology. 2002; 161: 1-16.

[18] De Wit H, Stewart J. Reinstatement of cocaine-reinforced responding in the rat. Psychopharmacology [Berl]. 1981; 75: 134-143.

[19] De Wit H, Stewart J. Drug reinstatement of heroin-reinforced responding in the rat. Psychopharmacology [Berl]. 1983; 79: 29-31.

[20] Bossert JM, Ghitza UE, Lu L, Epstein DH, Shaham Y. Neurobiology of relapse to heroin and cocaine seeking: an update and clinical implications. Eur J Pharmacol. 2005; 526[1-3]:36-50.

[21] Ahmed SH, Koob G. Transition from Moderate to Excessive Drug Intake: Change in Hedonic Set Point. Science. 1998; 282: 298-300.

[22] Ahmed SH, Walker JR, Koob G. Persistent Increase in the Motivation to Take Heroin in Rats with a History of Drug Escalation. Neuropsychopharmacology. 2000; 22: 413-421.

[23] Vanderschuren L, Everitt BJ. Behavioral and neural mechanisms of compulsive drug seeking. European Journal of Pharmacology. 2005; 526: 77-88.

[24] Pelloux Y, Everitt BJ, Dickinson A. Compulsive drug seeking by rats under punishment: effects of drug taking history. Psychopharmacology [Berl]. 2007; 194: 127-137.

[25] Economidou D, Pelloux Y, Robbins TW, Dalley JW, Everitt BJ. High Impulsivity Predicts Relapse to Cocaine-Seeking After Punishment-Induced Abstinence. Biol Psychiatry. 2009; 65: 851-856.

[26] Deroche-Gamonet V, Belin D, Piazza P. Evidence for addiction-like behavior in the rat. Science. 2004; 305: 1014-1017.

[27] Belin D, Mar A, Dalley J, Robbins TW, Everitt BJ High Impulsivity Predicts the Switch to Compulsive Cocaine-Taking. Science. 2008; 320: 1352-1355.

[28] Belin D, Berson N, Balado E, Piazza PV, Deroche-Gamonet V. High-Novelty-Preference Rats are Predisposed to Compulsive Cocaine Self-administration. Neuropsychopharmacology. 2011; 36: 569-579.

[29] Spealman RD, Goldberg SR. Drug Self-Administration by Laboratory Animals: Control by Schedules of Reinforcement. Annual Reviews in Pharmacology and Toxicology. 1978; 18: 313: 339.

[30] Goldberg SR, Kelleher RT, Morse WH. Second-order schedules of drug injection. Fed Proc. 1975; 34: 1771-1776.

[31] Stafford D, LeSage MG, Glowa JR. Progressive-ratio schedules of drug delivery in the analysis of drug self-administration: a review. Psychopharmacology. 1998; 139: 169-184.

[32] Schindler CW, Panlilio LV, Goldberg SR. Second-order schedules of drug self-administration in animals. Psychopharmacology [Berl]. 2002; 163: 327-344.

[33] Di Chiara G, Imperato A. Drugs abused by humans preferentially increase synaptic dopamine concentrations in the mesolimbic system of freely moving rats. ProcNatlAcadSciUSA. 1988; 85: 5274-5278.

[34] Bozarth MA, Wise RA. Intracranial self-administration of morphine into the ventral tegmental area in rats. Life Sci. 1981; 28: 551-555.

[35] Bozarth MA, Wise RA. Neural substrates of opiate reinforcement. Prog Neuropsychopharmacol Biol Psychiatry. 1983; 7: 569-575.

[36] Bozarth MA, Wise RA. Anatomically distinct opiate receptor fields mediate reward and physical dependence. Science. 1984; 224: 516-517.

[37] Bozarth MA, Wise RA. Toxicity associated with long-term intravenous heroin and cocaine self-administration in the rat. JAMA. 1985; 254: 81-83.

[38] Di Chiara G, Tanda G, Bassareo V, Pontieri F, Acquas E, Fenu S, Cadoni C, Carboni E. Drug addiction as a disorder of associative learning. rôle of nucleus accumbens shell/extended amygdala dopamine. Ann N Y Acad Sci. 1999; 877: 461-485.

[39] Everitt BJ, Parkinson JA, Olmstead M, Arroyo M, Robledo P, Robbins TW. Associative processes in addiction and reward. The rôle of amygdala-ventral striatal subsystems. Ann NYAcadSci. 1999; 877: 412-438.

[40] Everitt BJ, Dickinson A, Robbins TW. The neuropsychological basis of addictive behaviour. Brain Research Reviews. 2001; 36: 129-138.

[41] Everitt BJ, Belin D, Dalley J, Robbins TW. Dopaminergic mechanisms in drug-seeking habits and the vulnerability to drug addiction. In: Leslie Iversen SI, Stephen Dunnett, and Anders Bjorklund, editor. Dopamine Handbook. New York: Oxford University Press; 2010.

[42] Robbins TW, Everitt BJ. Drug addiction: bad habits add up. Nature. 1999; 398: 567-570.

[43] Robbins TW, Everitt BJ. Limbic-Striatal Memory Systems and Drug Addiction. Neurobiology of Learning and Memory. 2002; 78: 625-636.

[44] Robinson T, Berridge K. Incentive-sensitization and addiction. Addiction. 2001; 96: 103-114.

[45] Everitt BJ, Wolf ME. Psychomotor Stimulant Addiction: A Neural Systems Perspective. Journal of Neuroscience. 2002; 22: 3312-3320.

[46] Jones S, Bonci A. Synaptic plasticity and drug addiction. Curr Opin Pharmacol. 2005; 5: 20-25.

[47] Hyman SE, Malenka RC, Nestler EJ. Neural mechanisms of addiction: the rôle of reward-related learning and memory. Annu Rev Neurosci. 2006; 29: 565-598.

[48] Schultz W. Multiple Dopamine Functions at Different Time Courses. Annu Rev Neurosci. 2007; 30: 259-288.

[49] Schultz W. Behavioral dopamine signals. Trends in Neurosciences. 2007; 30: 203-210.

[50] Faure A, Reynolds SM, Richard JM, Berridge KC. Mesolimbic dopamine in desire and dread: enabling motivation to be generated by localized glutamate disruptions in nucleus accumbens. J Neurosci. 2008; 28: 7184-7192.

[51] Thomas MJ, Kalivas P, Shaham Y. Neuroplasticity in the mesolimbic dopamine system and cocaine addiction. Br J Pharmacol. 2008; 154: 327-342.

[52] Berridge KC, Robinson TE, Aldridge JW. Dissecting components of reward: 'liking', 'wanting', and learning. Curr Opin Pharmacol. 2009; 9[1]:65-73.

[53] Ettenberg A, Pettit HO, Bloom FE, Koob GF. Heroin and cocaine intravenous self-administration in rats: Mediation by separate neural systems. Psychopharmacology. 1982; 78: 204-209.

[54] Kelly PH, Roberts DC. Effects of amphetamine and apomorphine on locomotor activity after 6-OHDA and electrolytic lesions of the nucleus accumbens septi. Pharmacol Biochem Behav. 1983; 19: 137-143.

[55] Pettit HO, Ettenberg A, Bloom FE, Koob GF. Destruction of dopamine in the nucleus accumbens selectively attenuates cocaine but not heroin self-administration in rats. Psychopharmacology [Berl]. 1984; 84: 167-173.

[56] Badiani A, Belin D, Epstein D, Calu D, Shaham Y. Opiate versus psychostimulant addiction: the differences do matter. Nat Rev Neurosci. 2011; 12: 685-700.

[57] Robinson T, Kolb B. Persistent structural modifications in nucleus accumbens and prefrontal cortex neurons produced by previous experience with amphetamine. J Neurosci. 1997; 17: 8491-8497.

[58] Robinson T, Kolb B. Morphine alters the structure of neurons in the nucleus accumbens and neocortex of rats. Synapse. 1999; 33: 160-162.

[59] Robinson T, Kolb B. Alterations in the morphology of dendrites and dendritic spines in the nucleus accumbens and prefrontal cortex following repeated treatment with amphetamine or cocaine. Eur J Neurosci. 1999; 11: 1598-1604.

[60] Robinson T, Kolb B. Structural plasticity associated with exposure to drugs of abuse. Neuropharmacology. 2004; 47 Suppl 1: 33-46.

[61] Robinson TE, Leung AN, Northway WH, Blankenberg FG, Bloch DA, Oehlert JW, Al-Dabbagh H, Hubli S, Moss RB. Spirometer-triggered high-resolution computed tomography and pulmonary function measurements during an acute exacerbation in patients with cystic fibrosis. J Pediatr. 2001; 138: 553-559.

[62] Li Y, Kolb B, Robinson T. The location of persistent amphetamine-induced changes in the density of dendritic spines on medium spiny neurons in the nucleus accumbens and caudate-putamen. Neuropsychopharmacology. 2003; 28: 1082-1085.

[63] Wolf ME, Sun X, Mangiavacchi S, Chao SZ. Psychomotor stimulants and neuronal plasticity. Neuropharmacology. 2004; 47 Suppl 1: 61-79.

[64] Schmidt K, Krishnan B, Xia Y, Sun A, Orozco-Cabal L, Pollandt S, Centeno M, Genzer K, Gallagher JP, Shinnick-Gallagher P, Liu J. Cocaine withdrawal enhances long-

term potentiation induced by corticotropin-releasing factor at central amygdala glutamatergic synapses via CRF, NMDA receptors and PKA. Eur J Neurosci. 2006; 24: 1733-1743.

[65] Fu Y, Pollandt S, Liu J, Krishnan B, Genzer K, Orozco-Cabal L, Gallagher JP, Shinnick-Gallagher P Long-term potentiation [LTP] in the central amygdala [CeA] is enhanced after prolonged withdrawal from chronic cocaine and requires CRF1 receptors. J Neurophysiol. 2007; 97: 937-941.

[66] Bonci A, Borgland S. Role of orexin/hypocretin and CRF in the formation of drug-dependent synaptic plasticity in the mesolimbic system. Neuropharmacology. 2009; 56 Suppl 1: 107-111.

[67] Ahmed SH, Lutjens R, van der Stap LD, Lekic D, Romano-Spica V, Morales M, Koob GF, Repunte-Canonigo V, Sanna PP. Gene expression evidence for remodeling of lateral hypothalamic circuitry in cocaine addiction. Proc Natl Acad Sci U S A. 2005; 102: 11533-11538.

[68] Belin D, Deroche-Gamonet V, Jaber M. Cocaine-induced sensitization is associated with altered dynamics of transcriptional responses of the dopamine transporter, tyrosine hydroxylase, and dopamine D2 receptors in C57Bl/6J mice. Psychopharmacology [Berl]. 2007; 193: 567-578.

[69] Nestler EJ. Common molecular and cellular substrates of addiction and memory. Neurobiol Learn Mem. 2002; 78: 637-647.

[70] Koob G. Neuroadaptive mechanisms of addiction: studies on the extended amygdala. European Neuropsychopharmacology. 2003; 13: 442-452.

[71] Befort K, Filliol D, Ghate A, Darcq E, Matifas A, Muller J, Lardenois A, Thibault C, Dembele D, Le Merrer J, Becker JA, Poch O, Kieffer BL. Mu-opioid receptor activation induces transcriptional plasticity in the central extended amygdala. Eur J Neurosci. 2008; 27: 2973-2984.

[72] Feltenstein MW, See RE. The neurocircuitry of addiction: an overview. Br J Pharmacol. 2008; 154: 261-274.

[73] Corominas M, Roncero C, Casas M. Corticotropin releasing factor and neuroplasticity in cocaine addiction. Life Sci. 2009

[74] Marcinkiewcz CA, Prado MM, Isaac SK, Marshall A, Rylkova D, Bruijnzeel AW. Corticotropin-releasing factor within the central nucleus of the amygdala and the nucleus accumbens shell mediates the negative affective state of nicotine withdrawal in rats. Neuropsychopharmacology. 2009; 34: 1743-1752.

[75] Nestler EJ. The neurobiology of cocaine addiction. Sci Pract Perspect. 2005; 3: 4-10.

[76] Nestler EJ. Epigenetic mechanisms in psychiatry. Biol Psychiatry. 2009; 65: 189-190.

[77] Renthal W, Nestler EJ. Epigenetic mechanisms in drug addiction. Trends Mol Med. 2008; 14: 341-350.

[78] Maze I, Covington HE 3rd, Dietz DM, LaPlant Q, Renthal W, Russo SJ, Mechanic M, Mouzon E, Neve RL, Haggarty SJ, Ren Y, Sampath SC, Hurd YL, Greengard P, Tarakhovsky A, Schaefer A, Nestler EJ. Essential role of the histone methyltransferase G9a in cocaine-induced plasticity. Science. 2010; 327: 213-216.

[79] Russo SJ, Dietz DM, Dumitriu D, Morrison JH, Malenka RC, Nestler EJ. The addicted synapse: mechanisms of synaptic and structural plasticity in nucleus accumbens. Trends Neurosci. 2010

[80] Jedynak J, Uslaner J, Esteban J, Robinson T. Methamphetamine-induced structural plasticity in the dorsal striatum. Eur J Neurosci. 2007; 25: 847-853.

[81] Schoenbaum G, Shaham Y. The role of Orbitofrontal Cortex in Drug Addiction: A Review of Preclinical Studies. Biological Psychiatry. 2008; 63: 256-262.

[82] Winstanley CA, Green TA, Theobald DE, Renthal W, LaPlant Q, DiLeone RJ, Chakravarty S, Nestler EJ. DeltaFosB induction in orbitofrontal cortex potentiates locomotor sensitization despite attenuating the cognitive dysfunction caused by cocaine. Pharmacol Biochem Behav. 2008

[83] Kolb B, Gorny G, Li Y, Samaha AN, Robinson T. Amphetamine or cocaine limits the ability of later experience to promote structural plasticity in the neocortex and nucleus accumbens. Proc Natl Acad Sci U S A. 2003; 100: 10523-10528.

[84] Kolb B, Pellis S, Robinson T. Plasticity and functions of the orbital frontal cortex. Brain Cogn. 2004; 55: 104-115.

[85] Crombag H, Gorny G, Li Y, Kolb B, Robinson T. Opposite effects of amphetamine self-administration experience on dendritic spines in the medial and orbital prefrontal cortex. Cereb Cortex. 2005; 15: 341-348.

[86] Koob G, Le Moal M. Drug Abuse: Hedonic Homeostatic Dysregulation. Science. 1997; 278: 52-58.

[87] Koob G, Le Moal M. Drug addiction, dysregulation of reward, and allostasis. Neuropsychopharmacology. 2001; 24: 97-129.

[88] Koob GF, Le Moal M. Review. Neurobiological mechanisms for opponent motivational processes in addiction. Philos Trans R Soc Lond B Biol Sci. 2008; 363: 3113-3123.

[89] Tsankova N, Renthal W, Kumar A, Nestler EJ. Epigenetic regulation in psychiatric disorders. Nat Rev Neurosci. 2007; 8: 355-367.

[90] McClung CA, Nestler EJ. Neuroplasticity mediated by altered gene expression. Neuropsychopharmacology. 2008; 33: 3-17.

[91] Renthal W, Nestler EJ. Chromatin regulation in drug addiction and depression. Dialogues Clin Neurosci. 2009; 11: 257-268.

[92] Renthal W, Nestler EJ. Histone acetylation in drug addiction. Semin Cell Dev Biol. 2009; 20: 387-394.

[93] Ahmed SH. Validation crisis in animal models of drug addiction: beyond non-disordered drug use toward drug addiction. Neurosci Biobehav Rev. 2010; 35: 172-184.

[94] Clark R, Schuster CR, Brady JV. Instrumental conditioning of jugular self-infusion in the rhesus monkey. Science. 1961; 133: 1829-1830.

[95] Wise RA, Bozarth MA. A psychomotor stimulant theory of addiction. Psychol Rev. 1987; 94: 469-492.

[96] Robinson T, Berridge K. The neural basis of drug craving: an incentive-sensitization theory of addiction. Brain Research Reviews. 1993; 18: 247-291.

[97] APA. Diagnostic and Statistical Manual of Mental Disorders fourth edition, Text revision [DSM-IV TR]. Washington DC: American Psychiatric Association; 2000

[98] Shaham Y, Miczek K. Reinstatement?toward a model of relapse. Psychopharmacology. 2003; 168: 1-2.

[99] Shaham Y, Shalev U, Lu L, De Wit H, Stewart J. The reinstatement model of drug relapse: history, methodology and major findings. Psychopharmacology. 2003; 168: 3-20.

[100] Fuchs RA, Branham RK, See RE. Different neural substrates mediate cocaine seeking after abstinence versus extinction training: a critical rôle for the dorsolateral caudate-putamen. J Neurosci. 2006; 26: 3584-3588.

[101] Belin D, Everitt BJ. Cocaine-Seeking Habits Depend upon Dopamine-Dependent Serial Connectivity Linking the Ventral with the Dorsal Striatum. Neuron. 2008; 57: 432-441.

[102] O'Brien CP. A Range of Research-Based Pharmacotherapies for Addiction. Science. 1997; 278: 66-70.

[103] See RE, Elliott JC, Feltenstein MW. The role of dorsal vs ventral striatal pathways in cocaine-seeking behavior after prolonged abstinence in rats. Psychopharmacology [Berl]. 2007; 194: 321-331.

[104] Fuchs R, Tran-Nguyen LT, Specio SE, Groff RS, Neisewander JL. Predictive validity of the extinction/reinstatement model of drug craving. Psychopharmacology [Berl]. 1998; 135: 151-160.

[105] Shalev U, Grimm JW, Shaham Y. Neurobiology of Relapse to Heroin and Cocaine Seeking: A Review. Pharmacological Reviews. 2002; 54: 1-42.

[106] Capriles N, Rodaros D, Sorge RE, Stewart J. A role for the prefrontal cortex in stress- and cocaine-induced reinstatement of cocaine seeking in rats. Psychopharmacology [Berl]. 2003; 168: 66-74.

[107] Fuchs RA, Evans KA, Parker MP, See RE. Differential involvement of orbitofrontal cortex subregions in conditioned cue-induced and cocaine-primed reinstatement of cocaine seeking in rats. J Neurosci. 2004; 24: 6600-6610.

[108] Fuchs RA, Ramirez DR, Bell GH. Nucleus accumbens shell and core involvement in drug context-induced reinstatement of cocaine seeking in rats. Psychopharmacology [Berl]. 2008; 200: 545-556.

[109] Torregrossa MM, Tang XC, Kalivas PW. The glutamatergic projection from the prefrontal cortex to the nucleus accumbens core is required for cocaine-induced decreases in ventral pallidal GABA. Neurosci Lett. 2008; 438: 142-145.

[110] Zhou W, Kalivas P. N-Acetylcysteine Reduces Extinction Responding and Induces Enduring Reductions in Cue- and Heroin-Induced Drug-Seeking. Biological Psychiatry. 2008; 63: 338-340.

[111] Knackstedt LA, Kalivas PW. Glutamate and reinstatement. Curr Opin Pharmacol. 2009; 9: 59-64.

[112] Rocha A, Kalivas PW. role of the prefrontal cortex and nucleus accumbens in reinstating methamphetamine seeking. Eur J Neurosci. 2010; 31: 903-909.

[113] Kalivas P, Mcfarland K. Brain circuitry and the reinstatement of cocaine-seeking behavior. Psychopharmacology [Berl]. 2003; 168: 44-56.

[114] Kalivas P. Glutamate systems in cocaine addiction. Current Opinion in Pharmacology. 2004; 4: 23-29.

[115] LaLumiere RT, Kalivas PW. Glutamate release in the nucleus accumbens core is necessary for heroin seeking. J Neurosci. 2008; 28: 3170-3177.

[116] Kalivas PW. Perspective: the manifest destiny of cocaine research. Neuropsychopharmacology. 2009; 34: 1089-1090.

[117] Grimm JW, Hope BT, Wise RA, Shaham Y. Neuroadaptation. Incubation of cocaine craving after withdrawal. Nature. 2001; 412: 141-142.

[118] Lu L. Incubation of cocaine craving after withdrawal: a review of preclinical data. Neuropharmacology. 2004; 47: 214-226.

[119] Zernig G, Ahmed S, Cardinal R et al. Explaining the Escalation of Drug Use in Substance Dependence: Models and Appropriate Animal Laboratory Tests. Pharmacology. 2007; 80: 65-119.

[120] Ahmed S, Cador M. Dissociation of Psychomotor Sensitization from Compulsive Cocaine Consumption. Neuropsychopharmacology. 2006; 31: 563-571.

[121] Vanderschuren L, Everitt BJ. Drug Seeking Becomes Compulsive After Prolonged Cocaine Self-Administration. Science. 2004; 305: 1017-1019.

[122] McNamara R, Dalley JW, Robbins TW, Everitt BJ, Belin D. Trait-like impulsivity does not predict escalation of heroin self-administration in the rat. Psychopharmacology. 2010; 212: 453-464.

[123] Lenoir M, Ahmed S. Heroin-Induced Reinstatement is Specific to Compulsive Heroin Use and Dissociable from Heroin Reward and Sensitization. Neuropsychopharmacology. 2007; 32: 616-624.

[124] Corbit LH, Balleine B. The role of prelimbic cortex in instrumental conditioning. Behavioural Brain Research. 2003; 146: 145-157.

[125] Olmstead M, Parkinson J, Miles F, Everitt BJ, Dickinson A. Cocaine-seeking by rats: regulation, reinforcement and activation. Psychopharmacology. 2000; 152: 123-131.

[126] Olmstead M, Lafond M, Everitt BJ, Dickinson A. Cocaine seeking by rats is a goal-directed action. Behavioral Neuroscience. 2001; 115: 394-402.

[127] Zapata A, Minney VL, Shippenberg TS. Shift from goal-directed to habitual cocaine seeking after prolonged experience in rats. J Neurosci. 2010; 30: 15457-15463.

[128] Belin-Rauscent A, Everitt BJ, Belin D. Intrastriatal shifts mediate the transition from drug seeking actions to habits. Biological Psychiatry. 2012; In Press

[129] Goldberg SR, Spealman RD, Kelleher RT. Enhancement of drug-seeking behavior by environmental stimuli associated with cocaine or morphine injections. Neuropharmacology. 1979; 18: 1015-1017.

[130] Goldberg SR, Kelleher RT, Goldberg DM. Fixed-ratio responding under second-order schedules of food presentation or cocaine injection. J Pharmacol Exp Ther. 1981; 218: 271-281.

[131] Parkinson JA, Roberts AC, Everitt BJ, Di Ciano P. Acquisition of instrumental conditioned reinforcement is resistant to the devaluation of the unconditioned stimulus. QJExpPsycholB. 2005; 58: 19-30.

[132] Di Ciano P, Benham-Hermetz J, Fogg AP, Osborne GE. role of the prelimbic cortex in the acquisition, re-acquisition or persistence of responding for a drug-paired conditioned reinforcer. Neuroscience. 2007; 150: 291-298.

[133] Arroyo M, Markou A, Robbins TW, Everitt BJ. Acquisition, maintenance and reinstatement of intravenous cocaine self-administration under a second-order schedule of reinforcement in rats: effects of conditioned cues and continuous access to cocaine. Psychopharmacology [Berl]. 1998; 140: 331-344.

[134] Ito R, Dalley J, Robbins TW, Everitt BJ. Dopamine release in the dorsal striatum during cocaine-seeking behavior under the control of a drug-associated cue. J Neurosci. 2002; 22: 6247-6253.

[135] Ito R, Robbins TW, Everitt BJ. Differential control over cocaine-seeking behavior by nucleus accumbens core and shell. Nat Neurosci. 2004; 7: 389-397.

[136] Lee J, Di Ciano P, Thomas K, Everitt BJ. Disrupting Reconsolidation of Drug Memories Reduces Cocaine-Seeking Behavior. Neuron. 2005; 47: 795-801.

[137] Murray J, Belin D, Everitt BJ. Double dissociation of the dorsomedial and dorsolateral striatal control over the acquisition and performance of cocaine seeking. Neuropsychopharmacology. 2012; In Press

[138] Murray JE, Everitt BJ, Belin D. N-Acetylcysteine reduces early- and late-stage cocaine seeking without affecting cocaine taking in rats. Addict Biol. 2012; 17: 437-440.

[139] Di Ciano P, Everitt BJ. Direct Interactions between the Basolateral Amygdala and Nucleus Accumbens Core Underlie Cocaine-Seeking Behavior by Rats. Journal of Neuroscience. 2004; 24: 7167-7173.

[140] Corbit LH, Nie H, Janak PH. Habitual Alcohol Seeking: Time Course and the Contribution of Subregions of the Dorsal Striatum. Biol Psychiatry. 2012

[141] Murray J, Belin D, Everitt BJ. Double dissociation of the dorsomedial and dorsolateral striatal control over the acquisition and performance of cocaine seeking. Neuropsychopharmacology. 2012; In Press

[142] Vollstädt-Klein S, Wichert S, Rabinstein J, Bühler M, Klein O, Ende G, Hermann D, Mann K. Initial, habitual and compulsive alcohol use is characterized by a shift of cue processing from ventral to dorsal striatum. Addiction. 2010; 105: 1741-1749.

[143] Volkow ND, Wang GJ, Telang F, Fowler JS, Logan J, Childress AR, Jayne M, Ma Y, Wong C. Cocaine Cues and Dopamine in Dorsal Striatum: Mechanism of Craving in Cocaine Addiction. Journal of Neuroscience. 2006; 26: 6583-6588.

[144] Goodman WK, Price LH, Rasmussen SA, Mazure C, Fleischmann RL, Hill CL, Heninger GR, Charney DS. The Yale-Brown Obsessive Compulsive Scale. II. Validity. Arch Gen Psychiatry. 1989; 46: 1012-1016.

[145] Goodman WK, Price LH, Rasmussen SA, Mazure C, Fleischmann RL, Hill CL, Heninger GR, Charney DS. The Yale-Brown Obsessive Compulsive Scale. I. Development, use, and reliability. Arch Gen Psychiatry. 1989; 46: 1006-1011.

[146] Anton RF. Obsessive-compulsive aspects of craving: development of the Obsessive Compulsive Drinking Scale. Addiction. 2000; 95 Suppl 2: S211-7.

[147] Waldorf D, Reinarman C, Murphy S. Cocaine Changes: The Experience of Using and Quitting. Temple University Press; 1991

[148] Burman BD. The nonreimbursed patient. Rehab Manag. 1997; 10: 48-51.

[149] Cunningham JA, Lin E, Ross HE, Walsh GW. Factors associated with untreated remissions from alcohol abuse or dependence. Addict Behav. 2000; 25: 317-321.

[150] Dickinson A, Wood N, Smith J. Alcohol seeking by rats: Action or habit? The Quarterly Journal of Experimental Psychology: Section B. 2002; 55: 331-348.

[151] Miles F, Everitt BJ, Dickinson A. Oral cocaine seeking by rats: Action or habit? Behavioral Neuroscience. 2003; 117: 927-938.

[152] Heyne A, Wolffgramm J. The development of addiction to d-amphetamine in an animal model: same principles as for alcohol and opiate. Psychopharmacology [Berl]. 1998; 140: 510-518.

[153] Spanagel R, Holter SM. Long-term alcohol self-administration with repeated alcohol deprivation phases: an animal model of alcoholism? Alcohol Alcohol. 1999; 34: 231-243.

[154] Heyne A, May T, Goll P, Wolffgramm J. Persisting consequences of drug intake: towards a memory of addiction. J Neural Transm. 2000; 107: 613-638.

[155] Pearce JM, Dickinson A. Pavlovian counterconditioning: changing the suppressive properties of shock by association with food. J Exp Psychol Anim Behav Process. 1975; 1: 170-177.

[156] Azrin NH, Holz WC. Punishment. Operant behavior: Areas of research and application. 1966; 380-447.

[157] Cooper A, Barnea-Ygael N, Levy D, Shaham Y, Zangen A. A conflict rat model of cue-induced relapse to cocaine seeking. Psychopharmacology [Berl]. 2007; 194: 117-125.

[158] Smith SG, Davis WM. Punishment of amphetamine and morphine self-administration behavior. Psychol Rec. 1974; 24: 477-480.

[159] Corbit L, Balleine B. Instrumental and Pavlovian incentive processes have dissociable effects on components of a heterogeneous instrumental chain. Journal of Experimental Psychology: Animal Behavior Processes. 2003; 29: 99-106.

[160] Panlilio LV, Thorndike EB, Schindler CW. Reinstatement of punishment-suppressed opioid self-administration in rats: an alternative model of relapse to drug abuse. Psychopharmacology [Berl]. 2003; 168: 229-235.

[161] Robinson T, Berridge K. The psychology and neurobiology of addiction: an incentive-sensitization view. Addiction. 2000; 95: S91-S117.

[162] Robinson TE, Berridge KC. Review. The incentive sensitization theory of addiction: some current issues. Philos Trans R Soc Lond B Biol Sci. 2008; 363: 3137-3146.

[163] Dieckmann U, Doebeli M. On the origin of species by sympatric speciation. Nature. 1999; 400: 354-357.

[164] Hasegawa M, Yahara T, Yasumoto A, Hotta M. Bimodal distribution of flowering time in a natural hybrid population of daylily [Hemerocallis fulva] and nightlily [Hemerocallis citrina]. Journal of Plant Research. 2006; 119: 63-68.

[165] Ellenbroek BA, Cools AR. Apomorphine susceptibility and animal models for psychopathology: genes and environment. Behav Genet. 2002; 32: 349-361.

[166] Nesse RM, Berridge K. Psychoactive Drug Use in Evolutionary Perspective. Science. 1997; 278: 63-66.

[167] Belin D, Economidou D, Pelloux Y, Everitt BJ. Habit Formation and Compulsion. In: Olmstead MC, editor. Animal models of drug addiction. Humana Press; 2010. p. 337-378.

[168] Anthony JC, Warner LA, Kessler RC Comparative epidemiology of dependence on tobacco, alcohol, controlled substances, and inhalants: Basic findings from the National comorbidity Survey. Exp Clin Psychopharmacol. 1994; 2: 244-268.

[169] Kasanetz F, Deroche-Gamonet V, Berson N, Balado E, Lafourcade M, Manzoni O, Piazza PV. Transition to addiction is associated with a persistent impairment in synaptic plasticity. Science. 2010; 328: 1709-1712.

[170] Everitt BJ, Belin D, Economidou D, Pelloux Y, Dalley J, Robbins TW. Neural mechanisms underlying the vulnerability to develop compulsive drug-seeking habits and addiction. Philos Trans R Soc Lond B Biol Sci. 2008; 363: 3125-3135.

[171] Kreek M, Laforge K, Butelman E. Pharmacotherapy of addictions. Nat Rev Drug Discov. 2002; 1: 710-726.

[172] Kreek M, Nielsen D, Butelman E, Laforge K. Genetic influences on impulsivity, risk taking, stress responsivity and vulnerability to drug abuse and addiction. Nat Neurosci. 2005; 8: 1450-1457.

[173] Teichman M, Barnea Z, Rahav G. Sensation seeking, state and trait anxiety, and depressive mood in adolescent substance users. IntJAddict. 1989; 24: 87-99.

[174] Teichman M, Barnea Z, Ravav G. Personality and substance use among adolescents: a longitudinal study. BrJAddict. 1989; 84: 181-190.

[175] Zuckerman M. The sensation seeking motive. Prog Exp Pers Res. 1974; 7: 79-148.

[176] Zuckerman M. Sensation seeking and the endogenous deficit theory of drug abuse. NIDA Res Monogr. 1986; 74: 59-70.

[177] Zuckerman M. Sensation seeking and behavior disorders. Arch Gen Psychiatry. 1988; 45: 502-504.

[178] Kilpatrick DG, Sutker PB, Roitzsch JC, Miller WC. Personality correlates of polydrug abuse. PsycholRep. 1976; 38: 311-317.

[179] Pomerleau CS, Pomerleau OF, Flessland KA, Basson SM. Relationship of Tridimensional Personality Questionnaire scores and smoking variables in female and male smokers. J Subst Abuse. 1992; 4: 143-154.

[180] Schinka JA, Curtiss G, Mulloy JM. Personality variables and self-medication in substance abuse. JpersAssess. 1994; 63: 413-422.

[181] Wills TA, Vaccaro D, McNamara G. Novelty seeking, risk taking, and related constructs as predictors of adolescent substance use: an application of Cloninger's theory. J Subst Abuse. 1994; 6: 1-20.

[182] Wills TA, Windle M, Cleary SD. Temperament and novelty seeking in adolescent substance use: convergence of dimensions of temperament with constructs from Cloninger's theory. J Pers Soc Psychol. 1998; 74: 387-406.

[183] Scourfield J, Stevens DE, Merikangas KR. Substance abuse, comorbidity, and sensation seeking: gender differences. Compr Psychiatry. 1996; 37: 384-392.

[184] Sarramon C, Verdoux H, Schmitt L, Bourgeois M. [Addiction and personality traits: sensation seeking, anhedonia, impulsivity]. Encephale. 1999; 25: 569-575.

[185] Sher KJ, Bartholow BD, Wood MD. Personality and substance use disorders: a prospective study. J Consult Clin Psychol. 2000; 68: 818-829.

[186] Skinstad AH, Swain A. Comorbidity in a clinical sample of substance abusers. Am Jdrug Alcohol Abuse. 2001; 27: 45-64.

[187] Conway K, Swendsen JD, Rounsaville BJ, Merikangas KR. Personality, drug of choice, and comorbid psychopathology among substance abusers. Drug Alcohol Depend. 2002; 65: 225-234.

[188] Moeller FG, Dougherty DM, Barratt ES, Oderinde V, Mathias CW, Harper RA, Swann AC. Increased impulsivity in cocaine dependent subjects independent of antisocial personality disorder and aggression. Drug Alcohol Depend. 2002; 68: 105-111.

[189] Adams JB, Heath AJ, Young SE, Hewitt JK, Corley RP, Stallings MC. Relationships between personality and preferred substance and motivations for use among adolescent substance abusers. Am J Drug Alcohol Abuse. 2003; 29: 691-712.

[190] Conway K. Personality, substance of choice, and polysubstance involvement among substance dependent patients. Drug and Alcohol Dependence. 2003; 71: 65-75.

[191] O'Leary TA, Rohsenow DJ, Martin R, Colby SM, Eaton CA, Monti PM. The relationship between anxiety levels and outcome of cocaine abuse treatment. Am Jdrug Alcohol Abuse. 2000; 26: 179-194.

[192] Roberts A. Psychiatric comorbidity in white and African-American illicit substance abusers: evidence for differential etiology. ClinPsycholRev. 2000; 20: 667-677.

[193] Forsyth JP, Parker JD, Finlay CG. Anxiety sensitivity, controllability, and experiential avoidance and their relation to drug of choice and addiction severity in a residential sample of substance-abusing veterans. Addictive Behaviors. 2003; 28: 851-870.

[194] Zilberman ML, Tavares H, Hodgins DC, el-Guebaly N. The impact of gender, depression, and personality on craving. J Addict Dis. 2007; 26: 79-84.

[195] Petry NM. Discounting of delayed rewards in substance abusers: relationship to antisocial personality disorder. Psychopharmacology [Berl]. 2002; 162: 425-432.

[196] Hanson KL, Luciana M, Sullwold K. Reward-related decision-making deficits and elevated impulsivity among MDMA and other drug users. Drug Alcohol Depend. 2008; 96: 99-110.

[197] Franques P, Auriacombe M, Tignol J. [Addiction and personality]. Encephale. 2000; 26: 68-78.

[198] Zuckerman M, Neeb M. Sensation seeking and psychopathology. Psychiatry Res. 1979; 1: 255-264.

[199] Zuckerman M. The psychophysiology of sensation seeking. J Pers. 1990; 58: 313-345.

[200] Chandra PS, Krishna VA, Benegal V, Ramakrishna J. High-risk sexual behaviour & sensation seeking among heavy alcohol users. Indian J Med Res. 2003; 117: 88-92.

[201] Pellow S, Chopin P, File SE, Briley M. Validation of open: closed arm entries in an elevated plus-maze as a measure of anxiety in the rat. JneurosciMethods. 1985; 14: 149-167.

[202] Pellow S, File SE. Anxiolytic and anxiogenic drug effects on exploratory activity in an elevated plus-maze: a novel test of anxiety in the rat. PharmacolBiochemBehav. 1986; 24: 525-529.

[203] Pelloux Y, Costentin J, Duterte-Boucher D. Anxiety increases the place conditioning induced by cocaine in rats. Behav Brain Res. 2009; 197: 311-316.

[204] Homberg JR, van den Akker M, Raasø HS, Wardeh G, Binnekade R, Schoffelmeer AN, de Vries TJ. Enhanced motivation to self-administer cocaine is predicted by self-grooming behaviour and relates to dopamine release in the rat medial prefrontal cortex and amygdala. Eur J Neurosci. 2002; 15: 1542-1550.

[205] Bush D, Vaccarino F. Individual differences in elevated plus-maze exploration predicted progressive-ratio cocaine self-administration break points in Wistar rats. Psychopharmacology. 2007; 194: 211-219.

[206] Spanagel R, Montkowski A, Allingham K, Stöhr T, Shoaib M, Holsboer F, Landgraf R. Anxiety: a potential predictor of vulnerability to the initiation of ethanol self-administration in rats. Psychopharmacology [Berl]. 1995; 122: 369-373.

[207] Henniger MS, Spanagel R, Wigger A, Landgraf R, Holter SM. Alcohol self-administration in two rat lines selectively bred for extremes in anxiety-related behavior. Neuropsychopharmacology. 2002; 26: 729-736.

[208] Stewart SH, Karp J, Pihl RO, Peterson RA. Anxiety sensitivity and self-reported reasons for drug use. JsubstAbuse. 1997; 9: 223-240.

[209] Chakroun N, Doron J, Swendsen J. [Substance use, affective problems and personality traits: test of two association models.]. Encephale. 2004; 30: 564-569.

[210] Dilleen R, Pelloux Y, Mar AC, Molander A, Robbins TW, Everitt BJ, Dalley JW, Belin D. High anxiety is a predisposing endophenotype for loss of control over cocaine, but not heroin, self-administration in rats. Psychopharmacology [Berl]. 2012

[211] Conrod PJ, Pihl RO, Stewart SH, Dongier M. Validation of a system of classifying female substance abusers on the basis of personality and motivational risk factors for substance abuse. Psychol Addict Behav. 2000; 14: 243-256.

[212] Khantzian EJ. The self-medication hypothesis of substance use disorders: a reconsideration and recent applications. HarvRevPsychiatry. 1997; 4: 231-244.

[213] Paine TA, Jackman SL, Olmstead MC. Cocaine-induced anxiety: alleviation by diazepam, but not buspirone, dimenhydrinate or diphenhydramine. Behav Pharmacol. 2002; 13: 511-523.

[214] Müller CP, Carey RJ, Wilkisz M, Schwenzner S, Jocham G, Huston JP, De Souza Silva MA. Acute anxiolytic effects of cocaine: the rôle of test latency and activity phase. Pharmacol Biochem Behav. 2008; 89: 218-226.

[215] Dellu F, Mayo W, Vallée M, Maccari S, Piazza PV, Le Moal M, Simon H. Behavioral reactivity to novelty during youth as a predictive factor of stress-induced corticosterone secretion in the elderly--a life-span study in rats. Psychoneuroendocrinology. 1996; 21: 441-453.

[216] Blanchard MM, Mendelsohn D, Stamp JA. The HR/LR model: Further evidence as an animal model of sensation seeking. Neurosci Biobehav Rev. 2009; 33: 1145-1154.

[217] Cain M, Saucier D, Bardo M. Novelty seeking and drug use: Contribution of an animal model. Experimental and Clinical Psychopharmacology. 2005; 13: 367-375.

[218] Piazza PV, Deminiere JM, Le Moal M, Simon H. Factors that predict individual vulnerability to amphetamine self-administration. Science. 1989; 245: 1511-1513.

[219] Hooks MS, Jones GH, Smith AD, Neill DB, Justice JB. Individual differences in locomotor activity and sensitization. PharmacolBiochemBehav. 1991; 38: 467-470.

[220] Hooks MS, Jones GH, Smith AD, Neill DB, Justice JB. Response to novelty predicts the locomotor and nucleus accumbens dopamine response to cocaine. Synapse. 1991; 9: 121-128.

[221] Piazza PV, Rouge-Pont F, Deminiere JM, Kharoubi M, Le Moal M, Simon H. Dopaminergic activity is reduced in the prefrontal cortex and increased in the nucleus accumbens of rats predisposed to develop amphetamine self-administration. Brain Res. 1991; 567: 169-174.

[222] Misslin R, Cigrang M. Does neophobia necessarily imply fear or anxiety? Behavioural processes. 1986; 12: 45-50.

[223] Bevins RA, Klebaur JE, Bardo M. Individual differences in response to novelty, amphetamine-induced activity and drug discrimination in rats. Behav Pharmacol. 1997; 8: 113-123.

[224] Cain ME, Smith C, Bardo M. The effect of novelty on amphetamine self-administration in rats classified as high and low responders. Psychopharmacology [Berl]. 2004; 176: 129-138.

[225] Klebaur JE, Bevins RA, Segar TM, Bardo M. Individual differences in behavioral responses to novelty and amphetamine self-administration in male and female rats. Behavioural Pharmacology. 2001

[226] Bardo M, Neisewander JL, Pierce R. Novelty-induced place preference behavior in rats: effects of opiate and dopaminergic drugs. Pharmacol Biochem Behav. 1989; 32: 683-689.

[227] Dellu F, Mayo W, Piazza PV, Le Moal M, Simon H. Individual differences in behavioral responses to novelty in rats. Possible relationship with the sensation-seeking trait in man. Personality and Individual Differences. 1993; 15: 411-411.

[228] Piazza PV, Ferdico M, Russo D, Crescimanno G, Benigno A, Amato G. Circling behavior: ethological analysis and functional considerations. Behav Brain Res. 1989; 31: 267-271.

[229] Klebaur JE, Bardo M. Individual differences in novelty seeking on the playground maze predict amphetamine conditioned place preference. Pharmacol Biochem Behav. 1999; 63: 131-136.

[230] Kabbaj M. The search for the neurobiological basis of vulnerability to drug abuse: using microarrays to investigate the rôle of stress and individual differences. Neuropharmacology. 2004; 47: 111-122.

[231] Beckmann JS, Marusich JA, Gipson CD, Bardo MT. Novelty seeking, incentive salience and acquisition of cocaine self-administration in the rat. Behav Brain Res. 2010

[232] Dellu F, Piazza PV, Mayo W, Le Moal M, Simon H. Novelty-seeking in rats-- biobehavioral characteristics and possible relationship with the sensation-seeking trait in man. Neuropsychobiology. 1996; 34: 136-145.

[233] Zuckerman M, Eysenck S, Eysenck HJ. Sensation seeking in England and America: cross-cultural, age, and sex comparisons. J Consult Clin Psychol. 1978; 46: 139-149.

[234] Cloninger CR. A unified biosocial theory of personality and its rôle in the development of anxiety states: a reply to commentaries. Psychiatr Dev. 1988; 6: 83-120.

[235] Arnett J. Sensation seeking: a new conceptualization and a new scale. Personality and Individual Differences. 1994; 16: 289-296.

[236] Wohlwill JF. What are sensation seekers seeking. Behavioral and Brain Sciences. 1984; 7: 453.

[237] Beck LH, Bransome ED, Mirsky AF, Rosvold HE, Sarason I. A continuous performance test of brain damage. J Consult Psychol. 1956; 20: 343-350.

[238] Robbins TW. The 5-choice serial reaction time task: behavioural pharmacology and functional neurochemistry. Psychopharmacology. 2002; 163[3-4]:362-380.

[239] Bari A, Dalley J, Robbins TW. The application of the 5-choice serial reaction time task for the assessment of visual attentional processes and impulse control in rats. Nature Protocol. 2008; 3[5]:759-767.

[240] Dalley J, Cardinal R, Robbins TW. Prefrontal executive and cognitive functions in rodents: neural and neurochemical substrates. Neuroscience & Biobehavioral Reviews. 2004; 28: 771-784.

[241] Dalley J, Mar A, Economidou D, Robbins TW. Neurobehavioral mechanisms of impulsivity: Fronto-striatal systems and functional neurochemistry. Pharmacology Biochemistry and Behavior. 2008; 90: 250-260.

[242] Dalley JW, Fryer TD, Brichard L, Robinson ES, Theobald DE, Lääne K, Peña Y, Murphy ER, Shah Y, Probst K, Abakumova I, Aigbirhio FI, Richards HK, Hong Y, Baron JC, Everitt BJ, Robbins TW. Nucleus Accumbens D2/3 Receptors Predict Trait Impulsivity and Cocaine Reinforcement. Science. 2007; 315: 1267-1270.

[243] Diergaarde L, Pattij T, Poortvliet I, Hogenboom F, de Vries W, Schoffelmeer AN, De Vries TJ. Impulsive Choice and Impulsive Action Predict Vulnerability to Distinct Stages of Nicotine Seeking in Rats. Biological Psychiatry. 2008; 63: 301-308.

[244] Diergaarde L, Pattij T, Nawijn L, Schoffelmeer ANM, De Vries TJ. Trait impulsivity predicts escalation of sucrose seeking and hypersensitivity to sucrose-associated stimuli. Behavioral Neuroscience. 2009; 123: 794-803.

[245] Jentsch JD, Taylor JR. Impulsivity resulting from frontostriatal dysfunction in drug abuse: implications for the control of behavior by reward-related stimuli. Psychopharmacology. 1999; 146: 373-390.

[246] Molander AC, Mar A, Norbury A, Steventon S, Moreno M, Caprioli D, Theobald DE, Belin D, Everitt BJ, Robbins TW, Dalley JW. High impulsivity predicting vulnerability to cocaine addiction in rats: some relationship with novelty preference but not novelty reactivity, anxiety or stress. Psychopharmacology [Berl]. 2011; 215: 721-731.

[247] Evenden J, Meyerson B. The behavior of spontaneously hypertensive and Wistar Kyoto rats under a paced fixed consecutive number schedule of reinforcement. Pharmacol Biochem Behav. 1999; 63: 71-82.

Drug Addictions:
An Historical and Ethological Overview

Aude Belin-Rauscent and David Belin
INSERM U 1084, LNEC, Université de Poitiers,
INSERM AVENIR Team "Psychology of Compulsive Disorders", Poitiers,
France

1. Introduction

1.1 Preliminary considerations: Focus on cocaine and heroin

It is well established that several psychoactive substances can lead to addiction. These include legal drugs such as alcohol and nicotine which generate the major part of the addiction-related social and economical costs to modern societies (1), and a pleiad of illegal drugs amongst which cannabis, cocaine and heroin are the most commonly used.

When one wants to consider the harmful consequences of an addictive drug, both the dependence and physical harm potencies of the drug should be considered for these two aspects contribute to the deterioration of the user's life. A recent classification of the major classes of addictive drugs reveals that heroin and cocaine are clearly the most dangerous ones since both their addictive properties and physical harm potency are high (2). Cocaine and heroin are followed by barbiturates and street methadone, but tobacco is shown to have addictive property of the same magnitude as cocaine, thereby demonstrating that the legal status of a substance is not a predictive factor of least addictive properties.

In the present chapter, we will consider exclusively cocaine and heroin addictions, not only because these two drugs are clearly the most dangerous ones, but mainly because cocaine and heroin use have been increasing among western countries populations in the last ten years. This focus is one limitation of the general conclusions that will be provided in the following chapters that will also address alcoholism and food addiction that will be joined by another addiction, namely pathological gambling, in the clinical definition of addictions in the upcoming DSM-V. Thus, addictions are increasingly recognised as abnormal persistent maladaptive behaviours driven by specific, initially reinforcing, stimuli in the environment that are not anymore restricted to psychoactive substances.

1.2 Drug use: A behaviour as old as humankind?

Drug use seems to have entered human customs as early as the emergence of human societies. Evidences that recreational drug use has emerged early on after human sedentarisation, perhaps with the development of religious rites, can be found for several drugs and routes of administration.

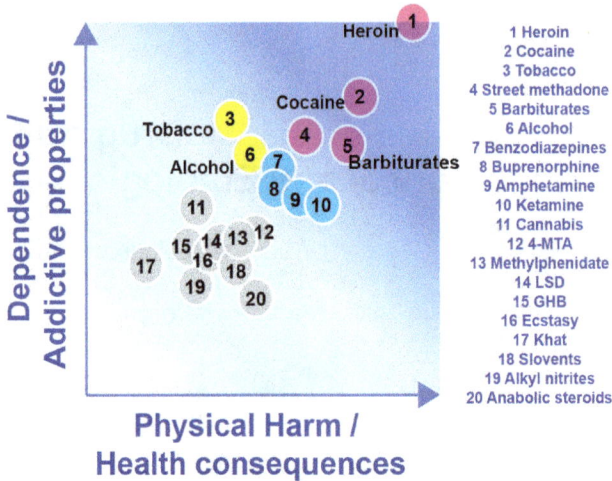

Fig. 1. Rational scale to assess the harm of drugs of potential misuse, after (2).

The addictive potential of a drug varies from substance to substance, and from individual to individual. Dose, frequency, pharmacokinetics of a particular substance, route of administration, and time are critical factors for physical harm and addictive potency. Heroin and cocaine are clearly the most dangerous ones since both their addictive properties and physical harm potency are high.

Thus, 5000 B.C. the sumerians used opium, as suggested by the fact that they had an ideogram for it which has been translated as HUL, meaning « joy » or « rejoicing » (3). A 3500 B.C. egyptian papyrus provides the earliest historical record of the production of alcohol in the description of a brewery (4).

Interestingly, 3000 B.C. is also the approximate date of the supposed origin of the use of tea in China. It is likely that coca leaf chewing began in the Andes at the same time since traces of coca have been found in mummies dating 3000 years back (5). The cocaine content of coca leaf is under 1% but after 1859, when cocaine was first isolated from coca leaf by Albert Niemann, cocaine was available legally in concentrations that were nearly 100% pure. Cocaine was first used recreationally in the 1860s, almost as soon as it was synthesised. A few years after its synthesis by Richard Willstätter in 1898 (6), cocaine appeared in cigarettes, ointments, nasal sprays, and tonics. The most popular cocaine-based product was Mariani Wine (Vin Mariani). It was a wine and cocaine mixture that was launched in 1863. Nearly all popular personalities of the day, including Queen Victoria, Thomas Edison and Pope Leon XIII endorsed it. Cocaine has also been popularised by Sigmund Freud who prescribed it for the treatment of digestive disorders, asthma, depression or opiate and alcohol dependence (7).

At the same time, more precisely in 1898, heroin (diacetylmorphine) was synthesized by Felix Hoffmann, 23 years after a first academic synthesis by Alder Wright. Akin to the launch of cocaine as a medicine, heroin was then introduced by Bayer as "safe preparation free from addiction-forming properties".

The broad availability of the pure form of cocaine and heroin has contributed to the marked development of addiction to these substances which, in their primary forms and routes of administration, were far less addictive. This phenomenon has been suggested to stem from a discrepancy between our brain and our modern environment, i.e, Nesse and Berridge wrote in 1997: «We are vulnerable to such fitness-decreasing incentives because our brains are not designed to cope with ready access to pure drugs, video games, and snack foods. Hundreds of generations of exposure would likely shape resistance to their allure and their deleterious effects» (8). This interesting consideration suggests that drug addiction may be a matter of mismatch between Human evolution and the recent revolution of human environment, a problem to which Evolution may be the best solution.

	All illicit drugs	Cannabis	Amphetamine-type stimulants		Cocaine	All opiates	Heroin
			Amphe-tamines	Ecstasy			
Number of users (in millions)	185.0	147.4	33.4	7.0	13.4	12.9	9.20
Proportion of global population (%)	3.1	2.5	0.6	0.1	0.2	0.2	0.15
Proportion of population 15 years and above (%)	4.3	3.5	0.8	0.2	0.3	0.3	0.22

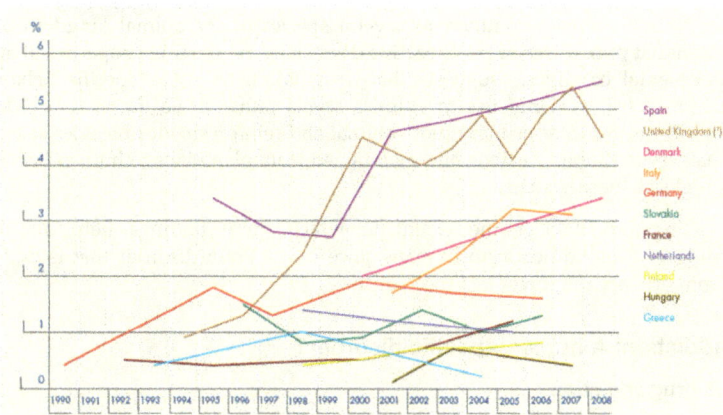

Fig. 2. Illicit drug use state at the beginning of the 21st century

Top panel: Annual prevalence of global, worldwide, illicit drug use over the period 1998-2001 (11). Bottom. A trend to increased cocaine use in European countries (10).

However, before these evolutionary, and rather fatalistic considerations, human societies have developed social and legal strategies to cope with addiction, as early as 10 years following the synthesis of heroin and cocaine. Indeed, the United States prohibited the importation of smoking opium (9) and the manufacture of heroin in 1909 and 1924, respectively, while the Harrison Narcotics Act of 1914 prohibited the use of cocaine. Since then law enforcement has limited, but not eradicated, heroin and cocaine use, as illustrated by figure 2 (EMCDDA) (10), the bottom panel of which shows a general increase in cocaine use within European countries over the past 20 years. Such a trend may induce an increase in the prevalence of drug-related health problems, and most importantly, of drug addiction.

1.3 Drug use: An evolutionary feature of animal kingdom

Drug use seems inherent to animal behaviour, perhaps because of the evolutionary selection of a reward system developed to maintain species survival, bringing animals towards sources of reinforcement. Thus spontaneous drug use has been observed in several species in the wild. Elephants would intoxicate with alcohol contained in ripe fruits and baboons would readily eat over-ripe fruits from the marula tree until they cannot walk anymore. Birds also use alcohol in that song thrush, for instance, struggle to fly after eating ripe grapes.

An exhaustive list of examples of spontaneous drug use in animal kingdom is beyond the scope of this chapter, but a last example should be enough to emphasise how broad are sources of intoxication in mammals: in the south of the United States, sheep and horses eat astragalus and then show hyperactive behaviour akin to human beings.

In experimental settings, it has been demonstrated that all drugs abused by humans are reinforcing in many species including planarians (12) and flies (13, 14), and they are readily self-administered by vertebrates such as mice (15-21) or rats (22-26), dogs (27, 28) and non human primates (29, 30).

Thus not only is drug used common to several species of the animal kingdom but the demonstration that pure forms of psychoactive drugs have reinforcing properties in animals under experimental conditions suggests that drug taking is not a specific behavioural feature of human beings. Drug use in animals seems rather to be the evidence that the neurobiological substrates of primary motivational and reinforcement processes selected by evolution have been shaped early on and maintained from planarians to human beings, and that drugs highjack these systems.

However, it remains unclear the extent to which these findings help inform our understanding of drug addiction in humans since it is a brain disorder that is clearly far removed from primary reinforcement mechanisms.

2. Drug addiction: A human-specific disorder?

2.1 What is drug addiction?

Drug addiction is a complex brain disorder (31), affecting the motivational (32, 33), learning (34-37) and behavioural control systems of the brain (38-40). Several definitions of drug addiction, ranging from the psychiatric to the social view have been presented by Koob and Le Moal (1) and will not be discussed any further.

Drug addiction is defined as a chronic relapsing compulsive habit characterised by loss of control over drug intake, maintained drug use despite adverse consequences (36, 41, 42) and the development of negative psycho-affective distress when access to the drug is prevented (42, 43).

Because the aetiology and pathophysiology of drug addiction remain unknown, this prominent psychiatric disorder is best defined by the clinical features of the DSM-IV (44) (figure 3). The diagnostic of drug addiction is currently based on a categorial dichotomous approach in that the patient must present at least three out of the seven clinical criteria listed in figure 5 to be said addicted to a substance.

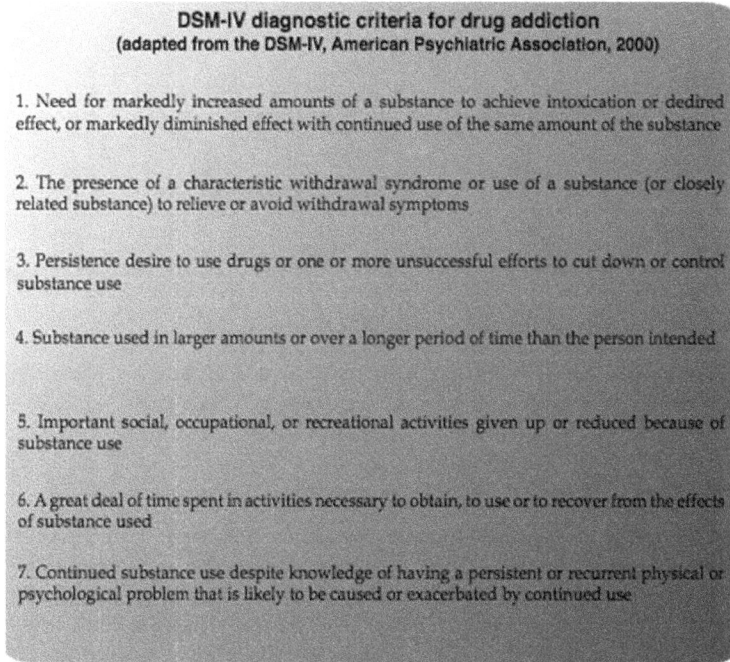

DSM-IV diagnostic criteria for drug addiction
(adapted from the DSM-IV, American Psychiatric Association, 2000)

1. Need for markedly increased amounts of a substance to achieve intoxication or dedired effect, or markedly diminished effect with continued use of the same amount of the substance

2. The presence of a characteristic withdrawal syndrome or use of a substance (or closely related substance) to relieve or avoid withdrawal symptoms

3. Persistence desire to use drugs or one or more unsuccessful efforts to cut down or control substance use

4. Substance used in larger amounts or over a longer period of time than the person intended

5. Important social, occupational, or recreational activities given up or reduced because of substance use

6. A great deal of time spent in activities necessary to obtain, to use or to recover from the effects of substance used

7. Continued substance use despite knowledge of having a persistent or recurrent physical or psychological problem that is likely to be caused or exacerbated by continued use

Fig. 3. Clinical features of drug addiction according to the DSM-IV-R (44).

The subject is diagnosed addicted to the substance if they show at least three out of the 7 clinical criteria over the last 12 months.

However, all addicted patients are not equally severely affected and a dimensional addiction severity scale has been developed to assess general behavioural, health and social drug-induced impairments (45-49).

Indeed, drug addicts do not only take drugs, they spend great amounts of time foraging for their drugs, compulsively take drugs, lose control over drug intake, and persist in taking drugs despite the many adverse consequences of doing so, including compromising their health, family relationships, friendships and work. Many drug addicts resort to criminal behaviour to obtain the funds necessary to sustain their compulsive drug use and the great majority eventually relapse to drug use even after prolonged periods of abstinence.

This negative behavioural picture illustrates how drug addiction is not merely a drug taking disorder. Indeed, among the individuals exposed to drugs, and there are many who occasionally drink only a glass or two of an alcoholic beverage, or smoke a cigarette or two, only 15 to 30% overall will switch from casual, 'recreational' drug use to drug abuse and drug addiction (1, 50) (figure 4).

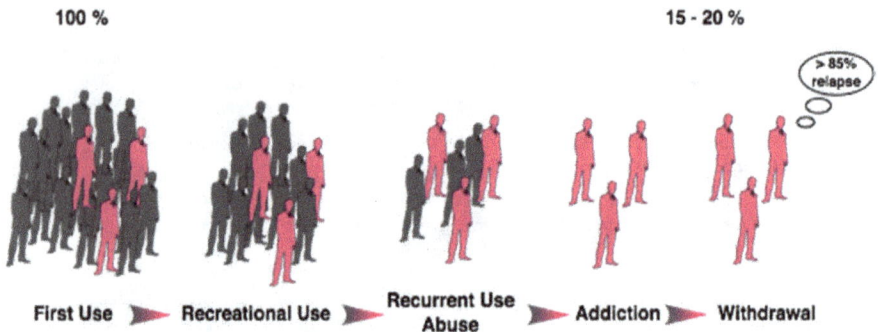

Fig. 4. We are not equally vulnerable to drug addiction

A substantial proportion of the general population experiences drugs at least once in a lifetime. Of the recreational users who control their drug intake, some will shift to more chronic drug use. Only a subgroup of these individuals will develop drug abuse and eventually drug addiction. Epidemiological studies reveal that of the individuals who have been exposed to addictive drugs, 15 to 20 % eventually develop addiction.

Despite considerable research we still do not understand why some individuals develop a compulsive use of drugs nor do we have effective treatments (51) to reduce the substantial social and economic burden (52); for review, see (1) of drug addiction (figure 5). Nevertheless, there is increasing evidence suggesting that drug addiction results from gradual adaptation processes in the brain of vulnerable subjects in response to chronic drug exposure. Not only do these between-systems adaptations trigger an emotional allostatic state (hedonic allostasis) (1, 53-55) characterised for instance by increased anxiety, irritability and depression but they may ultimately lead to a shift in the psychological mechanisms that govern drug seeking and drug taking behaviours, including habits (36, 37, 41, 42, 56, 57) as aberrant instrumental learning mechanisms controlled by Pavlovian cues, altered behavioural control (39, 58-60), decision-making and self-monitoring processes (61, 61).

Similarly, Everitt and colleagues have argued that, during the development of drug addiction, drug seeking is initially goal-directed but becomes habitual, and ultimately compulsive, thereby emphasizing the potential importance of maladaptive automatic instrumental learning mechanisms and their control by Pavlovian incentive processes, so called incentive habits (37, 42), in the emergence of compulsive drug use (35, 37, 42, 59). Additionally, drug-induced adaptations may also facilitate the shift from impulsivity to compulsivity that has been suggested to occur in the development of drug addiction (figure 6) whereby only vulnerable subjects would show a transition from impulse-related recreational drug use to compulsive drug intake (1).

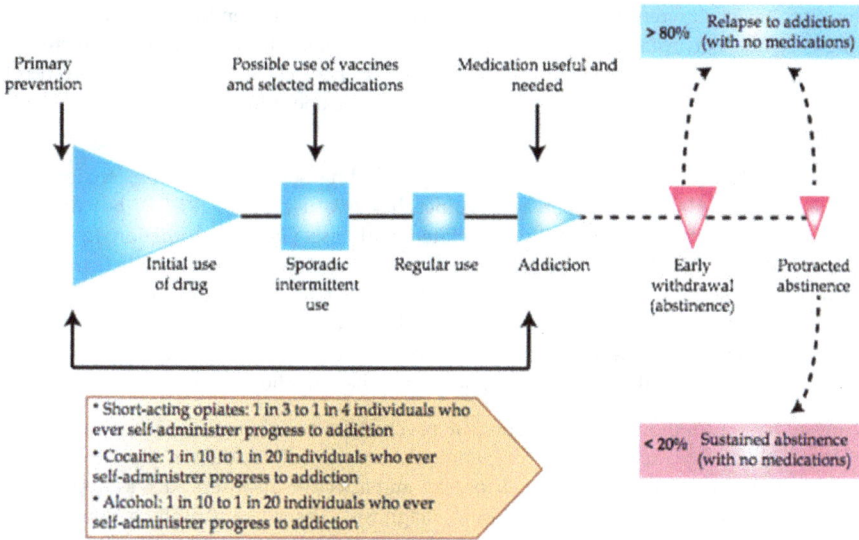

Fig. 5. Strategic targets of therapeutic treatment in the course of drug addiction (reproduced from (51))

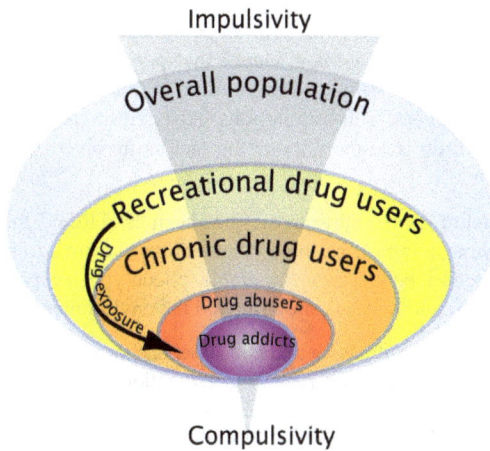

Fig. 6. A progressive shift from impulsivity to compulsivity in the development of drug addiction (42)

2.2 Behavioural and psychological profile of drug addicts

Besides their disinterest for alternative sources of reinforcement and their focus on the drug, drug addicts are characterised by several behavioural and cognitive deficits including impaired inhibitory control (62-67), decision making (68-75) and insight (76-78).

However, major differences can be observed between addicts depending on their preferred drug of abuse. For instance, although opiate and stimulant addicts both display increased sensation seeking (79-81) and impulsivity (82-87), they nevertheless differ in other respects, with heroin addicts showing greater anxiety than cocaine addicts (88), while the latter display higher impulsivity (62, 89, 90).

Thus not only are several personality traits, including sensation seeking, anxiety and impulsivity, associated with increased vulnerability to use drugs (91-94), but different personality traits are preferentially associated with use (95) and addiction to specific drugs (91, 92, 94, 96-103). It is therefore possible that heroin and cocaine addicts may self-medicate different personality characteristics or affective states (104-107), with impulsivity being preferentially self-medicated by cocaine use. However, as discussed in chapter 2 of this book, the relative contribution of a behavioural trait to the choice of a drug does not necessarily predict its implication in the transition to compulsive drug use.

Drug addicts also show several comorbid psychiatric disorders (108-111), as stated by O'Brien (112): «Psychiatric disorders commonly coexist with addictive disorders. These include anxiety disorders, psychotic disorders, and affective disorders such as depression. Although some of these so-called "dual diagnosis" cases are simply a coincidental occurrence of common disorders, the overlap is greater than would be expected by chance on the basis of population prevalences (109)». However, it remains unknown whether comorbid elements contribute to increased vulnerability to drug addiction (113) or whether chronic drug exposure facilitates the emergence of psychiatric comorbidity (for discussion see (112)). Similarly, while some personality, or behavioural, traits are triggered by chronic drug use, there is evidence that personality variables are associated with increased vulnerability to develop drug addiction (92, 114). This rather blur picture not only suggests that several sub-populations exist within drug addicts (115), but it clearly illustrates how little is known about the factors involved in the vulnerability to develop drug addiction.

To date a triadic model of contributing factors has been established that accounts well for both clinical and preclinical literature. Thus, vulnerability to drug addiction is suggested to result from the interaction between a vulnerable phenotype, or personality (being the interaction between genes and history), the drug and the environment (figure 7).

There is clearly a genetic vulnerability to addiction. Genetic factors may contribute up to 40% to the development of drug addiction (51). This estimation gives genetic factors a limited contribution to the vulnerability to drug addiction and highlights the importance of both the drug and the environment in the development of the pathology. There is indeed compelling evidence that life experiences and environments highly influence the effects of drugs of abuse and play a critical role in the transition from controlled to compulsive drug use (116, 117). For instance, drug addiction seems to be more frequent in people living in degraded areas or in people that undergo difficult experiences during their childhood. Such specific environmental conditions at either perinatal, developmental or adulthood stages may alter one's personality construction so that they become more vulnerable to use or abuse drugs (118). On the other hand, positive family relationships, friendships, involvement and attachment appear to somehow protect against the development of drug addiction (119, 120).

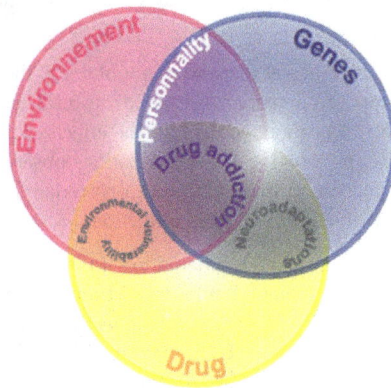

Fig. 7. Triad of influences underlying vulnerability to drug addiction

A number of interacting factors are hypothesised to influence the pathway to addiction, including biological determinants (genes), drug exposure and the environment. Genetic influences may account for up to 40% of the vulnerability for drug addiction

Thus, the present general strategies developed to treat addictions should perhaps be re-oriented towards a more patient-based medication strategy once better insights are gained in the understanding of the etiological and neurobiological substrates of individual vulnerabilities to addictions.

2.3 Biological correlates of drug addiction in humans: Insights from imaging studies

An exhaustive synthesis of the neurobiological correlates of drug addiction is beyond the scope of this chapter. Overall, drug exposure impacts both brain structure and function. Thus at the morphological level, drug addicts have decreased grey matter volumes in prefrontal (121-125) and cerebellar regions of the brain (126). Functionally, when presented with drug-related cues that induce craving, drug addicts show abnormal activation of limbic structures including the amygdala (127, 128), the insular (40, 129) and orbitofrontal cortices (39, 130) as well as cognitive prefrontal areas such as the cingulate (127, 128, 131) and dorsolateral prefrontal cortices (74).

Moreover, drug addicts are characterised by decreased levels of striatal D2/3 dopamine receptors (132-134) and reduced metabolism in the orbitofrontal cortex (132). These two alterations are highly correlated (132), thereby providing the orbitofrontal-limbic striatum circuit a prominent implication in addiction (134, 135), even though other networks, including the thalamo-cortical systems, have been identified to be impaired in drug addicts (136).

Interestingly, a growing body of evidence points towards an implication of non limbic striatal areas in the pathophysiology of drug addiction since dopamine transmission is specifically increased in the dorsal striatum of cocaine addicts experiencing craving in response to presentation of drug-associated cues (137, 138), providing a neurobiological evidence for a progressive involvement of dorsal striatum-dependent habits (139-141) in drug addiction (35-37, 41, 42).

A major limitation of human studies is that the data obtained, though clearly informative, are based on the comparison of current or former drug addicts and drug naive control subjects. Thereby, human studies cannot control for the effects of protracted drug exposure on the brain nor can they define whether the abnormalities observed in drug addicts are a pathological biological adaptation to drug exposure or predated drug use and hence are instead endophenotypes of vulnerability to drug addiction.

This is where the case for animal experimentation in addiction research is revealed compelling. Besides the aforementioned limitations, studies in human addicts are often prone to interpretative issues not least due to inter-subject variability in drug exposure, the frequent co-abuse of several drugs often in combination with alcohol, cannabis and nicotine, the regular occurrence of co-morbid brain disorders such as depression, conduct disorder and attention-deficit/hyperactivity disorder (ADHD) and the difficulty in controlling pre-morbid cognitive and intellectual abilities.

3. References

[1] Koob G, Le Moal M. Plasticity of reward neurocircuitry and the 'dark side' of drug addiction. Nat Neurosci. 2005; 8: 1442-1444.

[2] Nutt D, King LA, Saulsbury W, Blakemore C. Development of a rational scale to assess the harm of drugs of potential misuse. Lancet. 2007; 369: 1047-1053.

[3] Lindesmith AR. Addiction and opiates. Chicago: Aldine Pub. Co.; 1968: vii, 295.

[4] Fort J. The pleasure seekers; the drug crisis, youth, and society. Indianapolis: Bobbs-Merrill; 1969: 255.

[5] Rivera MA, Aufderheide AC, Cartmell LW, Torres CM, Langsjoen O. Antiquity of coca-leaf chewing in the south central Andes: a 3,000 year archaeological record of coca-leaf chewing from northern Chile. J Psychoactive Drugs. 2005; 37: 455-458.

[6] Humphrey AJ, O'Hagan D. Tropane alkaloid biosynthesis. A century old problem unresolved. Nat Prod Rep. 2001; 18: 494-502.

[7] Freud S. Uber coca. 1884; Centralbl Gesamte Ther: 289-314.

[8] Nesse RM, Berridge K. Psychoactive Drug Use in Evolutionary Perspective. Science. 1997; 278: 63-66.

[9] Kolb LC. Drug addiction. Bulletin of the New York Academy of Medicine. 1965; 41: 306.

[10] EMCDDA. The state of the drugs problem in Europe (annual report 2009).

[11] WHO. Neuroscience of psychoactive substance use and dependence. Geneva: World Health Organization; 2004

[12] Kusayama T, Watanabe S. Reinforcing effects of methamphetamine in planarians. Neuroreport. 2000; 11: 2511-2513.

[13] Li H, Chaney S, Roberts IJ, Forte M, Hirsh J. Ectopic G-protein expression in dopamine and serotonin neurons blocks cocaine sensitization in Drosophila melanogaster. CurrBiol. 2000; 10: 211-214.

[14] Wolf F, Heberlein U. Invertebrate models of drug abuse. J Neurobiol. 2002; 54: 161-178.

[15] Carney JM, Landrum RW, Cheng MS, Seale TW. Establishment of chronic intravenous drug self-administration in the C57BL/6J mouse. Neuroreport. 1991; 2: 477-480.

[16] Grahame NJ, Phillips TJ, Burkhart-Kasch S, Cunningham CL. Intravenous cocaine self-administration in the C57BL/6J mouse. Pharmacol Biochem Behav. 1995; 51: 827-834.

[17] Highfield DA, Mead AN, Grimm JW, Rocha BA, Shaham Y. Reinstatement of cocaine seeking in 129X1/SvJ mice: effects of cocaine priming, cocaine cues and food deprivation. Psychopharmacology (Berl). 2002; 161: 417-424.

[18] Cain ME, Denehy ED, Bardo M. Individual Differences in Amphetamine Self-Administration: The rôle of the Central Nucleus of the Amygdala. Neuropsychopharmacology. 2007; 33: 1149-1161.

[19] Thomsen M, Caine SB. Intravenous drug self-administration in mice: practical considerations. Behav Genet. 2007; 37: 101-118.

[20] van der Veen R, Piazza PV, Deroche-Gamonet V. Gene-environment interactions in vulnerability to cocaine intravenous self-administration: a brief social experience affects intake in DBA/2J but not in C57BL/6J mice. Psychopharmacology (Berl). 2007; 193: 179-186.

[21] Thomsen M, Han DD, Gu HH, Caine SB. Lack of cocaine self-administration in mice expressing a cocaine-insensitive dopamine transporter. J Pharmacol Exp Ther. 2009

[22] Pickens R, Harris WC. Self-administration of d-amphetamine by rats. Psychopharmacologia. 1968; 12: 158-163.

[23] Ettenberg A, Pettit HO, Bloom FE, Koob GF. Heroin and cocaine intravenous self-administration in rats: Mediation by separate neural systems. Psychopharmacology. 1982; 78: 204-209.

[24] Collins RJ, Weeks JR, Cooper MM, Good PI, Russell RR. Prediction of abuse liability of drugs using IV self-administration by rats. Psychopharmacology (Berl). 1984; 82: 6-13.

[25] Koob G, Le HT, Creese I. The D1 dopamine receptor antagonist SCH 23390 increases cocaine self-administration in the rat. NeurosciLett. 1987; 79: 315-320.

[26] Weissenborn R, Yackey M, Koob GF, Weiss F. Measures of cocaine-seeking behavior using a multiple schedule of food and drug self-administration in rats. Drug Alcohol Depend. 1995; 38: 237-246.

[27] Risner ME, Goldberg SR. A comparison of nicotine and cocaine self-administration in the dog: fixed-ratio and progressive-ratio schedules of intravenous drug infusion. J Pharmacol Exp Ther. 1983; 224: 319-326.

[28] Shannon HE, Risner ME. Comparison of behavior maintained by intravenous cocaine and d-amphetamine in dogs. JpharmacolExpTher. 1984; 229: 422-432.

[29] Deneau G, Yanagita T, Seevers MH. Self-administration of psychoactive substances by the monkey. Psychopharmacologia. 1969; 16: 30-48.

[30] Goldberg SR, Woods JH, Schuster CR. Morphine: Conditioned Increases in Self-Administration in Rhesus Monkeys. Science. 1969

[31] Leshner AI. Addiction is a brain disease, and it matters. Science. 1997; 278: 45-47.

[32] Robinson T, Berridge K. The psychology and neurobiology of addiction: an incentive-sensitization view. Addiction. 2000; 95: S91-S117.

[33] Kalivas P, Volkow N. The Neural Basis of Addiction: A Pathology of Motivation and Choice. American Journal of Psychiatry. 2005; 162: 1403-1413.

[34] Everitt B, Parkinson JA, Olmstead M, Arroyo M, Robledo P, Robbins TW. Associative processes in addiction and reward. The role of amygdala-ventral striatal subsystems. Ann NYAcadSci. 1999; 877: 412-438.

[35] Everitt BJ., Dickinson A, Robbins TW. The neuropsychological basis of addictive behaviour. Brain Research Reviews. 2001; 36: 129-138.

[36] Everitt BJ., Robbins TW. Neural systems of reinforcement for drug addiction: from actions to habits to compulsion. Nat Neurosci. 2005; 8: 1481-1489.

[37] Belin D, Jonkman S, Dickinson A, Robbins TW, Everitt BJ.. Parallel and interactive learning processes within the basal ganglia: Relevance for the understanding of addiction. Behavioural Brain Research. 2009; 199(1): 89-102.

[38] Volkow N, Fowler J. Addiction, a Disease of Compulsion and Drive: Involvement of the Orbitofrontal Cortex. Cerebral Cortex. 2000

[39] Goldstein RZ, Volkow ND. Drug addiction and its underlying neurobiological basis: neuroimaging evidence for the involvement of the frontal cortex. Am J Psychiatry. 2002; 159: 1642-1652.

[40] Goldstein RZ, Alia-Klein N, Tomasi D et al. Anterior cingulate cortex hypoactivations to an emotionally salient task in cocaine addiction. Proc Natl Acad Sci U S A. 2009; 106: 9453-9458.

[41] Robbins TW, Everitt BJ. Drug addiction: bad habits add up. Nature. 1999; 398: 567-570.

[42] Belin D, Everitt BJ. The Neural and Psychological Basis of a Compulsive Incentive Habit. In: Steiner H, tseng K, editors. Handbook of basal ganglia structure and function, 20. Elsvier, ACADEMIC PRESS; 2010.

[43] Koob G, Le Moal M. Addiction and the Brain Antireward System. Annu Rev Psychol. 2008; 59: 29-53.

[44] APA. Diagnostic and Statistical Manual of Mental Disorders fourth edition, Text revision (DSM-IV TR). Washington DC: American Psychiatric Association; 2000

[45] Mclellan A, Kushner H, Metzger D, Peters R. The Fifth Edition of the Addiction Severity Index. J Subst Abuse Treat. 1992

[46] McLellan AT, Cacciola JC, Alterman AI, Rikoon SH, Carise D. The Addiction Severity Index at 25: origins, contributions and transitions. Am J Addict. 2006; 15: 113-124.

[47] Rikoon S, Cacciola J, Carise D, Alterman A, Mclellan A. Predicting DSM-IV dependence diagnoses from Addiction Severity Index composite scores. Journal of Substance Abuse Treatment. 2006; 31: 17-24.

[48] Krenz S, Dieckmann S, Favrat B et al. French version of the addiction severity index (5th Edition): validity and reliability among Swiss opiate-dependent patients. French validation of the Addiction Severity Index. Eur Addict Res. 2004; 10: 173-179.

[49] Cacciola J, Alterman A, O'Brien CP, Mclellan A. The Addiction Severity Index in clinical efficacy trials of medications for cocaine dependence. NIDA ResMonogr. 1997; 175: 182-191.

[50] Anthony JC, Warner LA, Kessler RC. Comparative epidemiology of dependence on tobacco, alcohol, controlled substances, and inhalants: Basic findings from the National comorbidity Survey. Exp Clin Psychopharmacol. 1994; 2: 244-268.

[51] Kreek M, Laforge K, Butelman E. Pharmacotherapy of addictions. Nat Rev Drug Discov. 2002; 1: 710-726.

[52] Uhl G, Grow RW. The burden of complex genetics in brain disorders. Arch GenPsychiatry. 2004; 61: 223-229.

[53] Koob G, Moal ML. Drug Abuse: Hedonic Homeostatic Dysregulation. Science. 1997; 278: 52-58.

[54] Koob G, Le Moal M. Drug addiction, dysregulation of reward, and allostasis. Neuropsychopharmacology. 2001; 24: 97-129.

[55] Koob GF, Le Moal M. Review. Neurobiological mechanisms for opponent motivational processes in addiction. Philos Trans R Soc Lond B Biol Sci. 2008; 363: 3113-3123.

[56] Tiffany ST. A cognitive model of drug urges and drug-use behavior: rôle of automatic and nonautomatic processes. Psychol Rev. 1990; 97: 147-168.

[57] O'Brien CP, Mclellan A. Myths about the treatment of addiction. Lancet. 1996; 347: 237-240.

[58] Jentsch JD, Taylor JR. Impulsivity resulting from frontostriatal dysfunction in drug abuse: implications for the control of behavior by reward-related stimuli. Psychopharmacology. 1999; 146: 373-390.

[59] Everitt BJ, Belin D, Economidou D, Pelloux Y, Dalley J, Robbins TW. Neural mechanisms underlying the vulnerability to develop compulsive drug-seeking habits and addiction. Philos Trans R Soc Lond B Biol Sci. 2008; 363: 3125-3135.

[60] Kalivas PW. Addiction as a pathology in prefrontal cortical regulation of corticostriatal habit circuitry. Neurotox Res. 2008; 14: 185-189.

[61] Baumeister RF, Heatherton TF, Tice DM. Losing Control: How and Why People Fail at Self-Regulation. 1994.

[62] Kirby KN, Petry NM. Heroin and cocaine abusers have higher discount rates for delayed rewards than alcoholics or non-drug-using controls. Addiction. 2004; 99: 461-471.

[63] Mitchell C, Flaherty C. Differential effects of removing the glucose or saccharin components of a glucose–saccharin mixture in a successive negative contrast paradigm. Physiology & Behavior. 2005; 84: 579-583.

[64] Baler RD, Volkow ND. Drug addiction: the neurobiology of disrupted self-control. Trends Mol Med. 2006; 12: 559-566.

[65] Dom G, D'haene P, Hulstijn W, Sabbe B. Impulsivity in abstinent early- and late-onset alcoholics: differences in self-report measures and a discounting task. Addiction. 2006; 101: 50-59.

[66] Verdejo-Garcia A, Benbrook A, Funderburk F, David P, Cadet JL, Bolla KI. The differential relationship between cocaine use and marijuana use on decision-making performance over repeat testing with the Iowa Gambling Task. Drug Alcohol Depend. 2007; 90: 2-11.

[67] Verdejo-Garcia A, Lawrence AJ, Clark L. Impulsivity as a vulnerability marker for substance-use disorders: review of findings from high-risk research, problem

gamblers and genetic association studies. Neuroscience and biobehavioral reviews. 2008; 32: 777-810.

[68] Grant S, Contoreggi C, London ED. Drug abusers show impaired performance in a laboratory test of decision making. Neuropsychologia. 2000; 38: 1180-1187.

[69] Monterosso J, Ehrman R, Napier KL, O'Brien CP, Childress AR. Three decision-making tasks in cocaine-dependent patients: do they measure the same construct? Addiction. 2001; 96: 1825-1837.

[70] Bechara A, Damasio H. Decision-making and addiction (part I): impaired activation of somatic states in substance dependent individuals when pondering decisions with negative future consequences. Neuropsychologia. 2002; 40: 1675-1689.

[71] Bechara A, Dolan S, Hindes A. Decision-making and addiction (part II): myopia for the future or hypersensitivity to reward? Neuropsychologia. 2002; 40: 1690-1705.

[72] Hester R, Garavan H. Executive dysfunction in cocaine addiction: evidence for discordant frontal, cingulate, and cerebellar activity. J Neurosci. 2004; 24: 11017-11022.

[73] Bechara A. Decision making, impulse control and loss of willpower to resist drugs: a neurocognitive perspective. Nat Neurosci. 2005; 8: 1458-1463.

[74] Verdejo-Garcia A, Vilar-Lopez R, Perez-Garcia M, Podell K, Goldberg E. Altered adaptive but not veridical decision-making in substance dependent individuals. J Int Neuropsychol Soc. 2006; 12: 90-99.

[75] Vassileva J, Petkova P, Georgiev S et al. Impaired decision-making in psychopathic heroin addicts. Drug Alcohol Depend. 2007; 86: 287-289.

[76] Goldstein RZ, Craig AD, Bechara A et al. The neurocircuitry of impaired insight in drug addiction. Trends Cogn Sci. 2009; 13: 372-380.

[77] Naqvi NH, Bechara A. The hidden island of addiction: the insula. Trends Neurosci. 2009; 32: 56-67.

[78] Naqvi NH, Bechara A. The insula and drug addiction: an interoceptive view of pleasure, urges, and decision-making. Brain Struct Funct. 2010

[79] Allcock CC, Grace DM. Pathological gamblers are neither impulsive nor sensation-seekers. Aust N Z J Psychiatry. 1988; 22: 307-311.

[80] Gerra G, Angioni L, Zaimovic A et al. Substance use among high-school students: relationships with temperament, personality traits, and parental care perception. Subst Use Misuse. 2004; 39: 345-367.

[81] Maremmani I, Pacini M, Popovic D et al. Affective temperaments in heroin addiction. J Affect Disord. 2009; 117: 186-192.

[82] Madden GJ, Petry NM, Badger GJ, Bickel WK. Impulsive and self-control choices in opioid-dependent patients and non-drug-using control participants: drug and monetary rewards. Exp Clin Psychopharmacol. 1997; 5: 256-262.

[83] Kirby KN, Petry NM, Bickel WK. Heroin addicts have higher discount rates for delayed rewards than non-drug-using controls. J Exp Psychol Gen. 1999; 128: 78-87.

[84] Coffey SF, Gudleski GD, Saladin ME, Brady KT. Impulsivity and rapid discounting of delayed hypothetical rewards in cocaine-dependent individuals. Exp Clin Psychopharmacol. 2003; 11: 18-25.

[85] Bornovalova MA, Lejuez CW, Daughters SB, Zachary Rosenthal M, Lynch TR. Impulsivity as a common process across borderline personality and substance use disorders. Clin Psychol Rev. 2005; 25: 790-812.

[86] Clark L, Robbins TW, Ersche KD, Sahakian BJ. Reflection impulsivity in current and former substance users. Biol Psychiatry. 2006; 60: 515-522.

[87] Verdejo-Garcia AJ, Perales JC, Perez-Garcia M. Cognitive impulsivity in cocaine and heroin polysubstance abusers. Addict Behav. 2007; 32: 950-966.

[88] Lejuez CW, Paulson A, Daughters SB, Bornovalova MA, Zvolensky MJ. The association between heroin use and anxiety sensitivity among inner-city individuals in residential drug use treatment. Behav Res Ther. 2006; 44: 667-677.

[89] Bornovalova M, Daughters S, Hernandez G, Richards J, Lejuez C. Differences in impulsivity and risk-taking propensity between primary users of crack cocaine and primary users of heroin in a residential substance-use program. Experimental and Clinical Psychopharmacology. 2005; 13: 311-318.

[90] Lejuez CW, Bornovalova MA, Daughters SB, Curtin JJ. Differences in impulsivity and sexual risk behavior among inner-city crack/cocaine users and heroin users. Drug Alcohol Depend. 2005; 77: 169-175.

[91] Zuckerman M. Sensation seeking and the endogenous deficit theory of drug abuse. NIDA Res Monogr. 1986; 74: 59-70.

[92] Franques P, Auriacombe M, Tignol J. [Addiction and personality]. Encephale. 2000; 26: 68-78.

[93] Sher KJ, Bartholow BD, Wood MD. Personality and substance use disorders: a prospective study. J Consult Clin Psychol. 2000; 68: 818-829.

[94] Terracciano A, Lockenhoff CE, Crum RM, Bienvenu OJ, Costa PTJ. Five-Factor Model personality profiles of drug users. BMC Psychiatry. 2008; 8: 22.

[95] Adams JB, Heath AJ, Young SE, Hewitt JK, Corley RP, Stallings MC. Relationships between personality and preferred substance and motivations for use among adolescent substance abusers. Am J Drug Alcohol Abuse. 2003; 29: 691-712.

[96] Gossop M. Drug dependence, crime and personality among female addicts. Drug Alcohol Depend. 1978; 3: 359-364.

[97] Labouvie EW, McGee CR. Relation of personality to alcohol and drug use in adolescence. J Consult Clin Psychol. 1986; 54: 289-293.

[98] Greene RL, Adyanthaya AE, Morse RM, Davis LJ. Personality variables in cocaine- and marijuana-dependent patients. JpersAssess. 1993; 61: 224-230.

[99] Clapper RL, Martin CS, Clifford PR. Personality, social environment, and past behavior as predictors of late adolescent alcohol use. J Subst Abuse. 1994; 6: 305-313.

[100] Schinka JA, Curtiss G, Mulloy JM. Personality variables and self-medication in substance abuse. JpersAssess. 1994; 63: 413-422.

[101] Ball SA, Kranzler HR, Tennen H, Poling JC, Rounsaville BJ. Personality disorder and dimension differences between type A and type B substance abusers. J Pers Disord. 1998; 12: 1-12.

[102] Conway K, Swendsen JD, Rounsaville BJ, Merikangas KR. Personality, drug of choice, and comorbid psychopathology among substance abusers. Drug Alcohol Depend. 2002; 65: 225-234.

[103] Gerra G, Bertacca S, Zaimovic A, Pirani M, Branchi B, Ferri M. Relationship of personality traits and drug of choice by cocaine addicts and heroin addicts. Subst Use Misuse. 2008; 43: 317-330.

[104] Khantzian EJ, Mack JE, Schatzberg AF. Heroin use as an attempt to cope: clinical observations. AmJPsychiatry. 1974; 131: 160-164.

[105] Khantzian EJ. Addiction: self-destruction or self-repair? JsubstAbuse Treat. 1989; 6: 75.

[106] Khantzian EJ. Self-regulation factors in cocaine dependence--a clinical perspective. NIDA ResMonogr. 1991; 110: 211-226.

[107] Khantzian EJ. The self-medication hypothesis of substance use disorders: a reconsideration and recent applications. HarvRevPsychiatry. 1997; 4: 231-244.

[108] Khantzian EJ. Psychiatric illness in drug abusers. NenglJMed. 1980; 302: 869-870.

[109] Kessler RC, Nelson CB, McGonagle KA, Edlund MJ, Frank RG, Leaf PJ. The epidemiology of co-occurring addictive and mental disorders: implications for prevention and service utilization. Am J Orthopsychiatry. 1996; 66: 17-31.

[110] Skinstad AH, Swain A. Comorbidity in a clinical sample of substance abusers. Am Jdrug Alcohol Abuse. 2001; 27: 45-64.

[111] Gum AM, Cheavens JS. Psychiatric comorbidity and depression in older adults. Curr Psychiatry Rep. 2008; 10: 23-29.

[112] O'Brien CP. A Range of Research-Based Pharmacotherapies for Addiction. Science. 1997; 278: 66-70.

[113] Khantzian EJ. The self-medication hypothesis of addictive disorders: focus on heroin and cocaine dependence. Am J Psychiatry. 1985; 142: 1259-1264.

[114] Franques P. Sensation seeking as a common factor in opioid dependent subjects and high risk sport practicing subjects. A cross sectional study. Drug and Alcohol Dependence. 2003; 69: 121-126.

[115] Gunnarsdottir ED, Pingitore RA, Spring BJ et al. Individual differences among cocaine users. Addict Behav. 2000; 25: 641-652.

[116] Swadi H. Individual risk factors for adolescent substance use. Drug and Alcohol Dependence. 1999; 55: 209-224.

[117] Batts K, Grabill T, Galvin D, Schlenger W. Contextual and other factors related to workplace-based substance abuse prevention and earl intervention for adolescents and young adults [dissertation]. 2004.

[118] Khantzian EJ. A contemporary psychodynamic approach to drug abuse treatment. AmJDrug Alcohol Abuse. 1986; 12: 213-222.

[119] Jessor R, Jessor S. A social-psychological framework for studying drug use. NIDA Res Monogr. 1980; 30: 102-109.

[120] Jessor R, Chase JA, Donovan JE. Psychosocial correlates of marijuana use and problem drinking in a national sample of adolescents. Am J Public Health. 1980; 70: 604-613.

[121] Bartzokis G, Beckson M, Lu PH et al. Increased CSF volumes are associated with diminished subjective responses to cocaine infusion. Neuropsychopharmacology. 2000; 23: 468-473.

[122] Bartzokis G, Beckson M, Lu PH et al. Age-related brain volume reductions in amphetamine and cocaine addicts and normal controls: implications for addiction research. Psychiatry Res. 2000; 98: 93-102.

[123] Bartzokis G, Beckson M, Lu PH et al. Cortical gray matter volumes are associated with subjective responses to cocaine infusion. Am J Addict. 2004; 13: 64-73.

[124] Liu J, Liang J, Qin W et al. Dysfunctional connectivity patterns in chronic heroin users: an fMRI study. Neurosci Lett. 2009; 460: 72-77.

[125] Tanabe J, Tregellas JR, Dalwani M et al. Medial orbitofrontal cortex gray matter is reduced in abstinent substance-dependent individuals. Biol Psychiatry. 2009; 65: 160-164.

[126] Andersen BB. Reduction of Purkinje cell volume in cerebellum of alcoholics. Brain Res. 2004; 1007: 10-18.

[127] Childress AR, Mozley PD, McElgin W, Fitzgerald J, Reivich M, O'Brien CP. Limbic activation during cue-induced cocaine craving. Am J Psychiatry. 1999; 156: 11-18.

[128] Childress AR, Ehrman R, Wang Z et al. Prelude to Passion: Limbic Activation by "Unseen" Drug and Sexual Cues. PloS ONE. 2008; 3: e1506.

[129] Gray MA, Critchley HD. Interoceptive basis to craving. Neuron. 2007; 54: 183-186.

[130] Goldstein RZ, Tomasi D, Rajaram S, Cottone LA, Zhang L, Maloney T, Telang F, Alia-Klein N, Volkow ND. Role of the anterior cingulate and medial orbitofrontal cortex in processing drug cues in cocaine addiction. Neuroscience. 2007; 144: 1153-1159.

[131] Kaufman JN, Ross TJ, Stein EA, Garavan H. Cingulate hypoactivity in cocaine users during a GO-NOGO task as revealed by event-related functional magnetic resonance imaging. Jneurosci. 2003; 23: 7839-7843.

[132] Volkow ND, Fowler J, Wang G, Hitzemann R. Decreased dopamine D2 receptor availability is associated with reduced frontal metabolism in cocaine abusers. Synapse. 1993; 14: 169-177.

[133] Volkow ND, Chang L, Wang GJ, Fowler JS, Ding YS, Sedler M, Logan J, Franceschi D, Gatler J, Hitzemann R, Gifford A, Wong C, Pappas N. Low level of brain dopamine D2 receptors in methamphetamine abusers: association with metabolism in the orbitofrontal cortex. Am J Psychiatry. 2001; 158: 2015-2021.

[134] Koob GF, Volkow ND. Neurocircuitry of Addiction. Neuropsychopharmacology. 2009

[135] Fowler JS, Volkow ND, Kassed CA, Chang L. Imaging the addicted human brain. Sci Pract Perspect. 2007; 3: 4-16.

[136] Tomasi D, Goldstein R, Telang F, Maloney T, Alia-Klein N, Caparelli EC, Volkow ND. Thalamo-cortical dysfunction in cocaine abusers: implications in attention and perception. Psychiatry Res. 2007; 155: 189-201.

[137] Garavan H, Pankiewicz J, Bloom A, Cho JK, Sperry L, Ross TJ, Salmeron BJ, Risinger R, Kelley D, Stein EA. Cue-Induced Cocaine Craving: Neuroanatomical Specificity for Drug Users and Drug Stimuli. American Journal of Psychiatry. 2000; 157: 1789-1798.

[138] Volkow ND. Stimulant medications: how to minimize their reinforcing effects? Am J Psychiatry. 2006; 163: 359-361.

[139] Yin H, Mulcare S, Hilário MR, Clouse E, Holloway T, Davis MI, Hansson AC, Lovinger DM, Costa RM. Dynamic reorganization of striatal circuits during the acquisition and consolidation of a skill. Nat Neurosci. 2009; 12: 333-341.

[140] Yin H, Knowlton B. The role of the basal ganglia in habit formation. Nat Rev Neurosci. 2006; 7: 464-476.

[141] Yin H, Zhuang X, Balleine B. Instrumental learning in hyperdopaminergic mice. NeurobiolLearnMem. 2006

Pathophysiology of Addictions

3

Pathways Involved in the Cardiac Adaptive Changes Observed During Morphine Withdrawal

M.L. Laorden, M. V. Milanés and P. Almela
Department of Pharmacology, University of Murcia, Murcia,
Spain

1. Introduction

The development of opioid addiction involves complex adaptive changes in opioid receptors and associated signalling systems, leading to neuronal plasticity in the brain regions projecting to different systems including the cardiovascular system. So, adaptive changes also occur in peripheral tissues and cells expressing opioid receptors, such as in the heart (Pugsley, 2002).

The effects of drugs of abuse, especially cocaine, on the cardiovascular system, have been extensively documented in animal model and in human. There is emerging evidence that drug abuse might trigger a variety of cardiac disorders from arrhythmias to acute myocardial infarction, heart failure and even sudden cardiac death (Lippi et al., 2010). Thus, various types of cardiac arrhythmias have been described in heroin addicts. Moreover, street heroin addicts frequently die suddenly, and there is evidence that this is an arrhythmia-related event (Nerantzis et al., 2011).

The majority of studies dealing with morphine on the field of cardiology are oriented on clinical usage of this drug and current cardiovascular research has been limited to the evaluation of factors or pathways believed to contribute to its physiological actions, such as delta- and kappa-opioid receptors, cyclooxygenase-2, inducible nitric oxide synthase or reactive oxygen species (Huh et al., 2001; Wang et al., 2001; Jiang et al., 2006; Xu et al., 2011).

Given the importance of morphine in clinical practice for the treatment of pain, investigation of its impact on the heart at the molecular levels requires more attention. Therefore, in this chapter we will discuss our recent discoveries about the implication of different molecular pathways in the cardiac adaptive changes that occur during morphine withdrawal.

The noradrenergic pathways and the hypothalamo-pituitary-adrenocortical (HPA) axis, a system largely controlled by corticoticotropin-releasing factor (CRF) in the paraventricular nucleus (PVN) of the hypothalamus, comprise two major adaptation mechanisms to stress. Like stressors, morphine withdrawal activates HPA axis in rats, which results in neuronal activation of stress-related neurosecretory neurons in the parvocellular neurons of the PVN. The PVN is anatomically divided into three magnocellular and five parvocellular subdivisions. The parvocellular subdivisions comprise the dorsal, lateral, medial periventricular and anterior parvocellular subnuclei (fig. 1).

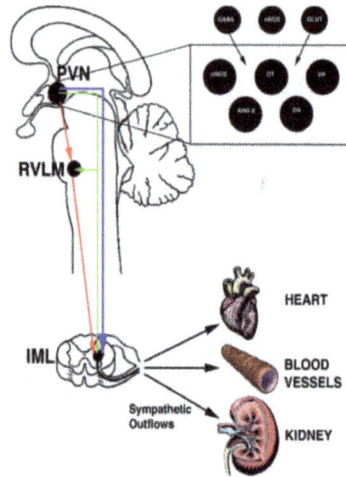

Fig. 1. Schematic illustrating the three main pathways by which the paraventricular nucleus of the hypothalamus (PVN) can influence sympathetic activity. Rostral ventrolateral medulla (RVLM), spinal intermediolateral cell column (IML). (Taken from Pyner, 2009).

These regions project to autonomic nuclei in the brain stem and spinal cord and are responsible for the activation of the sympathetic nervous system including cardiovascular regulation (Sawchenko and Swanson, 1982). In addition, the PVN receives afferent projections from several limbic structures that are implicated in behavioural and cardiovascular control, such as the medial amygdale, the prefrontal cortex and the lateral septum (Ongur et al., 1998; Risold and Swanson, 1997).

2. Hemodynamic variables during chronic morphine treatment and its withdrawal

Previous studies have demonstrated that chronic μ-opiod receptor stimulation decreases muscle sympathetic nerve activity (Kienbaum et al., 2001; 2002), NA plasma concentration (Kienbaum et al., 2001) and dopamine turnover in the heart (Rabadán et al., 1997). According to these data, we have demonstrated that chronic morphine treatment decreases two baseline cardiovascular parameters, mean arterial blood pressure (MAP) and heart rate (HR). However, μ-opioid receptor blockade by naloxone unmasks these effects, resulting in markedly increases in both parameters (fig. 2 and 3). In agreement with these data, naloxone administration to patients with chronic opioid abuse or to morphine dependent rats results in markedly increased muscle sympathetic nerve activity, NA plasma concentrations (Peart and Gross, 2006), NA and dopamine turnover (Almela et al., 2008; Milanés et al., 2000b) and total tyrosine hydroxylase (TH) expression (Almela et al., 2008). Altogether, these results suggest that an up-regulation of TH would be expected to increase the capacity of noradrenergic neurons to synthesize NA, which could contribute to the increase in NA turnover and in the hemodynamic changes seen in the heart during morphine withdrawal.

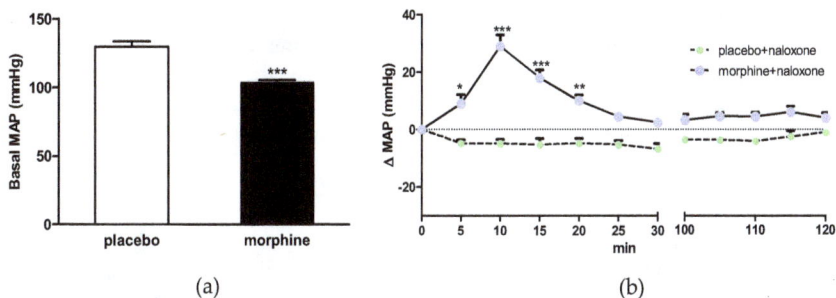

(a)   (b)

Fig. 2. Baseline mean arterial blood pressure (MAP) (mmHg) (A) in rats implanted with morphine or placebo pellets. Effects of naloxone (2 mg/kg s.c.) on changes in MAP (B). Naloxone was injected at time 0. Data are the mean±S.E.M. (n=5–7). ***P<0.001, **P<0.01, *P<0.05 versus placebo+naloxone.

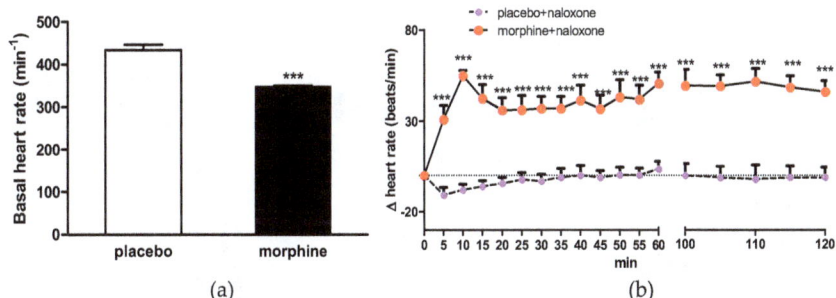

(a)   (b)

Fig. 3. Baseline heart rate (min−1) (A) in rats implanted with morphine or placebo pellets. Effects of naloxone (2 mg/kg s.c.) on changes in heart rate (B). Naloxone was injected at time 0. Data are the mean±S.E.M. (n=5–7). ***P<0.001, **P<0.01, *P<0.05 versus placebo+naloxone.

3. Evaluation of changes in pERK1/2 during morphine withdrawal

Extracellular signal-regulated kinase (ERK), one member of mitogen-activated extracellular kinase (MAPK) family, transduces a broad range of extracellular stimuli into diverse intracellular responses. ERK signalling pathway could be important as regulator of cardiac function (Michel et al., 2001) and neuronal plasticity (Adams et al., 2002). Recently, several studies have shown that this pathway contributes to naloxone-precipitated withdrawal in morphine dependent rats (Ren et al., 2004; Almela et al., 2007, 2008, 2011).

Our time course study showed that there was a significant elevation of phospho(p)ERK1 and phospho(p)ERK2 levels in the right (fig. 4) and left ventricle 30, 60, 90 or 120 min after naloxone administration to morphine dependent rats. We also studied the distribution of these proteins by immunohistochemical procedures and we observed high levels of pERK1/2 immunoreactivity in the right and left ventricle after naloxone administration to morphine-treated rats (fig. 5). The immunolabelling was mainly present in cytoplasmic compartments, suggesting a local activation of the protein. A nuclear staining was also observed in some myocytes, supporting a nuclear translocation of activated ERK proteins. These immunohistochemical results were consistent with western blot analyses (figure 4).

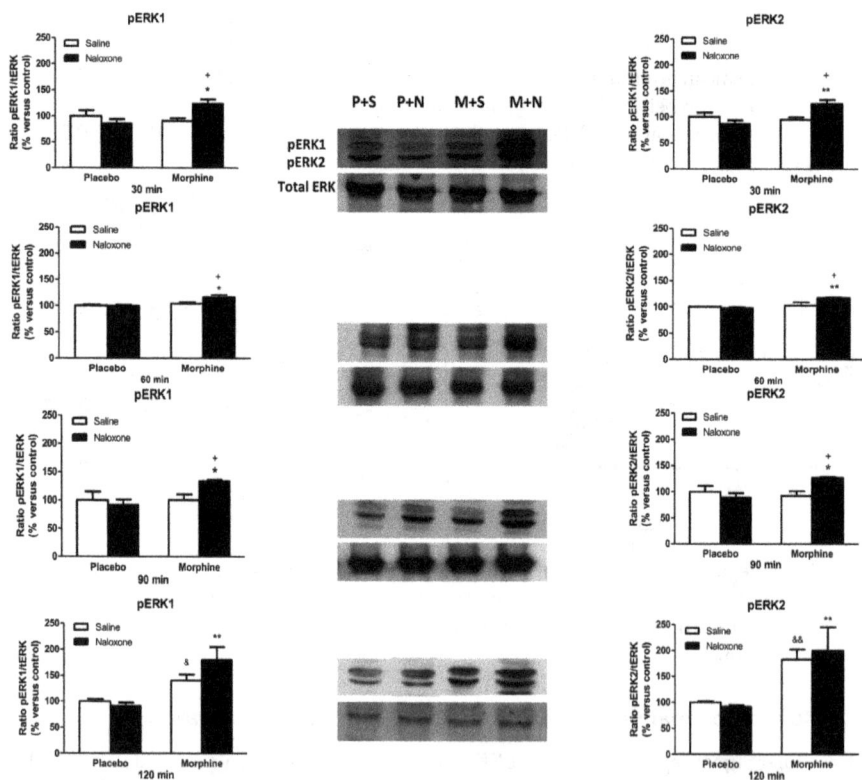

Fig. 4. Western-blotting analysis of phospho(p)ERK1 and phospho(p)ERK2 in the right ventricle 30, 60, 90 and 120 min after saline (S) or naloxone (N) administration to placebo- (P) or morphine- (M) pretreated rats. The immunoreactivity corresponding to pERK1 or pERK2 is expressed as a percentage of that in the control group defined as 100% value. Data are the mean±S.E.M. (n=5–6). **$P<0.01$, *$P<0.05$ versus the placebo group injected with naloxone; +$P<0.05$ versus the dependent group injected with saline instead of naloxone; &&$P<0.01$, &$P<0.05$ versus the placebo group receiving saline.

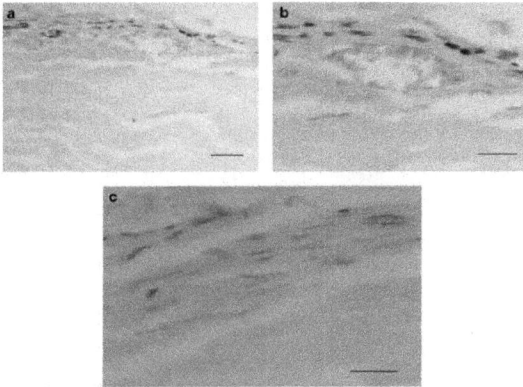

Fig. 5. Immunohistochemical detection of phospho(p)ERK1/2 in the left ventricular wall. Rats were made dependent on morphine for 7 days and on day 8 were injected with naloxone (2 mg/kg s.c.). 90 min after injections, rats were perfused and the right and left ventricle was processed for pERK1/2 immunohistochemistry. Scale bar 30 μm (a), 20 μm (b, c).

4. Tyrosine hydroxylase phosphorylation

TH, the rate limiting enzyme in the synthesis of catecholamines, plays important roles in the regulation of sympathetic nervous system and its impact on cardiac function (Rao et al., 2007). In particular, increases in the phosphorylation of Ser40 and Ser31 accelerate TH activity, thereby stimulating production of neurotransmitter in catecholamines terminals (Kumer and Vrana, 1996; Dunkley et al., 2004). TH expression is subjected to intricate regulation by a number of mechanisms, including transcriptional and post-transcriptional processes (Kumer and Vrana, 1996; Mallet, 1999). Short-term regulation of catecholamine biosynthesis occurs through the modulation of the state of phosphorylation of TH. TH phosphorylation and activation is the primary mechanism responsible for the maintenance of catecholamine levels in tissues after catecholamine secretion. TH can be phosphorylated at serine (Ser) residues 8, 19, 31 and 40 by a variety of PKs (Campbell et al., 1986). PKA and PKC phosphorylate TH only at Ser40 (Roskoski et al., 1987; Funakoshi et al., 1991). ERK1 and ERK2 were shown to phosphorylate Ser31 in situ (Haycock et al., 1992). The phosphorylation of Ser40 increases the enzyme's activity in vitro, in situ and in vivo. Phosphorylation at Ser31 also increases the activity but to a much lesser extent than Ser40 phosphorylation. The phosphorylation of TH at Ser19 or Ser8 has no direct effect on TH activity (Dunkley et al., 2004) (fig. 6).

Previous studies have shown that naloxone-induced morphine withdrawal results in an increased NA turnover at heart level (Milanés et al., 2000a). This enhancement in NA turnover could be due to changes in the state of phosphorylation of TH, which are critically involved in the regulation of catecholamines synthesis and function. Therefore, we have studied the expression and phosphorylation at Ser31 and Ser40 during morphine withdrawal at different time points. Rats withdrawn from morphine presented an increase in total TH expression (fig. 7) and in TH phosphorylated at Ser31 (fig. 8) and Ser40 (fig. 9), together with an enhancement of TH activity (fig. 10). This activation of TH could be responsible for the increase in the hemodynamic parameters described above.

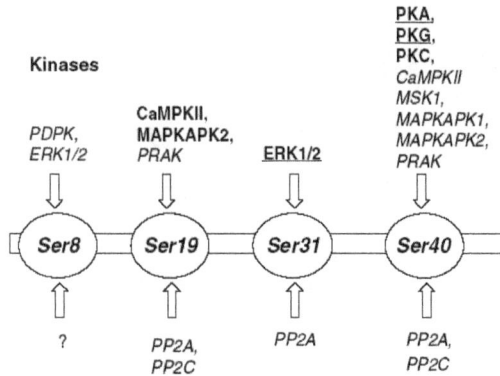

Fig. 6. The protein kinases (PK) and protein phosphatases (PP) capable of modulating tyrosine hydroxylase (TH) phosphorylation in vitro and in situ (Taken from Dunkley et al., 2004).

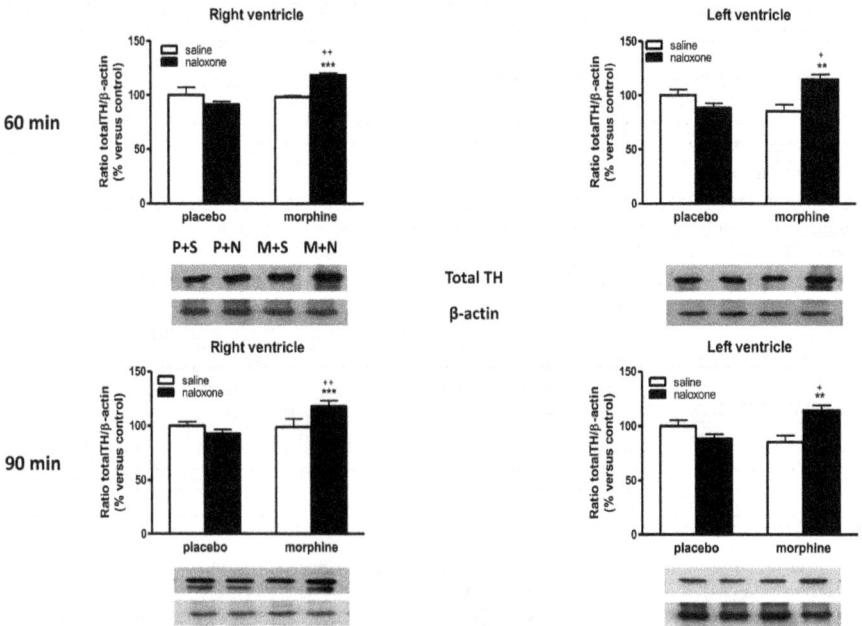

Fig. 7. Western blotting analysis of TH immunoreactivity levels in the right and left ventricle 60 or 90 min after saline (S) or naloxone (N) administration to placebo– (P) or morphine– (M) treated rats. The immunoreactivity corresponding to total TH is expressed as a percentage of that in the control group (P+S; defined as 100%). Data are the mean±S.E.M (n=4–6). **P<0.01, ***P<0.001 versus the group receiving saline instead of naloxone; +P<0.05, ++P<0.01 versus the group pretreated with placebo instead of morphine.

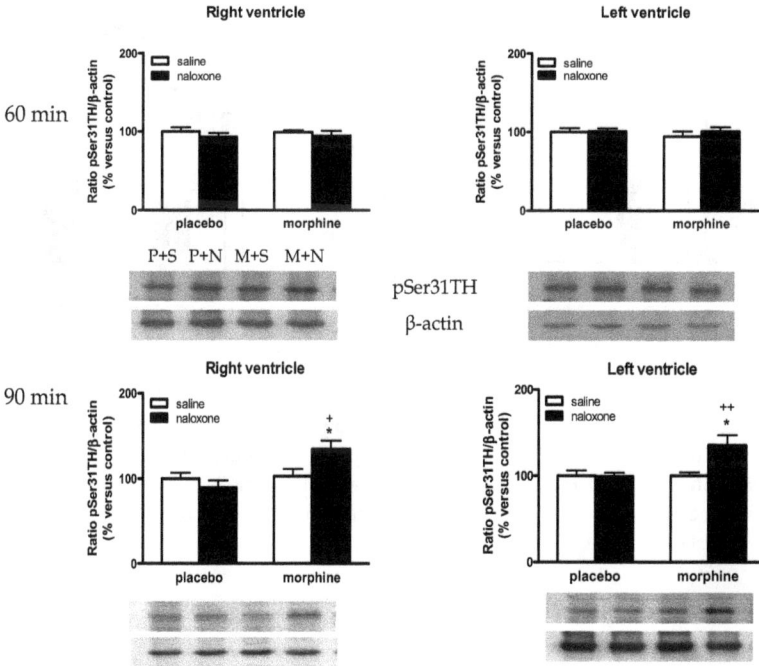

Fig. 8. Western blotting analysis of phospho(p)Ser31TH in the right and left ventricle 60 or 90 min after saline (S) or naloxone (N) administration to placebo- (P) or morphine- (M) treated rats. The immunoreactivity corresponding to pSer31TH is expressed as a percentage of that in the control group (P+S; defined as 100%). Data are the mean±S.E.M. (n=4-6). *P<0.05 versus the group receiving saline instead of naloxone; ++P<0.01, +P<0.05 versus the group pretreated with placebo instead of morphine.

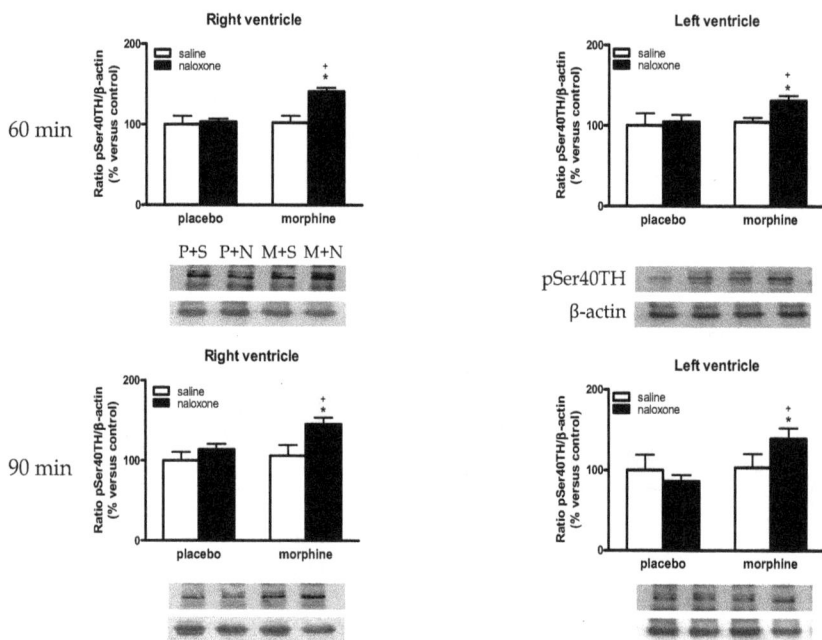

Fig. 9. Western blotting analysis of phospho(p)Ser40 TH in the right and left ventricle 60 or 90 min after saline (S) or naloxone (N) administration to placebo- (P) or morphine- (M) treated rats. The immunoreactivity corresponding to pSer40TH is expressed as a percentage of that in the control group (P+S; defined as 100%). Data are the mean±S.E.M. (n=4–6). *P<0.05 versus the group receiving saline instead of naloxone; +P<0.05 versus the group pretreated with placebo instead of morphine.

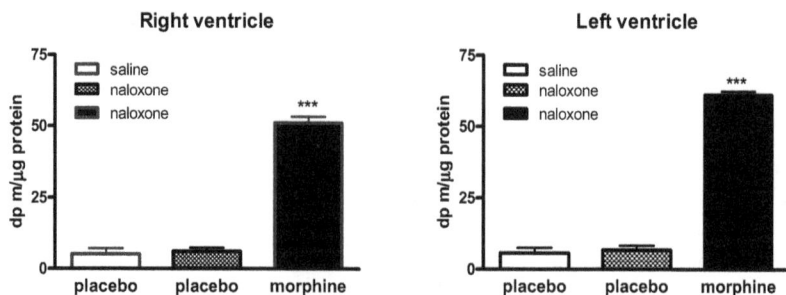

Fig. 10. TH activity in right and left ventricle from placebo or morphine dependent rats 90 min after s.c. administration of saline or naloxone. Data are the mean±S.E.M. (n=4–6). ***P<0.001 versus the group pretreated with placebo instead of morphine.

5. Changes in c-Fos expression

c-Fos immunoreactivity was examined by western blot and immunohistochemistry. Western blot analysis showed that after naloxone injection to rats chronically treated with morphine, there was a significant induction of c-Fos immunoreactivity in the right and left ventricle. Immunohistochemical analysis corroborated these results. Thus, rats dependent on morphine and given naloxone showed a significant induction of c-Fos immunoreactivity in the right ventricle, septum and left ventricle (fig. 11). This increase of c-Fos could contribute to activate TH synthesis through its activity on the AP-1 sequence present in the TH gene promoter region.

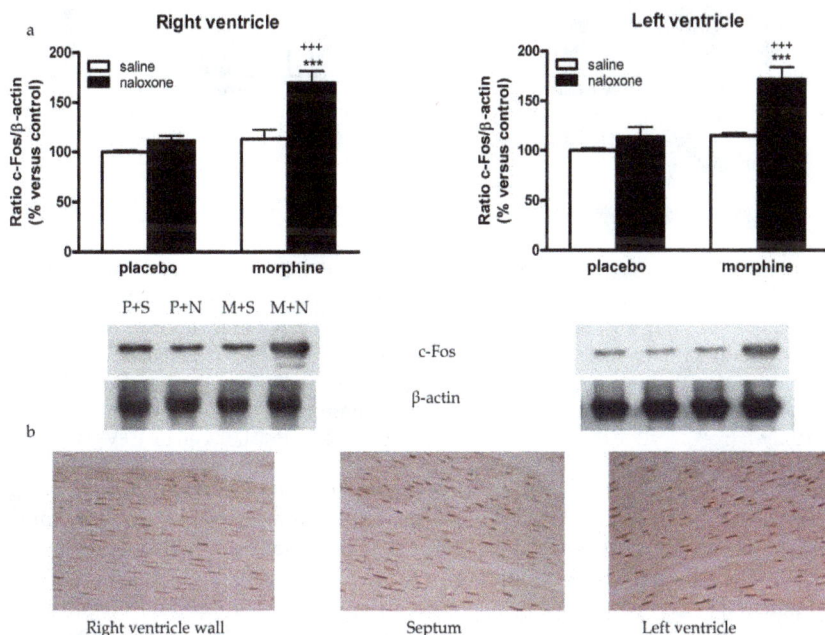

Fig. 11. (a) Representative immunoblots of c-Fos in samples isolated from placebo (P) or morphine (M) dependent rats 90 min after s.c. administration of saline (S) or naloxone (N). For quantification, optical densities of c-Fos immunoreactive bands were measured, normalized to the background values, and expressed as percentage of controls, defined as 100% value. Data are the mean±S.E.M. (n=4-6). +++P<0.001 versus M+S; ***P<0.001 versus P+N. (b) Photomicrographs of c-Fos immunoreactvity in the right and left ventricular wall and in the septum, after naloxone-precipitated withdrawal. Scale bar 58 μm.

6. Implication of ERK and PKA in the cardiac adaptive changes observed during morphine withdrawal

To assess the relative contribution of ERK and PKA to the regulation of c-Fos and TH, we examined morphine withdrawal-induced c-Fos expression in animals receiving SL327, a selective ERK inhibitor or HA-1004, a selective PKA inhibitor. SL327 administration before naloxone to rats chronically treated with morphine significantly diminished the increase in c-Fos levels in both ventricles (fig. 12).

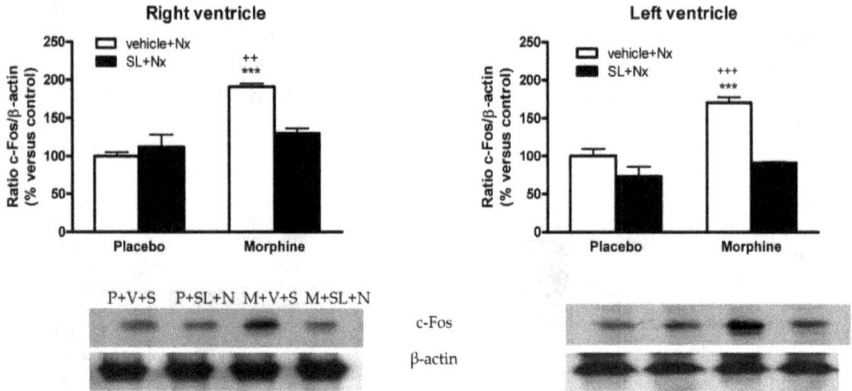

Fig. 12. Morphine withdrawal stimulates c-Fos expression in the right and left ventricle. Representative immunoblots of c-Fos in the right and left ventricle tissue isolated from placebo (P) or morphine (M) dependent rats, 90 min after s.c. administration of naloxone (Nx, N) in the absence (vehicle, veh, V, DMSO) or presence of SL327 (SL, 100 mg/kg) 1 h before naloxone. c-Fos immunoreactive bands were measured, normalized to the background values and expressed as percentages of controls. Data correspond to mean±S.E.M. (n=4). $^{+++}P<0.001$, $^{++}P<0.01$ versus M+SL+N; $^{***}P<0.001$ versus P+V+N.

However, chronic inhibition of PKA concurrently with morphine treatment did not modify c-Fos induction during morphine withdrawal (fig. 13). These results reveal that ERK but not PKA is an important pathway mediating c-Fos induction. However, previous results from our laboratory showed that inhibition of PKC also produced an inhibition of c-Fos expression in the heart (Almela et al., 2006) suggesting that the transcriptional regulation of c-Fos seems to be under a combined control of an ERK-dependent and-independent pathway. On the other hand, the expression of c-Fos, mainly due to phosphorylation of ERK1/2, was not antagonized by propranolol or prazosin (González-Cuello et al., 2004), suggesting that the activation of ERK and c-Fos expression is not due to an indirect mechanism via sympathetic activation.

In addition, our results showed that SL327 blocks the increase in TH phosphorylated at Ser31 observed in the right and left ventricle after the injection of naloxone to morphine dependent rats (fig. 14). The only protein kinase reported to phosphorylate TH at Ser31 in vitro was ERK (Haycock et al., 1992; Lindgren et al., 2002). In situ phosphorylation of TH at Ser31 increases TH activity and catecholamine synthesis (Haycock, 1992). Given that TH is phosphorylated on a specific serine residue (Ser31) by the ERK, it is possible that activation of ERK1/2 in the heart provides a way in which TH is regulated under morphine dependence.

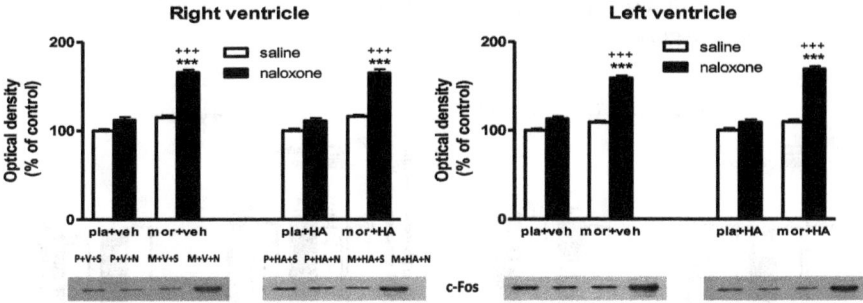

Fig. 13. Western blotting analysis of c-Fos immunoreactivity levels in the right and left ventricle after naloxone-precipitated withdrawal in vehicle- (veh, V) infused rats and in animals chronically administered with HA-1004 (HA). Animals received s.c. implantation of placebo (pla, P) or morphine (mor, M) pellets for 7 days and concomitantly were infused with vehicle or HA-1004 (40 nmol/day). On day 8, rats were injected with saline (S) or naloxone (N, 5 mg/kg, s.c.) and were decapitated 90 min later. The immunoreactivity corresponding to c-Fos is expressed as a percentage of that in the control group (P+V+S; defined as 100% value). Data are the mean±SEM (n=4-6). ***p<0.001 versus the group receiving saline instead of naloxone; +++p<0.001 versus the group pretreated with placebo instead of morphine.

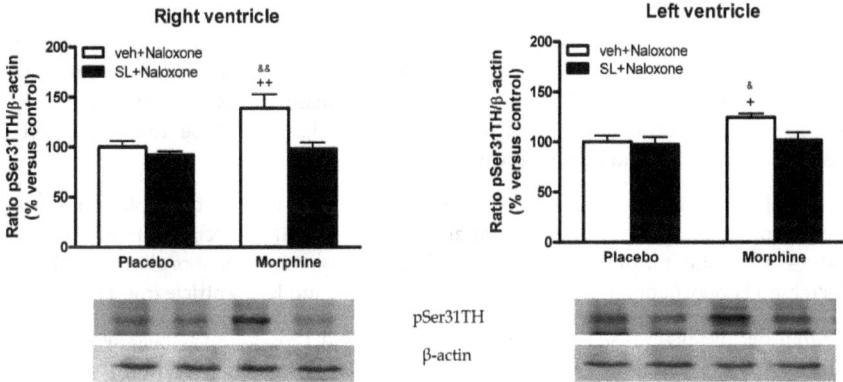

Fig. 14. Phospho(p)Ser31TH immunoblots in right and left ventricle from placebo or morphine dependent rats 90 min after s.c. administration of naloxone in the absence or presence of SL327 (SL, 100 mg/kg, i.p.), 1 h before naloxone. pSer31TH immunoreactive bands were measured, normalized to the background values and expressed as percentage of controls. Data are the mean±S.E.M. (n=4-6). ++P<0.01 versus the group pretreated with placebo instead of morphine; &&P<0.01 versus morphine+SL+naloxone.

Similarly, HA-1004 blocked the enhancement of TH phosphorylated at Ser40 in the heart after morphine withdrawal (fig. 15), suggesting that different pathways are implicated in the postranscriptional regulation of TH.

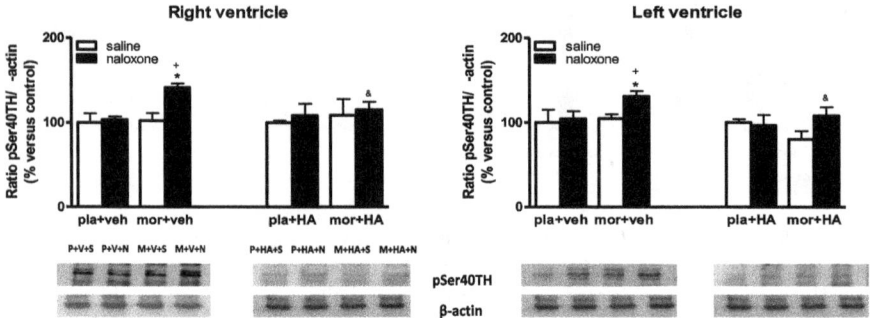

Fig. 15. Western blotting analysis of phospho(p)Ser40TH in the right ventricle 60 min after saline (S) or naloxone (N) administration to placebo- (pla, P) or morphine- (mor, M) treated rats receiving vehicle (veh, V) or HA-1004 (HA). The immunoreactivity corresponding to pSer40TH is expressed as a percentage of that in the control group (P+V+S; defined as 100%). Data are the mean±S.E.M. (n=4–6). *P<0.05 versus the group receiving saline instead of naloxone; +P<0.05 versus the group pretreated with placebo instead of morphine; &P<0.05 versus the group receiving vehicle instead of HA-1004.

7. Crosstalk between PKA and ERK

It is now appreciated that crosstalk among various signal pathways plays an important role in activation of intracellular and intranuclear signal transduction cascades. In our study, chronic treatment with HA-1004 antagonized the increase in ERK1/2 phosphorylation observed during morphine withdrawal in the heart (fig. 16). These results suggest a crosstalk between PKA and ERK pathways.

To assess the contribution of PKA to the regulation of TH, we examined TH phosphorylated at Ser31 during morphine withdrawal in animals receiving the selective inhibitor of PKA HA-1004. This inhibitor prevents the ability of naloxone-precipitated morphine withdrawal to increase TH phosphorylated at Ser31 levels in the right and left ventricle (fig. 17).

Although the mechanism of crosstalk between PKA and ERK pathways has not yet been clarified, it is possible that PKA pathway facilitates MEK1/2 that activates the ERK1/2 pathway (Obama et al., 2007; Stork and Schmitt, 2002). The activated ERK pathway increases the phosphorylation of proteins related to morphine dependence, including TH. Using phosphorylation state-specific antibodies directed toward TH at Ser31, we have shown that HA-1004 blocked the increase in the level of TH phosphorylation at Ser31 induced after naloxone injection to morphine dependent rats in the right and left ventricle. These data suggest that crosstalk between PKA and ERK pathways is a key regulatory design necessary to regulate the Ser31 phosphorylation of TH.

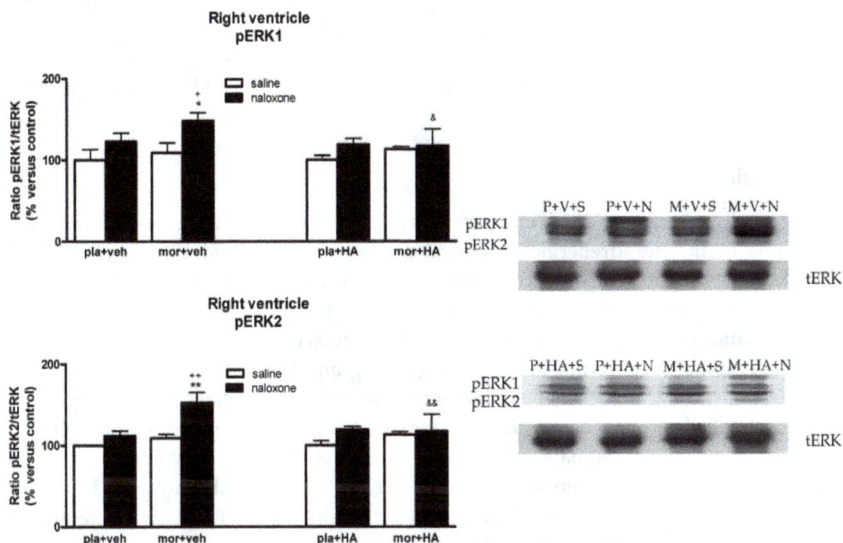

Fig. 16. Western blotting analysis of phospho(p)ERK1 and phospho(p)ERK2 immunoreactivity levels in the right ventricle 60 min after saline (S) or naloxone (N) administration to placebo- (pla, P) or morphine- (mor, M) treated rats receiving vehicle (veh, V) or HA-1004 (HA). The immunoreactivity corresponding to pERK1 or pERK2 is expressed as a percentage of that in the control group (P+V+S; defined as 100% value). Data are the mean±S.E.M. (n=4-6). **$P<0.01$, *$P<0.05$ versus the dependent group receiving saline instead of naloxone. ++$P<0.01$, +$P<0.05$ versus the group pretreated with placebo instead of morphine injected with naloxone. &&$P<0.01$, &$P<0.05$ versus the group receiving vehicle instead of HA.

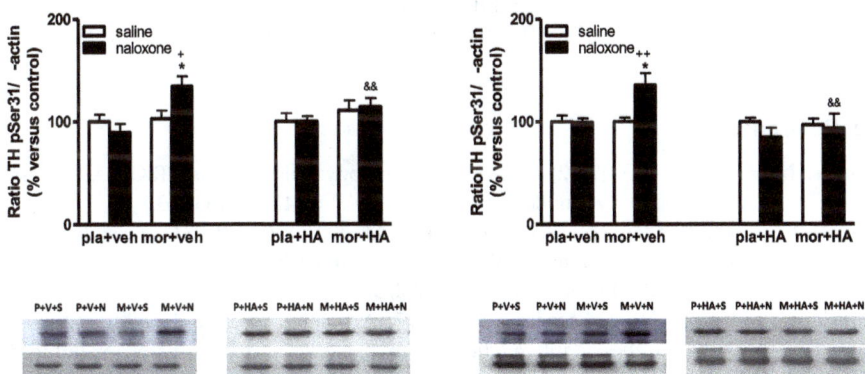

Fig. 17. Western blotting analysis of phospho(p)Ser31TH in the right and left ventricle 90 min after saline (S) or naloxone (N) administration to placebo- (pla, P) or morphine- (mor, M)

treated rats receiving vehicle (veh, V) or HA-1004 (HA). The immunoreactivity corresponding to pSer31TH is expressed as a percentage of that in the control group (P+V+S or P+HA+S; defined as 100% value). Data are the mean±S.E.M. (n=4–6). *$p<0.05$ versus the dependent group receiving saline instead of naloxone; ++$P<0.01$, +$P<0.05$ versus the group pretreated with placebo instead of morphine injected with naloxone. &&$P<0.01$ versus the group receiving vehicle instead of HA.

8. Conclusion

Naloxone administration after chronic morphine treatment, triggers neurochemical adaptations in the noradrenergic system and enhances PKA and ERK pathways. The functional consequences of this activation include an increase in TH activation and NA turnover and an enhancement in c-Fos expression. Many pathways implicated in the adaptive changes observed during withdrawal are subject to feedback mechanisms that can either amplify or suppress their own signalling and there is considerable signalling from one pathway to another, a phenomenon known as crosstalk. Consequently, the responses that cells mount to specific environmental conditions depend on the sum of the intensity and duration of signals from several pathways and how they interact with each other. Although the mechanism of crosstalk between PKA and ERK pathways has not yet been clarified, it is possible that PKA pathway facilitates MEK1/2 that activates the ERK1/2 pathway (Obama et al., 2007; Stork and Schmitt, 2002). The activated ERK pathway increases the phosphorylation of proteins related to morphine dependence, including TH. Our data suggest that crosstalk between PKA and ERK pathways is a key regulatory design necessary to regulate the phosphorylation of TH. These findings provide a new explanation to understand the complex mechanisms implicated in the adaptive changes observed during morphine withdrawal and could be useful for future treatment strategies.

9. Acknowledgment

This work was supported by Ministerio de Educación y Ciencia (Grants SAF 2010-17907), Fundación Séneca, CARM (15405/PI/10) and Instituto de Salud Carlos III (RETICS: RD06/001/1006).

10. References

Adams, J.P. & Sweatt, J.D. (2002) Molecular psychology: roles for the ERK MAP kinase cascade in memory. *Annu Rev Pharmacol Toxicol*, Vol. 42, pp. 135-163.

Almela, P.; Cerezo, M.; Milanés, M.V. & Laorden, M.L. (2006) Role of PKC in regulating of Fos and TH expression after naloxone induced morphine withdrawal in the heart. *Naunyn-Schmiedeberg's Arch Pharmacol*, Vol. 372, pp. 374-382.

Almela, P.; Milanés, M.V. & Laorden, M.L. (2007) Activation of ERK signaling pathway contributes to the adaptive changes in rat hearts during naloxone-induced morphine withdrawal. *Br J Pharmacol*, Vol. 151, pp. 787-797.

Almela, P.; Milanés, M.V. & Laorden, M.L. (2008) The PKs PKA and ERK 1/2 are involved in phosphorylation of TH at serine 40 and 31 during morphine withdrawal in rat hearts. *Br J Pharmacol*, Vol. 155, pp. 73-83.

Almela P.; Martínez-Laorden E.; Atucha N.M.; Milanés M.V. & Laorden M.L. (2011) Naloxone-precipitated morphine withdrawal evokes phosphorylation of heat shock protein 27 in rat heart through extracellular signal-regulated kinase. *J Mol Cell Cardiol*, Vol. 51, pp. 129-39.

Armour, J.A. (1991) Intrinsic cardiac neurons. *J Cardiovasc Electrophysiol*, Vol. 2, pp. 331–341.

Campbell, D.G.; Hardie, D.G. & Vulliet, P.R. (1986) Identification of four phosphorylation sites in the N-terminal region of tyrosine hydroxylase. *J Biol Chem*, Vol. 261, pp. 10489–10492.

Cerezo, M.; Milanés, M.V. & Laorden, M.L. (2005) Alterations in protein kinase A and different protein kinase C isoforms in the heart during morphine withdrawal. *Eur J Pharmacol*, Vol. 522, pp.9-19.

Childers, S.R. (1991) Opioid receptor-coupled second messengers systems. *Life Sci*, Vol. 48, pp. 1991-2003.

Dunkley, P.; Bobrovskaya, L.; Graham, M.E., von Nagy-Felsobuki, E.I. & Dickson, P.W. (2004) Tyrosine hydroxylase phosphorylation: Regulation and consecuences. *J Neurochem*, Vol. 91, pp. 1025-1043.

Funakoshi, H.; Okuno, S. & Fujisawa, H. (1991). Different effects on activity caused by phophorylation of tyrosine hydroxylase at serine 40 by three multifunctional protein kinases. *J Biol Chem*, Vol. 266, pp. 15614–15620.

González-Cuello, A.; Milanés, M.V.; Avilés, M. & Laorden, M.L. (2004) Changes in c-fos expression in the rat heart during morphine withdrawal. Involvement of alpha2-adrenoceptors. *Naunyn-Schmiedeberg's Arch Pharmacol*, Vol. 370, pp. 17-25.

Haycock, J.W.; Ahn, N.G.; Cobbe, M.H. & Krebs, E.G. (1992) ERK 1 and ERK 2, two microtubule-associated protein 2 kinases, mediate the phosphorylation of tyrosine hydroxylase at serine-31 in situ. *Proc Natl Acad Sci USA*, Vol. 89, pp. 2365-2369.

Huh, J.; Gross, G.J.; Nagase, H. & Liang, B.T. (2001) Protection of cardiac myocytes via delta(1)-opioid receptors, protein kinase C, and mitochondrial K(ATP) channels. *Am J Physiol Heart Circ Physiol*, Vol. 280, pp. H377-383.

Hussain, M.; Drago, G.A.; Bhogal, M.; Colyer, J. & Orchard, C.H. (1999) Effects of the protein kinase A inhibitor H-89 on Ca^{2+} regulation in isolated ferret ventricular myocytes. *Pflugers Arch*, Vol. 437, pp. 529-537.

Jiang, X.; Shi, E.; Nakajima, Y. & Sato, S. (2006) COX-2 mediates morphine-induced delayed cardioprotection via an iNOS-dependent mechanism. *Life Sci*, Vol. 78, pp. 2543-2549.

Johnson, S.M. & Fleming, W.W. (1989) Mechanisms of cellular adaptive sensitivity changes: Aplication to opioid tolerance and dependence. *Pharmacol Rev*, Vol. 41, pp. 435-488.

Kamp, T.J. & Hell, J.W. (2000) Regulation of cardiac L-type calcium channels by protein kinase A and protein kinase C. *Circ Res*, Vol. 87, pp. 1095-1102.

Kienbaum, P.; Heuter, T.; Michel, M.C.; Scherbaum, N.; Gastpar, M. & Peters, J. (2001) Chronic μ-opioid receptor stimulation in humans decreases muscle sympathetic nerve activity. *Circulation*, Vol. 103, pp. 850-855.

Kienbaum, P.; Heuter, T.; Scherbaum, N.; Gastpar, M. & Peters, J. (2002) Chronic μ-opioid receptor stimulation alters cardiovascular regulation in humans: differential effects on muscle sympathetic and heart rate responses to arterial hypotension. *J Cardiovasc Pharmacol*, Vol. 40, pp. 363-369.

Koob, G.F. & Bloom, F.E. (1988) Cellular and molecular mechanisms of drug dependence. *Science*, Vol. 242, pp. 715-723.

Kumer, S.C. & Vrana, K.E. (1996) Intricate regulation of tyrosine hydroxylase activity and gene expression. *J Neurochem*, Vol. 67, pp. 443-462.

Lindgren, N.; Goiny, M.; Herera-Marschitz, M.; Haycock, J.W.; Hökfelt, T. & Fisone, G. (2002) Activation of extracellular signals-regulated kinases 1 and 2 by depolarization stimulates tyrosine-hydroxylase phosphorylation and dopamine synthesis in rat brain. *Eur J Neurosci*, Vol. 15, pp. 769-773.

Lippi, G.; Plebani, M. & Cervellin, G. (2010) Cocaine in acute myocardial infarction. *Adv Clin Chem*, Vol. 51, pp. 53-70.

Mallet, J. (1999) Tyrosine hydroxylase from cloning to neuropsychiatric disorders. *Brain Res Bull*, Vol. 50, pp. 381–382.

Michel, M.C.; Li, Y. & Heusch, G. (2001) Mitogen-activated protein kinases in the heart. *Naunyn-Schmiedeberg´s Arch Pharmacol*, Vol. 363, pp. 245-266.

Milanés, M.V.; Fuente, T.; Marín, M.T. & Laorden, M.L. (1999) Catecholaminergic activity and 3´,5´-cyclic adenosine monophosphate concentrations in the right ventricle after acute and chronic morphine administration in the rat. *Br J Anaesth*, Vol. 83, pp. 784-788.

Milanés, M.V.; Fuente, T. & Laorden, M.L. (2000a) Catecholaminergic activity and 3´,5´-cyclic adenosine monophosphate levels in heart right ventricle after naloxone induced withdrawal. *Naunyn-Schmiedeberg´s Arch Pharmacol*, Vol. 361, pp. 61-66.

Milanés, M.V. & Laorden, M.L. (2000b) Changes in catecholaminergic pathways innervating the rat heart ventricle during morphine dependence. Involvement of A1 and A2 adrenoceptors. *Eur J Pharmacol*, Vol. 397, pp. 311-318.

Milanés, M.V.; Martínez, M.D.; González-Cuello, A. & Laorden, M.L. (2001) Evidence for a peripheral mechanism in cardiac opioid withdrawal. *Naunyn-Schmiedeberg's Arch Pharmacol*, Vol. 364, pp. 193–198.

Nerantzis, C.E.; Koulouris, S.N.; Marianou, S.K.; Pastromas, S.C., Koutsaftis, P.N. & Agapitos, E.B. (2011) Histologic findings of the sinus node and the perinodal area in street heroin addicts, victims of sudden unexpected death. *J Forensic Sci*, Vol. 56, pp. 645-648.

Obama, Y.; Horgan, A. & Sork, J.S. (2007) The requirement of Ras and Rap1 for the activation of ERKs by cAMP, PACAP, and KCL in cerebellar granule cells. *J Neurochem*, Vol. 101, pp. 470-482.

Ongur, D.; An, X. & Price, J.L. (1998) Prefrontal cortical projections to the hypothalamus in macaque monkeys. *J Comp Neurol*, Vol. 401, pp. 480-505.

Peart, J.N. & Gross, G.J. (2006) Cardioprotective effects of acute and chronic opioid treatment is mediated via different signalling pathways. *Am J Physiol Heart Circ Physiol*, Vol. 291, pp. H1746-53.

Pugsley, M.K. (2002) The diverse molecular mechanism responsible for the actions of opioids on the cardiovascular system. *Pharmacol Ther*, Vol. 93, pp. 51-75.

Pyner, S. (2009) Neurochemistry of the paraventricular nucleus of the hypothalamus: implications for cardiovascular regulation. *J Chem Neuroanat*, Vol. 38, pp. 197-208.

Rabadán, J.V.; Milanés, M.V. & Laorden, M.L. (1997) Effects of chronic morphine treatment on catecholamines content and mechanical response in the rat heart. *J Pharmacol Exp Ther*, Vol. 280, pp. 32-37.

Rabadán, J.V.; Milanés, M.V. & Laorden, M.L. (1998) Changes in right atrial catecholamine content in naive rats and after naloxone-induced withdrawal. *Br J Anaesth*, Vol. 80, pp. 354-359.

Rao F.; Zhang L.; Wessel J.; Zhang K.; Wen G.; Kennedy B.P.; Rana B.K.; Das M.; Rodriguez-Flores J.L.; Smith D.W.; Cadman P.E.; Salem R.M.; Mahata S.K.; Schork N.J.; Taupenot L.; Ziegler M.G. & O'Connor D.T. (2007) Tyrosine hydroxylase, the rate-limiting enzyme in catecholamine biosynthesis: discovery of common human genetic variants governing transcription, autonomic activity, and blood pressure in vivo. *Circulation*, Vol. 116, pp. 993-1006.

Ren, X.; Noda, Y.; Mamiya, T.; Nagai, T. & Nabeshima, T.A. (2004) Neuroactive steroid, dehydroepiandrosterone sulfate, prevents the development of morphine dependence and tolerance via c-Fos expression linked to the extracellular signal-regulated protein kinase. *Behav Brain Res*, Vol. 152, pp. 243-250.

Risold, P.Y. & Swanson, L.W. (1997) Connections of the rat lateral septal complex. *Brain Res Rev*, Vol. 24, pp. 115-195.

Roskoski, R.J.; Vulliet, P.R. & Glass, B.D. (1987) Phosphorylation of tyrosine hydroxylase by cyclic GMP-dependent protein kinase. *J Neurochem*, Vol. 48, pp. 840-845.

Sawchenko, P.E. & Swanson, L.W. (1982) Immunohistochemical identification of neurons in the paraventricular nucleus of the hypothalamus that project to the medulla or to the spinal cord in the rat. *J Comp Neurol*, Vol. 205, pp. 260-272.

Self, D.W. & Nestler, E.J. (1995) Molecular mechanisms of drug reinforcement and addiction. *Ann Rev Neurosci*, Vol. 18, pp. 463-495.

Stork, P. & Schmitt, J. (2002) Crosstalk between cAMP and MAP kinase signalling in the regulation of cell proliferation. *Trends Cell Biol*, Vol. 12, pp. 258-266.

Sugden, P.H. & Bogoyevitch, M.A. (1995) Intracellular signalling through protein kinases in the heart. *Cardiovasc Res*, Vol. 30, pp. 478-492.

Wang, G.Y.; Wu, S.; Pei, J.M.; Yu, X.C. & Wong, T.M. (2001) Kappa- but not delta-opioid receptors mediate effects of ischemic preconditioning on both infarct and arrhythmia in rats. *Am J Physiol Heart Circ Physiol*, Vol. 280, pp. H384-391.

Xu, J.; Tian, W.; Ma, X.; Guo, J.; Shi, Q.; Jin, Y.; Xi, J. & Xu, Z. (2011) Mechanism underlying morphine-induced Akt activation: Roles of protein phosphatases and reactive oxygen species. *Cell Biochem Biophys*, Vol. 61, pp. 303-311.

4

Food Addiction, Obesity and Neuroimaging

Karen M. von Deneen[1] and Yijun Liu[2]
[1]*Xidian University,*
[2]*University of Florida,*
[1]*China*
[2]*USA*

1. Introduction

This chapter will be dedicated to addressing various aspects of food addiction (where food is portrayed as being an addictive substance). It will encompass our group's and colleagues' newest neuroimaging research results and methods with respect to the findings of other researchers in the field. The chapter will attempt to elucidate the mechanisms of food addiction (FA) leading to obesity. It will begin with a brief introduction on the major points relating to obesity and FA. The first section will address the neurobiology and neurophysiology of addiction as well as the causes of obesity and its global impacts, concluding with therapeutic measures and future research.

2. Food addiction and obesity: Health problems

Obesity-related deaths rank second in the world (Mokdad et al., 2004). Obesity is linked with stroke, heart disease, diabetes mellitus, osteoarthritis, and certain cancers (Raman, 2002). Developing countries have also been affected by this global epidemic (Zemmet, 2000). The number of adults over the age of 20 with a BMI over 30 has increased rapidly over the past 20 years (Pi-Sunyer, 2002). Although the etiology of obesity has been predominantly correlated with eating behavior, other factors such as individual preferences, mental disorders, genetic makeup, or addictive tendencies have been suggested to play contributing roles (von Deneen and Liu, 2011). Among some known etiological factors, the intrauterine environment plays a role in placing children at risk for becoming obese and having diabetes and high cholesterol levels (Blumenthal & Gold, 2010). McMillen et al. (2009) suggested that specific periods during pregnancy predisposed individuals to obesity, therefore maternal nutrition and perinatal lifestyle played a major role in fetal programming. Over-nutrition during pregnancy led to larger offspring or gestational diabetes associated with obesity, while breastfeeding could counter the effects of obesity (Martorell et al., 2001).

New insights into the obesity issue involved developing an FA model that states food is eaten for pleasure and hedonistic intake of food can be linked with drug addiction and eating disorders.

This section will assess childhood obesity etiology, metabolic syndrome, dietary and behavioral causes with a specific impetus on the Han Chinese population (von Deneen et al.,

2011). Obesity particularly in China has led to worldwide attention and is becoming a pandemic disease resulting from a shift in energy balance caused by altered genes, a sedentary lifestyle, and neurohormonal imbalances as a result of Western influence. Obesity is spreading to low income and middle-income countries, such as China, as a result of novel dietary habits, promoting chronic diseases and premature mortality (Cecchini et al., 2010). Work-related activities declined, whereas leisure time is dominated by television/computer programs and other physically inactive pursuits (Popkin, 2001). The vicious obesity cycle begins with excess adipose leading to chronic low grade inflammation that results in insulin resistance (IR) along with hypertension, atherosclerosis, dyslipidemia and type 2 diabetes mellitus (T2DM), which are consistent findings of metabolic syndrome (MetS) (Achike et al., 2011). Studies have shown that obesity can be linked to lower ghrelin concentrations in obese individuals (Groschl et al., 2005). As a result, ghrelin levels have been found to be negatively correlated with body fat and waist circumference (WC) (Fagerberg, Hulten & Hulthe, 2003).

Metabolic syndrome (MetS) is defined as "a combination of clinical disorders that increase the risk for diabetes and cardiovascular disease, including atherosclerosis, stroke and hypertension" (Achike et al., 2011). The components of MetS include abdominal fat, atherogenic dyslipidemia, hypertension, pro-inflammatory state, pro-thrombic state and IR with or without glucose intolerance (Grundy et al., 2004). Obesity, dyslipidemia and hyperglycemia are all risk factors for colorectal cancer (Giovannucci, 2002). Increased plasma free fatty acids (FFA) in obese Chinese people acted as an important link between obesity and IR, and plasma FFA levels were negatively correlated with insulin sensitivity (Li et al., 2005). The Chinese were five times more likely to have a family history of T2DM than non-Chinese subjects (Xu et al., 2010). Finally, in middle-aged and elderly Chinese living in northeast China, there was a higher incidence of MetS and cardiovascular disease, especially atherosclerosis (Liu et al., 2010), which is increasing as influenced by a Westernized lifestyle (Mi et al., 2008).

2.1 Social and cultural influence on obesity

Parents and extended family members play a crucial role in shaping their children's eating and exercise habits (Rhee, 2008). This is a global phenomenon, but the best example to describe the state the world is in with regards to obesity is China. Even though the Western world (first world countries) has had the greatest problems with obesity and FA, China is following in its footsteps. Approximately 22% of Chinese parents regarded their children as being underweight even if their children weren't. Meanwhile, 23% of overweight children were perceived by their parents as being normal (Shi et al., 2007). Parental assessment of the weights of their children was associated with the physical appearance of the parents themselves (Huang, Becerra & Oda, 2007). Overweight daughters were more likely to be criticized by their mothers (Maynard et al., 2003). Chinese parents tended to misperceive their sons' weights more than their daughters'. Mothers had a better ability to discriminate their children's size. This gender difference could be related to social values and status (Campbell et al., 2006), hence exacerbating the obesity problem. For example, girls with slim and graceful bodies were deemed acceptable by Chinese society, while overweight boys were regarded as "strong and healthy" (Maynard et al., 2003). Parents' and other family members' 'pressure to eat' strategy was correlated with children's caloric consumption (Drucker et al., 1999). Another important factor leading to childhood obesity is that a high portion of Hong-Kong school children spend too many hours watching television (TV) and playing computer or video games (Kong & Chow, 2010). Overweight or obese adolescents had a tendency to view TV programs and become less physically active. In China, access to Westernized TV programming and food advertising has increased (Hong, 1998). Advertisements for food products, such as soft drinks and salty snacks, constituted more than 80% of commercials in China (Ji & McNeal, 2001). According to mothers surveyed in urban areas in China, many children have their own spending money, and they often use this money to buy snacks and beverages (Zhang & Harwood, 2004). Chinese parents stated that their children influenced most of their purchases, especially of snacks (McNeal & Yeh, 1997). This can be witnessed in most Chinese cities with large supermarkets today. Food products and restaurant chains seen in TV programs and commercials provide food cues to children, thus enhancing the need to snack while watching TV (Coon et al., 2001). TV is present in almost every Chinese household, and TV advertising in China increasingly promotes high-calorie foods (Parvanta et al., 2010). Low-income families spend more hours watching TV than their counterparts (Livingstone, 2002). However, snacks seen on TV tended to be purchased more by those with higher incomes (Wang et al., 2008b). All in all, this evidence portrays that non-physical entertainment does play a major role in weight management in young people all over the world.

China can be portrayed as a "double burden of malnutrition" where under-nutrition coexists with obesity (Popkin et al., 1995). The food selection and consumption in China has resulted in a diet that is more energy-dense and laden with saturated animal fat and processed sugars, and is low in complex carbohydrates, fiber, fresh fruits and vegetables (Zhai et al., 2009). Underprivileged individuals tend to stock up on non-nutritious, high-calorie foods as low-budget staples, whereas nutrient-rich foods and high-quality diets are consumed by more affluent customers (Jones et al., 2007). In China, sugar-sweetened beverages (SSB) are a major food source with a high glycemic index (Murakami et al., 2006), thus are easily exploitable as a form of addictive substance. Another study found associations between frequent SSB intake and obesity predominantly in Chinese women, while lack of exercise, smoking, and high meat consumption increased the risk for greater weight gain in both genders (Ko et al., 2010). One study found that overweight children and adolescents consumed more energy, protein, and fat and ate fewer carbohydrates than did the controls (Guldan, 2010). They consumed less grain, fewer vegetables, more fruits, meats and cooking oil, eggs, fish, milk, and legumes. Those who ate at least 25g of cooking oil, 200g of meat, and 100g of dairy products had a higher chance of being overweight (Li et al., 2007).

From a recent cross-sectional survey done in Jiangsu Province, researchers found that a higher socio-economic status and urban residency were associated with energy-dense foods such as animal and dairy products, soft drinks, Western food, and increased snacking/breakfast skipping behaviors (Shi et al., 2005). Rural and lower income students normally consumed rice porridge, a traditional, thin breakfast gruel. However, they also preferred hamburgers, ice cream, milk, fruits, chocolate, and SSB (Shi et al., 2005). The traditional Chinese high-glycemic diet consists of a variety of high-glycemic staple rice products such as boiled rice, rice congee, and glutinous rice which pose adverse cardiovascular and MetS risks (Ding & Malik, 2008). When the Chinese population was lean and active, this diet did not pose as much risk. However, China today has an obesity epidemic and a dietary transition shifting toward more processed foods such as SSB (Ding & Malik, 2008).

The reason is that these foods are "appetizing, convenient and ready to eat, portable, affordable in single portions," and widely marketed for the younger generation, allowing them to be addicted to these foods. These addictive substances include soft drinks, biscuits, snacks, and fast-food sandwiches (Guldan, 2010). Higher incomes in China allow families to purchase SSB, snacks, and fast food. Supermarkets are packed with highly-processed, energy-dense, nutrient-poor, and lower-priced foods. Preferences include polished grains/white rice products, because Chinese consumers are unaware of the benefits from whole grains (Guldan, 2010). Another major dietary component is glutamate, which is a major taste ingredient of dietary protein described as 'Umami' (Kurihara & Kashiwayangani, 2000). Increasing concern with the rise of obesity in Westernized nations with the addition of monosodium glutamate (MSG) to commercially prepared foods is evident (Shi et al., 2010). There was a positive association between MSG consumption and the socio-economic status in rural China (Shi et al., 2010). Along those lines, Kazaks, Uyghurs and Mongolians are the major minorities in Xinjiang. The Kazaks have been reported to have hypertension (Jumabay et al., 2001), while obesity is common in the Uyghurs and Mongolians (Wang et al., 2006). Significant differences in mean blood pressure between Han, Kazaks, Uyghurs and Tibetan ethnic groups were deemed to be caused by different diet-related habits. It is well-known that alcohol, high-sodium foods and meat are traditionally popular among these groups, which are associated with surviving the cold weather in Xinjiang. Traditionally among Kazaks, Uyghurs and Mongolians in Xinjiang, alcohol consumption is paired with eating large amounts of animal fat or salty dishes, which could lead to an increase in fibrinogen levels. Males in particular traditionally drink spirits to deal with the cold. Additionally, salted milk tea is consumed in large amounts; vegetables are also rare in this region, hence they are not commonly consumed (Xi & Mi, 2009).

Eating disorders ranged from 1.3% to 5.21% among young Chinese females (Fu et al., 2005). However, these data do not represent the entire population. Currently, there is little knowledge about weight control concerns and behaviors in China. Body mass index (BMI), dieting, and eating disorder symptoms are not clearly defined (Fan et al., 2010). Another important study of adolescents in China found a strong association between smoking and the belief that smoking was important in weight control (Ge et al., 1994).

Overall, there are numerous problems arising from this epidemic such as psychosocial, emotional, neurological, cardiovascular, endocrine, musculoskeletal, gastrointestinal and pulmonary issues (Ebbeling, Pawlak & Ludwig, 2002). The costs of healthcare "associated with being overweight or obese projected exceed 850 billion dollars annually by 2030 in United States alone (Wang et al., 2008a)." As a result, this leads to a significant financial burden.

3. Biology and neurobiology of food intake

Food consumption is regulated via peripheral signals and central neuronal circuits (Wang et al., 2009) including the hypothalamus (HYP), amygdala (AMY), hippocampus (HIPP), insula, orbitofrontal cortex (OFC), and striatal brain regions (Dagher, 2009). These pathways regulate mechanisms of food reward, environmental stimuli perception, and integration of homeostasis of energy and gastrointestinal tract contents with food availability (Dagher, 2009). Most importantly, midbrain dopamine (DA) reward circuits motivate food ingestion and hedonistic sensations resulting from eating (Dagher, 2009) as well as brain opioid peptides (Barbano et al., 2005), which in turn work in tandem with other circuits responsible for enforcing feeding behaviors and weight regulation (Wang et al., 2009), as seen in Figure 1.

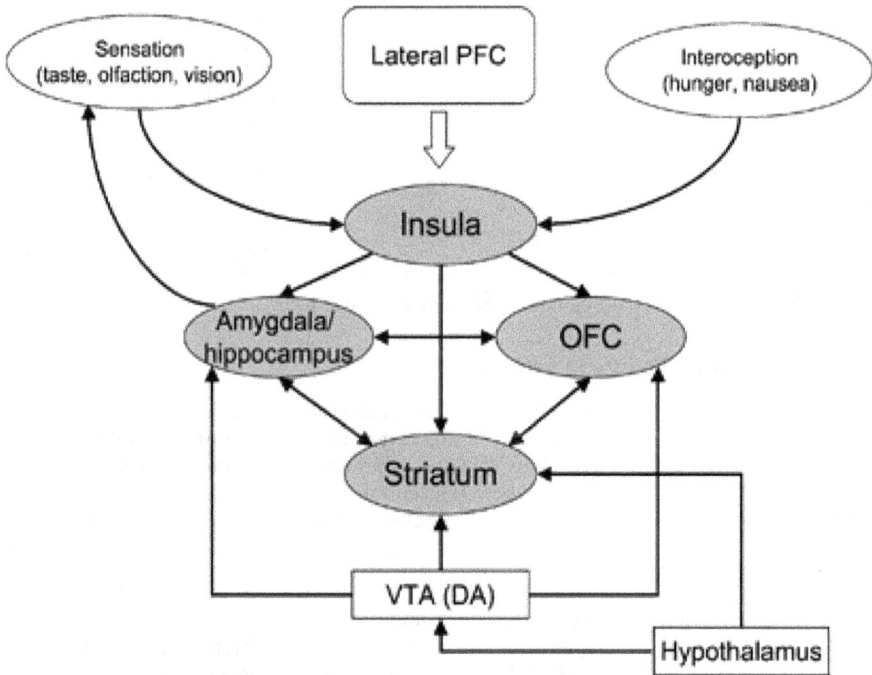

Fig. 1. A generalized brain network for regulation of hunger as depicted from Dagher (2009). PFC, prefrontal cortex; OFC, orbitofrontal cortex; VTA, ventral tegmental area; DA, dopamine.

The HYP and its circuits include orexin (ORX) and melanin concentrating hormone producing neurons in the lateral HYP as well as neuropeptide Y (NPY)/agouti related protein and alpha-melanocyte stimulating hormone producing neurons in the arcuate nucleus (ARC) known as the principal homeostatic brain regions responsible for regulating body weight (Wang et al., 2009). At the cellular level, important factors involved in communicating with the ARC in hunger regulation include ORX, melanin, NPY, and alpha-melanocyte-stimulating hormone (Wang et al., 2009). Ghrelin, leptin, insulin, and peptide YY all regulate hunger, satiety, and metabolism by stimulating neurons in the HYP (Wang et al., 2009). Ghrelin interacts with HYP depending on food intake, while leptin relays information to the HYP as well with regards to adipose storage (Wang et al., 2009). Insulin and peptide YY regulate metabolic changes (Wang et al., 2009). A useful summary of the neuropeptides that have the most dramatic influence on weight and eating regulation is listed in Table 1 and is also described in more detail by Wang et al. (2009).

Stimulate feeding	Inhibit feeding
Decrease energy expenditure	Increase energy expenditure
Anandamide	Calcitonin, Amylin, Bombesin,
	Somatostatin, Cytokines
β-endorphin	Cholecystokinin
Dynorphin	CRF
GABA	Dopamine
Galanin	Insulin
Ghrelin	Leptin
GHRH	Neurotensin
Neuropeptide Y	Serotonin
Norepinephrine	TRH, MSH, Glucagon,
	Enterostatin

Table 1. Neuropeptides That Regulate Food Intake (Sahu & Kalra, 1993)

4. Food addiction: Failure in self-regulation

Overeating and obesity are related to other substance addictions, not only in terms of overlapping neural substrates, but also in terms of genetic and environmental influences on eating behaviors and the implications that these influences have on treatment (Joranby, Pineda & Gold, 2005). The interaction between central satiety signals and reward responses to food stimuli with regards to failure in self-regulation will be discussed.

There are two primary circuits depicting reward behavior. The first one is the connected regions of the prefrontal cortex and the AMY. The second one is the limbic system involving the AMY, HYP, septal nuclei, ventral striatum, and dopaminergic innervations (Augustine, 1996). In most addictions, long-term is associated with drastic physiological alterations in the reward circuitry (Goldstein & Volkow, 2002) such as down-regulation of motivation, higher cognition and self-monitoring. Most importantly, emotions are correlated with the strength of the addiction (Shapira et al., 2003). One study found that hunger signals in the right OFC caused cravings and memories of food in fasting patients (Morris & Dolan, 2001). In more detail, those that fasted recognized previously viewed food faster. This is interesting because it implies dissociable roles of the OFC and left AMY in recognition of previously viewed food, while the nucleus accumbens (NA_c) responds to internal reward (Morris & Dolan, 2001).

4.1 Homeostatic substrates of over-eating

Hyperphagia is primarily due to continuous stimulation of NPY receptors (Kalra & Kalra, 1996). An imbalance of NPY signaling at a local level in the hypothalamus (ARC and paraventricular nucleus (PVN)) results in unregulated eating (Kalra & Kalra, 2004a). The neurotransmitter γ-aminobutyric acid (GABA) has also been known to enhance feeding behavior via its receptors, causing decreased melanocortin signaling to the PVN, which in turn results in hyperphagia (Cowley et al., 2001). Furthermore, it is possible that mutations or disturbances of α-melanocyte stimulating hormone (α-MSH) and other peptides involved in satiety can lead to hyperphagia and obesity (Kalra et al., 1999). Finally, in the case of abnormal hypothalamic function that accounts for a variety of eating disorders, it may lead to hyperglycemia, which in turn causes other endocrine problems (Liu & Gold, 2003). This may be explained by one dietary example where fructose was consumed. Fructose promotes insulin production but blocks its release (Sato et al., 1996). Insulin is known to inhibit feeding by increasing leptin which in turn leads to weight gain (Saad et al., 1998).

Hence, this would be a good model to explain why individuals with FA are obese and are more vulnerable to develop addiction-like behavior towards high carbohydrate foods containing high fructose corn syrup.

From a neurohormonal perspective, glutamate is believed to be the neurotransmitter responsible for transmitting information between the areas depicted above, although the exact mechanism is still not understood (Swanson & Petrovich, 1998). It may be plausible that potential feeding mechanisms involve direct glutamatergic connections from the basolateral amygdala (BLA) to the lateral hypothalamic area (LHA), although the exact LHA neurons involved in this process remain unidentified. Nevertheless, it may be safe to assume that BLA outputs could influence LHA subsystems required for feeding initiation. For example, groups of LHA neurons express two recently discovered neuropeptides, melanin-concentrating hormone (MCH) and ORX, which are regulated by the hunger–satiety state and are linked to initiation of feeding (Elmquist, Elias & Saper, 1999). There is still more information with regards to the interaction between ORX and FA that is outside the realm of this chapter, so refer to Kalra & Kalra (2004b). However, hunger caused by food cues is an adaptive mechanism for survival, but at the same time, learned cues can serve as a harmful force to promote overindulgence in food despite satiety. These particular learned cues can overcome specific satiety signals in order to promote continued eating (De Castro, 1997).

4.2 Metabolic substrates

The gene-environment interaction, as part of the metabolic substrates contributing to obesity, is defined as "the response or the adaptation to an environmental agent, a behavior, or a change in behavior is conditional on the genotype of the individual" (Bouchard, 2009). For example, in Fujian province, the rate of obesity has increased due to poor nutrition before and during pregnancy, economic development, urbanization and improved living standards (McAuley et al., 2001). The genetic loci associated with obesity are: *NEGR1, SEC16B-RASAL2, TMEM18, SFRS10-ETV5-DGKG, GNPDA2, NCR3-AIF1-BAT2, LGR4-LIN7CBDNF, MTCH2, BCDIN3DFAIM2, SH2B1-ATP2A1, KCTD15,* and *FTO* (fat mass and obesity associated) (Scuteri et al., 2007). The *FTO* gene is present in all tissues and encodes a non-heme (FeII)-dioxygenase that adapts to hypoxia, lipolysis, or DNA methylation (Gerken et al., 2007). This key protein may serve as a link between the central nervous system and energy homeostasis. *FTO* variants (rs8050136 and rs9939609) were associated with obesity and body mass index (BMI) in Hong Kong, Taiwan, and Singapore populations (Frayling et al., 2007). Further research needs to be done on obesity susceptibility genes for clinical applications. One study found a relationship between *FTO* SNP rs8050136 and BMI. It showed that the combined genetic risk of single-nucleotide polymorphisms (SNPs) may be useful in predicting obesity (Cheung et al., 2010). The A allele was indeed linked to obesity in Chinese adults (Li et al., 2010). Future studies need to be done if there is a link between FA and these obesity genes as well as with other addictions. For further discussion on this topic, please refer to these specific studies (Chen et al., 2009; Ruiz et al., 2010).

Prader-Willi syndrome (PWS) is the primary model for failure in self-regulation and the most important metabolic substrate with regards to hedonic food addiction (von Deneen, Gold & Liu, 2009). Our group has worked in both of these areas and believes that there are many shared neurohormonal pathways as well as distinct differences that may clue researchers in on why certain individuals overeat and become obese. Neuroimaging studies have shown that highly palatable food has characteristics similar to that of drugs of abuse. Many of the brain changes reported for hedonic eating and obesity are also seen in various forms of addictions (von Deneen et al., 2011). Most importantly, overeating and obesity may have an acquired drive such as for alcohol or drugs, and motivation and incentive craving, wanting, and liking occur after early and repeated exposures to stimuli. The acquired drive for great food and relative weakness of the satiety signal would cause an imbalance in drive and hunger centers of the HYP and their regulation. Prader-Willi may be a genetic model of the disease we are seeing on a daily basis. New hypotheses can yield new screening tests for new treatments.

4.3 Increased drive

Volkow & Fowler (2000) believe that reward circuits (NAc, AMY) have been central to drug addiction mechanisms, where the addictive state also involves disruption of circuits involved with compulsive behaviors and with increased drive. Intermittent activation of reward circuitry involving DA leads to dysfunction of the OFC via the striato-thalamo-orbitofrontal circuit. The OFC is hypermetabolic in proportion to the intensity of the craving seen after last cocaine use or during drug-induced craving (Volkow & Fowler, 2000). Since the OFC is directly involved with drive and compulsive repetitive behaviors, abnormal activation in addicted individuals could explain compulsive drug use despite adverse reactions. This indicates that pleasure by itself cannot maintain compulsive substance abuse and drugs that could interfere with the activation of the striato-thalamo-orbitofrontal circuit could be beneficial in the treatment of drug addiction (Volkow & Fowler, 2000).

Carbohydrates, as one of the most commonly abused food substances in FA, have been found to have an interesting psychological effect. For instance, women who craved and sought high-carbohydrate foods did so to alleviate negative feelings and emotions, showing that this food group depicts compulsive behavior (Corsica & Pelchat, 2010). More so, being chronically or acutely stressed led to consumption of high-fat or sugary foods, predisposing these individuals to bingeing and a failure in dieting (Dagher & Robbins, 2009; Dagher, 2009). An interesting concept is the "refined food hypothesis" in which processed foods such as sugars, fat, salt, flour, and caffeine are the source of addiction (Ifland et al., 2009) as well as salty foods which mimic opiate agonists (Cocores & Gold, 2009). Finally, interesting findings have shown that motivation circuits relating to drinking alcohol and eating fat lead to the release of hypothalamic orexigenic peptides, such as ghrelin, which increase the consumption of these foods and raise triglyceride levels (Barson et al., 2009). In a study utilizing rats, the level of triglycerides predicted increased caloric consumption and orexigenic peptide expression following a high-fat meal (Karatayev et al., 2009).

Drugs and food exert their reinforcing effects in part by increasing DA in limbic regions, which may explain how drug abuse/addiction relates to obesity (Volkow et al., 2008). Eating craved food and drug addiction result in reward circuitry activation involving DA pathways. However, these actions activate these pathways in different ways. FA affects reward circuitry through endogenous opioids and cannabinoids, while drugs share the same circuitry through direct effects on DA neurons or via indirect effects through neurotransmitters (Volkow & Wise, 2005). Overstimulation of DA leads to more compulsive behavior and loss of control of food and drug intake due to increased availability of DAD2 receptors in the striatum (Volkow & Li, 2004). However, FA can be considered more complex than drug abuse due to involvement of peripheral, endocrine and central pathways outside of the reward circuitry (Levine, Kotz & Gosnell, 2003).

The fundamental idea of the reward system hypothesis is that there must be an explicit emotional state connected with the addiction, such as seen in PWS. The stronger the emotional link, the stronger the addiction. There exist a couple of primary circuits for the reward system. The first one involves a reciprocal connection between the prefrontal areas of the brain and the AMY. The second is the limbic system that links the AMY with the HYP and septal nuclei. The Papez limbic system also joins the HYP with the hippocampus and thalamus (Joranby, Pineda & Gold, 2005). Therefore, the reward system hypothesis states that appetizing food and addictive behaviors compete for reward regions such as the NA$_C$. The act of overeating and obesity can lead to decreasing food reward and addiction (Kleiner et al., 2004). On the other hand, obesity is a "reward deficiency syndrome" (Blum et al., 1996). Most importantly, increased activation in the somatic parietal areas in food addicted individuals suggests that enhanced activity in these regions involves sensory processing of food, making food even more rewarding (Wang et al., 2001), which is not typical in PWS cases. The reward hypothesis was best explained through sugar-dependent rat studies (Avena, Long & Hoebel, 2005; Rada, Avena & Hoebel, 2005; Avena, Rada & Hoebel, 2008). These rats had a disrupted Acetylcholine (ACh) response to hunger, ingested greater amounts of sugar, and produced more DA than control rats (Avena, Long & Hoebel, 2005). This may explain why PWS and obese individuals may be addicted to certain palatable foods that cause a delayed, prolonged increase in ACh levels. In drug addiction, the ventral striatum and midbrain were associated with immediate rewards and the hippocampus responded to reward consequences. The globus pallidus, thalamus, and subgenual cingulate were associated with immediate rewards, while the caudate, insula, and ventral prefrontal cortex (vPFC) responded to reward consequences (Elliott, Friston & Dolan, 2000). The mesolimbic reward system is a common pathway that food and drugs follow in order to reinforce craving behavior (Tartar, Ammerman & Ott, 1998). This pathway is also affected by PWS causing aberrant reward circuitry (James et al., 2007). We are still unable to differentiate the reward system mechanisms in PWS and other addictions.

There are specific circuits and networks in the brain that regulate cravings, appetite, and cue-induced ingestion of addictive foods. The NA$_C$ and DA are specifically responsible for food reward and motivated eating (Cardinal et al., 2002). There are a variety of pathways that depict appetite and food craving regulation (Kalra & Kalra, 2004b). The ability of food-related cues and a food-associated environment to induce eating in healthy humans can shed light on why PWS individuals overeat and become obese. In animal models, brain regions consisting of the BLA, medial prefrontal cortex (mPFC), and LHA act as a network to regulate eating by learned, motivational cues (Elmquist, Elias & Saper, 1999). The AMY has been shown to be crucial in cue-enhanced eating (Arana et al., 2003). The OFC is also involved in food-related cues (Arana et al., 2003). The mPFC regulates eating due to environmental cue pressure (O'Doherty, 2004). Activations of the AMY and medial OFC occur when food-deprived individuals are shown food items, and greater activations are seen when food items are viewed (Arana et al., 2003). Our group has seen similar activations in PWS (James et al., 2007). The ventral mPFC has a significant role in appetite influenced by motivational cues, as reported by our group in PWS patients who had increased blood oxygen level-dependent (BOLD) responses in the ventral mPFC while viewing pictures of food (James et al., 2007). This would explain the excessive hunger due to increased reward values when viewing food, as well as the importance of the frontal cortex in its role in food responses. This data is also supported by findings of our group (James et al., 2002). Similarly, regions of the PFC may also participate in brain networks involved in cue-induced drug cravings. Other regions overlapping the ventral mPFC are also activated by chocolate- and nicotine-associated contextual cues in rats (Schroeder, Binzak & Kelley, 2001). The ventral mPFC was correlated with decreased consumption of high caloric, sweet and fatty foods, as in the case of PWS. A dysfunctional ventral mPFC could mechanistically depict feeding behavior in PWS or obese humans relevant to overeating, appetite, cues and cravings (O'Doherty et al., 2000). This may be a key point as to why food addicted obese individuals continue to overeat despite satiety. In PWS patients, obsession and preoccupation with food, lack of satiation, and incessant food seeking are typical behaviors as compared to normal obese humans (Ogura et al., 2008). PWS adults show preference for sweet or high carbohydrate foods over any other type of food. This is sometimes the case in normal obese individuals (Ogura et al., 2008). PWS patients will often eat the most desirable foods first, such as sweet, high caloric foods, and the least preferred foods last. Oftentimes, this is a ritualistic procedure in which the PWS-afflicted individual will gather the food and line it up in order of preference and ingest it sequentially (Singh et al., 2008). PWS cases are most susceptible to visual cues, thus passing by a bakery or restaurant, or even seeing sweet or highly palatable foods on television, will cause an enormous increase in craving and appetite despite satiety as compared to normal obese people. PWS patients will often have tantrums and aberrant behavior after seeing or smelling delicious, inviting food (Singh et al., 2008), which is highly uncommon in non-PWS individuals. In PWS, food cues (visual) have a very high emotional attachment and significance leading to bingeing episodes (Simmons, Martin & Barsalou, 2005). PWS is a biological model for hyperphagia and the reward system utilized to explain human obesity using functional magnetic resonance imaging (fMRI). Neuroimaging would be the most logical tool in precisely locating the brain regions responsible for controlling appetite and for being the reward centers specifically for FA (Tataranni & DelParigi, 2003). Using food-related pictures or other visual means to elicit brain responses has been a standard method of determining valid mechanisms that delineate the path to obesity (Jansen, 1998). Hence, the fMRI-supported hypothesis that PWS is a naturally occurring human model for FA or loss of control of eating or absence of satiety would be crucial for further studies. In the end, what remains is how logical and effective past, present, and future research can aid and treat abnormal eating behavior and brain responses to internal and external food cues in individuals afflicted with obesity.

4.4 Increased incentive

Compulsive drug-seeking and drug-taking behaviors are not always motivated by pleasure or by the desire to relieve withdrawal. The question remains, why do addicts compulsively seek drugs? Several groups have attempted to address this question by proposing the concept of "incentive–sensitization" (Robinson & Berridge, 1993; Berridge & Robinson, 1995). The essential concepts of the incentive–sensitization theory are: (1) potentially addictive drugs produce long-term adaptations in neural systems, hence altering the brain; (2) the brain systems that are altered are involved in the process of incentive motivation and reward; (3) the critical neuroadaptations for addiction hypersensitize these brain reward systems to drugs and drug-associated stimuli; and (4) the brain systems that become sensitized do not mediate the pleasurable effects of addictive substances, but instead they mediate a subcomponent of the reward system known as incentive salience or "wanting" (Robinson & Berridge, 1993; Berridge & Robinson, 1995; Berridge & Robinson, 1998).

A study has shown that low D2 receptor availability places people at risk for FA and obesity (Allison et al., 1999). In morbidly obese individuals, prefrontal regions were responsible for the correlation between D2 receptor availability and glucose metabolism (Volkow et al., 2008). Food cues increased striatal DA production which in turn caused increased hunger and craving for that particular food; this indicated regulation by the NA_C (Volkow et al., 2002). The four major circuits involved in drug and food addictions are reward/saliency, motivation/drive, learning/conditioning and inhibitory control/emotional regulation/executive function (Volkow et al., 2008). Disruption of these circuits leads to decreased motivation for good behavior and potentiates bad behavior that ends with negative results (weight gain in FA and drug overdose in substance abuse). This results in linking new memories of expected pleasurable responses when consuming the addictive substance or viewing similar stimuli (Volkow et al., 2008).

4.5 Food addiction as an addiction

Food addiction results from craving certain food or food-substances so as "to obtain a state of heightened pleasure, energy or excitement (Tartar, Ammerman & Ott, 1998)." It is important to understand the general pathophysiology of obesity in that metabolic alterations are not necessarily a cause of this disease, as seen in other eating disorders. Investigations into non-drug related addictions such as gambling, sex and food have provided insightful findings in understanding the neural mechanisms behind the addiction process (Comings et al., 2001; Bancroft & Vukadinovic, 2004; Petry, 2006; Warren & Gold, 2007; Avena et al., 2008; Cocores & Gold, 2009; Blumenthal & Gold, 2010; Liu et al., 2010; Potenza et al., 2012) .

FA is a chronic relapsing disorder associated with food cravings or food-related substances that lead to euphoria (Gold & Stembach, 1984) or amend negative emotions (Ifland et al., 2009). As a result, the new DSM-V (http: //www.dsm5.org) will revise the category 'Eating Disorders' to 'Eating and Feeding Disorders.' Most food addicts crave carbohydrates or specific foods (Spring et al., 2008). FA is predominantly influenced by compulsive behavior instigated by emotional and environmental factors such as stress, pressure from family to be thinner, religious traditions, etc. (Gold, 1999). Most importantly, FA is related to drug addiction in that DA levels regulate this type of psychological dependence by activating DA pathways responsible for addictive behavior (Warren & Gold, 2007; Wang et al., 2009; Blumenthal & Gold, 2010). In one study, Wang et al. (2009) stated that drug addiction hijacks neurobiological pathways that regulate reward, motivation, decision-making, learning, and memory. Withdrawal results in anti-reward effects due to a loss of brain reward system function and stress when the addictive substance is not available (Dackis & O'Brien, 2005; Koob, 2009).

High-fat and high-sugar foods are being exploited by developed and developing countries (Davis & Carter, 2009) resulting in increased numbers of food addicts. These foods are linked to increasing neurochemicals such as DA (Liu et al., 2010), as demonstrated in animal studies (Rada & Hoebel, 2005), which can be applied to fMRI studies that have shown delayed satiety in obese people, meaning they consume more food despite being full than do normal individuals (Liu et al., 2000). Sugar craving caused a decrease in serotonin levels as well (Wurtman & Wurtman, 1995). As a result, FA is associated with the formation of pathological brain pathways that are reinforced by abnormal eating patterns and behaviors.

Current research in FA and other disorders has shown that there were similar neurobiological pathways as those found in drug addiction (Berry & Mechoulam, 2002; Gearhardt et al., 2009a; Wang et al., 2009; Blumenthal & Gold, 2010). Animal studies attributed addiction to specific foods (Avena et al., 2004; Avena et al., 2005; Avena et al., 2008), although humans have a tendency to respond to external food cues (Benarroch et al., 2007; James et al., 2007; von Deneen et al., 2009). Food and drugs cause DA to be released from dopaminergic neurons, originating from the mesencephalon and projecting to forebrain structures in the ventral striatum depending on the amount of reward obtained (Volkow et al., 2002; Volkow et al., 2008). Brain regions known to be associated with reward circuitry include the OFC, AMY, insula, striatum, anterior cingulate cortex (ACC), and dorsolateral prefrontal cortex (DLPFC) (McBride et al., 2006; Franklin et al., 2007). FA can be diagnosed using the Yale Food Addiction Scale (YFAS) based on the Diagnostic Statistical Manual (DSM)-IV-TR substance dependence criteria. This would then allow direct comparison between FA and drug abuse (Gearhardt et al., 2009b). There are numerous current reviews that would be helpful references in explaining the neurobiology and neurophysiology of addiction (please see Detar, 2011; Avena et al., 2102; Urban & Martinez, 2012).

4.6 Neuroimaging of addiction: Main findings

Most imaging projects studied DA involvement in the process of drug addiction because the ability of drugs of abuse to increase limbic DA is considered crucial for their reinforcing effects (Koob et al., 1994; Di Chiara, 1999). However, increased DA does not account for the process of addiction, since drugs of abuse increase DA in non-addicted as well as addicted subjects (Goldstein & Volkow, 2002). In the case of cocaine addiction, drug-induced DA increases and the intensity of self-reports of the drug's reinforcing properties is smaller in addicted subjects (Volkow et al., 1997). This means DA involvement in drug addiction is likely to be mediated by changes in neurocircuitry modulated by DA, including the frontal cortex. Current structural/volumetric MRI studies depicted morphological changes in the frontal lobe in various forms of drug addiction (Goldstein & Volkow, 2002). In one study, frontal lobe volume losses were shown in cocaine-dependent subjects (Liu et al., 1998; Franklin et al., 2002), alcoholic subjects (Jernigan et al., 1991; Pfefferbaum et al., 1997), and heroin-dependent subjects (Liu et al., 1998). The latter study indicated there were negative correlations between normalized prefrontal volumes and prolonged cocaine or heroin use, meaning there was a cumulative effect of substance abuse on frontal volumes. DA activation, as seen during amphetamine administration, also prevented inhibition of the AMY by the medial prefrontal cortex (Rosenkranz & Grace, 2001). A similar process may be occurring in human drug addiction, in which prefrontal top-down processes are diminished (see Miller & Cohen, 2001). Therefore, if the frontal cortex and its functions become down-regulated in human drug addiction, the motivational, higher cognitive, and self-monitoring processes become affected (Goldstein & Volkow, 2002).

5. Neuroimaging of food addiction: Main findings

This section will briefly examine the neural correlates of addictive-like eating behavior using fMRI as compared to those with substance dependence (Gearhardt et al., 2011c). Other studies of interest relating to FA deal with the addiction potential of hyperpalatable foods (Gearhardt et al., 2011a), the public health and policy implications of FA (Gearhardt et al., 2011b), the diagnostic criteria for FA (Gearhardt et al., 2009a), and the psychological correlates of obesity (Friedman & Brownell, 1995).

Researchers may benefit from functional neuroimaging results depicting shared neural and hormonal pathways to determine similarities between substance abuse and hedonistic overeating, such as in FA and drug abuse individuals who continue to have cravings despite a dysfunctional satiety signal (Zhang et al., 2011). Functional neuroimaging studies have further revealed that good or great smelling, looking, tasting, and reinforcing food has characteristics similar to that of drugs of abuse (James et al., 2002; James et al., 2007). Many of the brain changes in fMRI studies showed that both food and drugs activated the AMY, insula, OFC, and striatum (Jonas & Gold, 1986; Matsuda et al., 1999). Food and drug cravings also showed signal activation in the HIPP, insula, and caudate (Matsuda et al., 1999).

In Brownell's group study (Gearhardt et al., 2011c), the relationship between high food addiction scores and blood oxygen level–dependent (BOLD) functional magnetic resonance imaging activation in response to receiving palatable food was evaluated. FA scores were positively correlated with activation in the ACC, medial OFC, and AMY when anticipating eating highly palatable food such as a chocolate milkshake. There was greater activation in the DLPFC and caudate when anticipating highly palatable food and decreased activation in the lateral OFC when eating palatable foods (Gearhardt et al., 2011c). These regions are associated with positive rewards from food cues (Rolls, 2000) and satiety (Small et al., 2001). Similar patterns of neural activation were seen in substance dependence (Gearhardt et al., 2011c) in response to visual cues. Another interesting finding showed that the urge to cease consumption of a palatable food or drug is suppressed in the lateral OFC (Berridge & Kringelbach, 2008; Schoenbaum & Shaham, 2008). There has been some thought that food addicts eat compulsively but have compensatory behaviors to reduce weight (Fuhrer et al., 2008). Recent functional neuroimaging studies have found abnormal brain activations in obese people. We found that before food intake, obese men had significantly increased baseline activity in the left putamen, left posterior insula, left medial temporal cortex and bilateral parietal cortex relative to lean men using a regional homogeneity (ReHo) analysis method. In this method, we measured temporal homogeneity of the regional BOLD signals. Decreased activity was also found in the medial orbitofrontal lobe, left DPFC, right inferior temporal lobe and right cerebellum in the obese subjects. After food intake, the obese men had remarkably elevated brain activity in the left putamen and bilateral parietal lobe, and reduced activity in the left superior frontal lobe and bilateral middle temporal lobe. These results indicated that, either before or after food intake, obese men might have a stronger desire to eat. This study provided strong evidence supporting the hypothesis that there is hypo-functioning reward circuitry in obese individuals, in which the prefrontal cortex may fail to inhibit the striatum and insula, and consequently lead to overeating and obesity.

This study (Zhang et al., unpublished results) found a difference in BOLD activation between obese individuals versus controls especially in the left hemisphere as shown in Figure 2. It has been shown that a higher BMI was correlated with decreased gray matter in the left OFC and right cerebellum (Walther et al., 2010), indicating that obese individuals have limited inhibitions than controls (Baylis & Moore, 1994). In this study (Zhang et al., unpublished results), obese men had decreased neural activity in the left DLPFC prior to liquid ingestion, meaning they could not inhibit their hunger and found eating to be more desirable. The obese men also had higher activation in the left insula indicating that the insula could have affected satiety and eating (Zhang et al., unpublished results). Furthermore, greater ReHo activation in the bilateral parietal cortex in obese individuals showed that food was more palatable and enjoyable (Volkow, Fowler & Wang, 2004). Overall, it was found that the obese have hypo-functioning reward circuitry where the medial prefrontal cortex (MPFC) and left DLPFC fail to inhibit the left putamen and insula causing overeating (Zhang et al., unpublished results). fMRI was thus useful in determining the mechanisms of obesity with regards to neural activity.

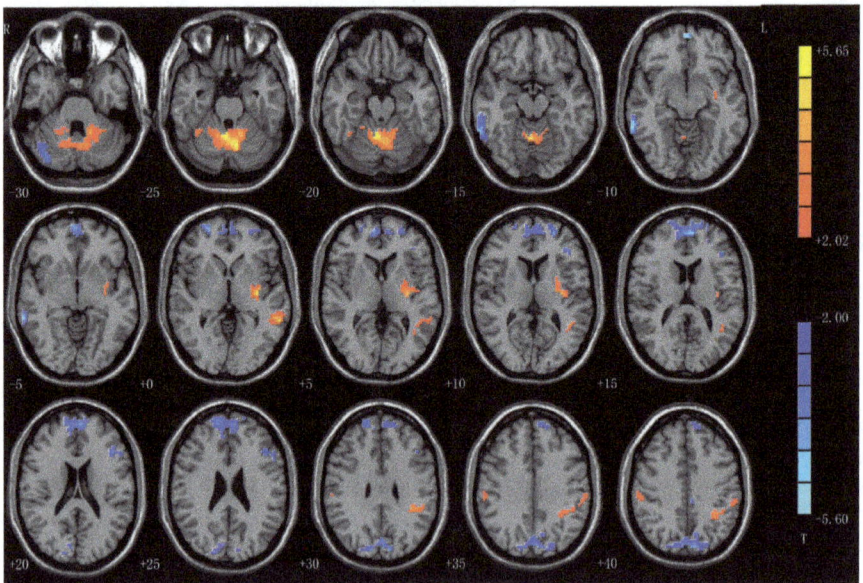

Fig. 2. A T-statistical difference map between obese subjects and controls before liquid ingestion ($p<0.05$, corrected). Warm and cold colors indicate obese subject-related ReHo increases and decreases, respectively (Zhang et al., unpublished).

6. Food addiction versus drug addiction

This section will introduce similarities and differences between food and drugs of abuse (Blumenthal & Gold, 2010). The DSM fifth edition has been prepared to address addiction with new terminologies and approaches. For example, the term substance dependence was replaced with substance-use disorder. This is defined as 'A maladaptive pattern of substance-use leading to clinically significant impairment or distress, as manifested by two (or more) of the listed criteria occurring within a 12-month period (http://www.dsm5.org/ProposedRevisions/Pages/Substance-RelatedDisorders.aspx).' Substance-abuse disorder progresses from bingeing to withdrawal, and finally leading to craving the substance (Koob & Volkow, 2010). This cyclic behavior can be sustained and entertained by stress. Substance-use disorder stems from taking over neurobiological pathways regulating reward, motivation, decision-making, learning and memory in order to become responsive to the drug of choice (Everitt & Robbins, 2005; Wise, 2006; Belin et al., 2009; Hyman et al., 2009; Wang et al., 2009). Various neural networks, such as in the dorsolateral striatum, AMY, OFC and midbrain, regulate drug-seeking behavior which depends on feelings associated with using and craving that particular drug (Zapata et al., 2003; Belin & Everitt, 2008; Everitt et al., 2008; Koob, 2009). For a thorough review of this process and the neural structures involved, please see Robbins & Everitt (1999). Furthermore, DA seems to be the essential regulator of dependence, particularly in stimulants, while alcohol, opioids, and nicotine act upon opioid receptors (Koob & Volkow, 2010). This can be seen in individuals with Parkinson's disease who become addicted to dopamine-containing medications (Dagher & Robbins, 2009).

A general figure (Figure 3) of the neurobiology of addiction is provided below.

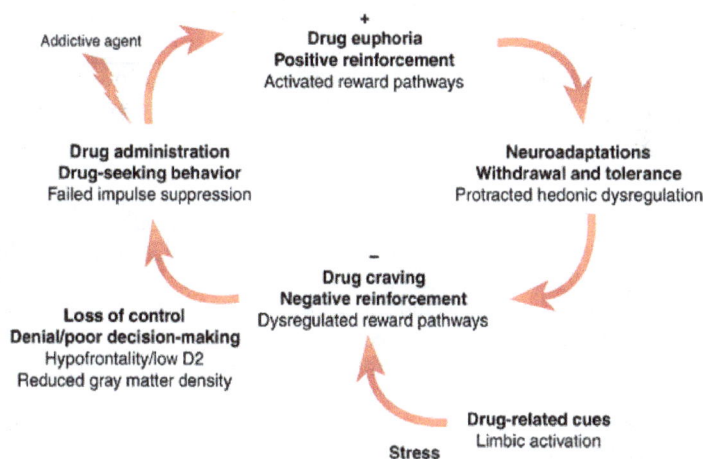

Fig. 3. Neurobiology of addiction that can be applied to food addiction as depicted by Dackis & O'Brien (2005).

The figure clearly depicts how the cycle of drug addiction is positively reinforced by euphoria from drug intake and negatively reinforced during withdrawal, craving for the drug and hedonic dysregulation. This cycle becomes more uncontrollable as the brain becomes more addicted. Drug-related cues and stress increase this craving leading to a loss of control stemming from dysfunction of the prefrontal cortex. Neuronal mechanisms for these components of addiction have been delineated in animal models and human neuroimaging studies (Dackis & O'Brien, 2005).

Accumulating evidence has shown that there are many shared neural and hormonal pathways as well as distinct differences that may help researchers find why certain individuals overeat and become addicted. The FA criteria that provide this evidence are listed in Table 2 below.

Tolerance	Starting out with a single cookie, gradually increasing to several or a whole box
Withdrawal symptoms	Habitually eating to relieve depression, anxiety, and other emotional states; unpleasant physical sensations when cutting back on carbohydrates
Taking in larger amounts or for a longer duration	Intending to eat a single serving but instead eating a whole package; binges extending several hours
Attempts to cut back	Frequent attempts to eat 'correctly'(e.g. avoid overeating or eating certain foods)
Excessive time spent pursuing, using, or recovering from use	Frequent thinking about food, planning intake, preparing, and/or resting or sleeping after excessive intake
Reduction/discontinuation of important activities because of use	Eating instead of spending time with friends; feeling too sick after overeating to do anything
Continued use despite consequences	Overeating in spite of overweight, physical illness, and/or distress about overeating

Table 2. Food addiction characteristics compared with substance abuse criteria based on Ifland et al. (2009).

Most importantly, overeating and obesity may have an acquired drive such as drug addiction with respect to motivation and incentive craving, wanting, and liking which occur after early and repeated exposures to stimuli. The acquired drive for great food and relative weakness of the satiety signal would cause an imbalance between the drive and hunger/reward centers in the brain described earlier and their regulation when conditioned via visual cues (Liu et al., 2010). As mentioned before, FA can be defined as a chronic relapsing problem caused by various fundamental factors that encourage craving for food or food-related substances so as "to obtain a state of heightened pleasure, energy, or excitement (Tartar, Ammerman & Ott, 1998)." An example of this would be carbohydrate cravers that have learned to consume high carbohydrate foods to improve their mood caused by a drop in serotonin levels (Spring et al., 2008). Most FA and eating disorders are the result of loss of control, impulsive and/or compulsive behavior stemming from emotional and environmental conditions and a psychological dependence on food. Abnormal eating behaviors along with other addictions affect the levels of DA in the mesolimbic dopaminergic system (Mogenson, 1982; Blum et al., 1996; Goldstein & Volkow, 2002; Everitt & Robbins, 2005). FA is defined by a system as follows: bingeing consists of "unusually large bouts of intake" (Colantuoni et al., 2001); withdrawal is "indicated by signs of anxiety and behavioral depression" (Colantuoni et al., 2002); craving is "measured during sugar abstinence as enhanced by responding to sugar" (Avena, Long & Hoebel, 2005); and cross-sensitization results "from sugar to drugs of abuse" (Avena et al., 2004). Furthermore, bingeing is also defined as "escalation of intake with a high proportion of intake at one time, usually after a period of voluntary abstinence or forced deprivation" (Avena, Rada & Hoebel, 2008). FA consists of sensitization and tolerance phases, which initiate addiction (Koob & Le Moal, 2005). Withdrawal resulting from the addictive food or foods has been known to be caused by alterations in the opioid system (Colantuoni et al., 2002). This phase consists of two parts, in which DA decreases and ACh is released from the NA$_C$.

When sugar was analyzed with regards to withdrawal symptoms, it was stated that it was capable of producing DA, ACh, and opioids similar to most narcotic substances (Avena, Rada & Hoebel, 2008). Withdrawal is marked by anxiety (File et al., 2004) and depression (Avena, Rada & Hoebel, 2008). For more information on using sugar as an addictive substance please refer to the following references (Colantuoni et al., 2001; Colantuoni et al., 2002; Avena et al., 2004; Avena et al., 2005; Avena, Rada & Hoebel, 2008). Food craving can happen after a prolonged period of abstinence since "craving" is better defined by "increased efforts to obtain a substance of abuse or its associated cues as a result of dependence and abstinence" (Avena, Rada & Hoebel, 2008). Cross-sensitization is the last phase of FA and is predominantly defined as "an increased locomotor response to a different drug or substance" (Avena, Rada & Hoebel, 2008). All of these definitions play a major role in helping define and classify food (especially sugar) as a true addictive substance in comparison to the criteria for drug dependence as shown at least in rats (Haddock et al., 2000). People becoming addicted to food may be overweight and may possibly have leptin resistance as well that leads to overeating (Liu & Gold, 2003).

Finally, the most problematic group for an increase in addictive behavior and obesity has been young adults and adolescents in the past 30 years (Dietz, 2001). One study showed that binge eating and drug abuse were linked (Ross & Ivis, 1999). Interestingly, those that smoked had an increased body mass index (BMI) than non-smokers, and they were also at a risk for gaining weight when not using drugs (Hodgkins et al., 2004). Therefore, it is reasonable to conclude that teenagers used food to replace the reinforcement behavior of drug addiction to compensate for the reward systems of the brain. Eating disorders are a form of addiction in a way that individuals are obsessed with body image and compulsively crave certain foods such as in binge eating.

6.1 Intervention and prevention

Besides altering the endocrine makeup of individuals affected by FA via drug therapies, alternative and complementary approaches could play a major role in the intervention and possible prevention of obesity. Decreasing access to highly palatable and addicting foods is necessary (and restriction to all foods and small inanimate objects for patients with PWS) (von Deneen, Gold & Liu, 2009). Management includes 24 hour or constant supervision, planned physical activities, a strict diet (≤ 1200 cal/day) divided into structured, portioned meals at set times, and a static, predictable way of life (Benarroch et al., 2007). Encouraging afflicted groups to exercise or do other enjoyable activities will discourage them from their usual eating behaviors, as well as maintaining a highly controlled eating environment and food regimen with strict, consistent and reinforced rules. There are two common types of non-medicinal methods to decreasing body weight and/or improving the health condition of the individual. The first one is the undieting approach which discourages the use of food restriction or dieting due to its ineffectiveness and possible health risks (Foster, 2001). The second type is isolated dieting in which one consumes less of a particular type of food or food group such as seen in the Adkins diet where carbohydrates are almost completely eliminated from the diet. Experimental treatments in animals may have practical application in treatment and prevention of obesity. There is a possibility such drugs can be marketed for use in human medicine. Another suggested experimental treatment is the aid of central leptin gene therapy (Kalra & Kalra, 2002), where an injection of recombinant adeno-associated virus vector encoding leptin into the HYP of prepubertal and adult rats resulted in weight gain and suppressed diet-induced obesity. The explanation was that it promoted loss of fatty deposits caused by a decrease in NPY and an increase in MCH and thermogenesis. This is a novel approach that may not be suitable for humans at this point. Indeed, disrupting NPYergic signaling at multiple loci without affecting normal hypothalamic function would be ideal, but more research needs to be done in this area (Kalra & Kalra, 2004a). Another experimental method is based on the theory that ACh inhibits feeding through the M1 receptors if a muscarinic agonist, arecholine, is injected into the NA_C. This can be reversed by using an M1 antagonist pirenzapine (Rada & Hoebel, unpublished). Thus, it would be interesting to determine if arecholine would be a safe and effective method to prevent hyperphagia in individuals with FA and PWS patients. Some studies showed that taste aversion was a very useful therapy in which ACh levels were increased while decreasing DA levels (Mark et al., 1995). Others have found that baclofen, a GABA-B agonist, is useful for those that over-indulge on fatty foods (Buda-Levin, Wojnicki & Corwin, 2005). Other treatments utilized naloxone (an opioid antagonist) to block the opioid system, and rimonabant (a CB1 receptor antagonist) to block the cannabinoid system (Kenny, 2011); these systems have been shown to reinforce feeding behavior, and when used together, they act synergistically to treat obesity (Berry & Mechoulam, 2002). The still-investigational drug is Lorcaserin, a combination of benzazepine and hydrochloride, two neurological agents. Lorcaserin is a selective 5-HT2C receptor agonist, working through the serotonin system, which regulates appetite, mood, and motor behavior. Two other investigational obesity drugs target the DA reward system-Contrave, which is a combination of bupropion and naltrexone, and Qnexa, which combines phentermine and topiramate (Solinas & Goldberg, 2005).

7. Conclusion

Obesity continues to place a tremendous burden on healthcare systems. Our current and future research on the neurobiological systems that motivate appetitive behavior strongly suggests that an acquired drive for highly energy-dense, reinforcing foods is contributing to weight gain. The limitations of current treatments compel healthcare professionals to develop more effective ways based on neurobiological addiction models to curb the obesity epidemic.

Future studies should examine the relation between FA, hunger, and reward circuitry response with food intake and anticipated intake. The use of fMRI technology directly measures DA release or its receptors. It will be important to examine induced DA release and D2 receptor availability in those with FA. Other neurotransmitters are also likely to play an important role. Thus, future studies connecting FA and neural activation associated with these neurotransmitters will also be important. Understanding the mechanisms of hedonic eating is essential for developing and implementing treatment and management strategies that address the root causes of obesity. In addition, cognitive factors such as social environment, emotional state, or intentional efforts to control consumption can also influence food intake. Most of what we know about these regulatory systems is derived from animal models, but our understanding of the control of eating behavior in humans is very limited. Consistent with the biological imperative to identify and consume food, neuroimaging studies have begun to document the responsiveness of the human brain to food cues such as odors and/or taste samples of food (Wang et al., 2004; Rosenbaum et al., 2008). Future positron emission tomography (PET) and fMRI studies will provide neurobiological insights in brain alterations during addiction. fMRI is ideal for investigating activation in regions involved in a specific function, because scans can detect these simultaneously. It also provides temporal-spatial resolution and anatomical accuracy to be able to describe the interaction between major CNS components. This allows the monitoring of dynamic activities in the brain while processing visual cues (Zhang et al., 2011). Our group has future studies planned to determine brain responses when viewing photographs of food and non-food objects, where we will specifically examine brain regions important to the regulation of appetite and food intake in overweight and normal individuals. For example, one such fMRI study is to scan young healthy subjects of normal weight to measure different brain activation by visual images of highly rewarding-foods (high caloric foods such as hamburgers and chips) compared with images of non-rewarding objects during various physiological states; in particular, we are interested in effects of fast food-branding on the brain and the effects in Chinese children with and without exposure to the Golden Arches (McDonald's®) or the Kentucky Colonel (KFC®). The study tests the hypothesis of 'food addiction' that the fast food brands such as McDonald's® may have reinforcing effects in the brain and such effects may be related to children's drive to eat (Zhang et al., 2011). Using the Chinese population who has never been exposed to such food brands as controls (this CANNOT be done in the USA), this study would have a strong impact in the areas of addiction and obesity. Another research paradigm proposed is mostly based on a bottom-up approach to test the relationship between chronic subcutaneous recombinant leptin injections and weight loss (Benoit et al., 2004). fMRI techniques are powerful tools to probe leptin neurological function in modulation of human ingestive behavior and are ideal for investigating the concerted activity among the ensemble of regions involved in a specific function, because scans can detect all regions of brain activation simultaneously. Many recent studies have employed fMRI techniques to gain neuroanatomical insights into the effects of leptin in brain processing hunger, satiety and food reward in obese human subjects (Farooqi et al., 2007; Baicy et al., 2007). As a result, we propose to assess brain activation in response to acute subcutaneous leptin injection by examining the resting-state and exposure to stimuli consisting of food cues using an fMRI experiment (Zhang et al., 2011). We will also attempt to correlate the fMRI leptin brain response with weight gain based on a cafeteria diet. Positive results from this study will provide an invaluable diagnostic guideline for initiating early adulthood nutritional and behavioral intervention on an individualized basis to temper obesity development. This would constitute a realistic and meaningful cost-effective approach. An obesity-prevention strategy will help curb rising obesity treatment-related health expenditures. Positive study outcomes will also highlight a technological breakthrough for fMRI investigation of region-specific neural activity in an acutely stimulated brain reactive state rather than in a chronically adapted state following long-term drug treatment or other types of intervention. Thus, we hope to illuminate promising methods that use visual food cues to investigate mechanisms of human eating behavior, and to facilitate a more unified and reproducible approach to neuroimaging studies of FA and obesity. Results from this study can go far beyond obesity studies and could extend to the field of pharmacological research (Zhang et al., 2011). Furthermore, more research needs to be conducted world-wide especially in the Chinese population. Obesity in China is a multifactorial disease where intervention is not always clear-cut or applicable. For instance, specific gene therapy may be available in the future to prevent childhood and adulthood weight gain and endocrine disorders. Lifestyle and behavioral changes need to be addressed and applied to prevent unhealthy physiques. Alternative medicine intervention, such as acupuncture and Traditional Chinese Medicine remedies, may be most appropriate for this part of the world. Overall, obesity is preventable and now is the ideal time in implementing current scientific methods and techniques to battle this epidemic (von Deneen & Liu, 2011).

8. Acknowledgment

This research was supported by the Project for the National Key Basic Research and Development Program (973) under Grant Nos. 2011CB707702 and 2012CB518501, the National Natural Science Foundation of China under Grant Nos. 30930112, 30970774, 60901064, 30873462, 81000640, 81000641, 81071217, 81101036, 81101108 and 31150110171, the Fundamental Research Funds for the Central Universities and the Knowledge Innovation Program of the Chinese Academy of Sciences under Grant No. KGCX2-YW-129.

9. References

Achike, FI.; To, NH.; Wang, H. & Kwan, CY. (2011). Obesity, metabolic syndrome, adipocytes and vascular function: a holistic viewpoint. *Clin Exp Pharmacol Physiol*, Vol.38, No.1, pp. 1-10.

Allison, DB.; Mentore, JL.; Heo, M.; Chandler, LP.; Cappelleri, JC.; Infante, MC. & Weiden, PJ. (1999). Antipsychotic-induced weight gain: a comprehensive research synthesis. *Am. J. Psychiatry*, Vol.156, pp. 686-696.

Arana, FS.; Parkinson, JA.; Hinton, E.; Holland, AJ.; Owen, AM. & Roberts, AC. (2003). Dissociable contributions of the human amygdala and orbitofrontal cortex to incentive motivation and goal selection. *J Neurosci*, Vol.23, No.29, pp. 9632-9638.

Augustine, JR. (1996). Circuitry and functional aspects of the insular lobe in primates including humans. *Brain Research. Brain Research Reviews*, Vol.22, pp. 229-244.

Avena, NM.; Carrillo, CA.; Needham, L.; Leibowitz, SF. & Hoebel, BG. (2004). Sugar-dependent rats show enhanced intake of unsweetened ethanol. *Alcohol*, Vol.34, No.2-3, pp. 203-209.

Avena, NM.; Gold, JA.; Kroll, C. & Gold, MS. (2012). Further developments in the neurobiology of food and addiction: update on the state of the science. *Nutrition*, Vol.28, No.4, pp. 341-343.

Avena, NM.; Long, KA. & Hoebel, BG. (2005). Sugar-dependent rats show enhanced responding for sugar after abstinence: evidence of a sugar deprivation effect. *Physiol Behav*, Vol.84, No.3, pp. 359-362.

Avena, NM.; Rada, P. & Hoebel, BG. (2008). Evidence for sugar addiction: behavioral and neurochemical effects of intermittent, excessive sugar intake. *Neurosci Biobehav Rev*, Vol.32, No.1, pp. 20-39.

Baicy, K.; London, ED.; Monterosso, J.; Wong, ML.; Delibasi, T.; Sharma, A. & Licinio, J. (2007). Leptin replacement alters brain response to food cues in genetically leptin-deficient adults. *Proc Natl Acad Sci USA*, Vol.104, No.46, pp. 18276-18279.

Bancroft, J. & Vukadinovic, Z. (2004). Sexual addiction, sexual compulsivity, sexual impulsivity, or what? Toward a theoretical model. *J Sex Res*, Vol.41, No.3, pp. 225-234.

Barbano, MF.; Stinus, L.; Cador, M. & Ahmed, SH. (2005). Mesolimbic dopamine drives the diurnal variation in opiate-induced feeding. *Pharmacol Biochem Behav*, Vol.81, No.3, pp. 569-574.

Barson, JR.; Karatayev, O.; Chang, GQ.; Johnson, DF.; Bocarsly, ME.; Hoebel, BG. & Leibowitz, SF. (2009). Positive relationship between dietary fat, ethanol intake, triglycerides, and hypothalamic peptides: counteraction by lipid-lowering drugs. *Alcohol*, Vol.43, pp. 433–441.

Baylis, GC. & Moore, BO. (1994). Hippocampal lesions impair spatial response selection in the primate. *Exp Brain Res*, Vol.98, pp. 110-118.

Belin, D. & Everitt, BJ. (2008). Cocaine seeking habits depend upon dopamine-dependent serial connectivity linking the ventral with the dorsal striatum. *Neuron*, Vol.57, No.3, pp. 432-441.

Belin, D.; Jonkman, S.; Dickinson, A.; Robbins, TW. & Everitt, BJ. (2009). Parallel and interactive learning processes within the basal ganglia: relevance for the understanding of addiction. *Behav Brain Res*, Vol.199, No.1, pp. 89-102.

Benarroch, F.; Hirsch, HJ.; Genstil, L.; Landau, YE. & Gross-Tsur, V. (2007). Prader-Willi syndrome: medical prevention and behavioral challenges. *Child Adolesc Psychiatr Clin N Am*, Vol.16, No.3, pp. 695-708.

Benoit, SC.; Clegg, DJ.; Seeley, RJ. & Woods, SC. (2004). Insulin and leptin as adiposity signals. *Recent Prog Horm Res*, Vol.59, pp. 267-285.

Berridge, KC. & Kringelbach, ML. (2008). Affective neuroscience of pleasure: reward in humans and animals. *Psychopharmacology (Berl)*, Vol.199, No.3, pp. 457-480.

Berridge, KC. & Robinson, TE. (1995). The mind of an addicted brain: neural sensitization of wanting versus liking, *Current Directions in Psychological Science*, Vol.4, pp. 71–76.

Berridge, KC. & Robinson, TE. (1998). What is the role of dopamine in reward: hedonic impact, reward learning, or incentive salience? *Brain Research Reviews*, Vol.28, pp. 309–369.

Berry, EM. & Mechoulam, R. (2002). Tetrahydrocannabinol and endocannabinoids in feeding and appetite. *Pharmacol Ther*, Vol.95, No.2, pp. 185-190.

Blum, K.; Sheridan, PJ.; Wood, RC.; Braverman, ER.; Chen, TJ.; Cull, JG. & Comings, DE. (1996). The D2 dopamine receptor gene as a determinant of reward deficiency syndrome. *J R Soc Med*, Vol.89, No.7, pp. 396-400.

Blumenthal, DM. & Gold, MS. (2010). Neurobiology of food addiction. *Current Opinion in Clinical Nutrition and Metabolic Care*, Vol.13, No.4, pp. 359–365.

Bouchard C. (2009). Childhood obesity: are genetic differences involved? *Amer J Clin Nut,* Vol.89, pp. 1494S-1501S.

Buda-Levin, A.; Wojnicki, FH. & Corwin, RL. (2005). Baclofen reduces fat intake under binge- type conditions. *Physiol Behav,* Vol.86, No.1-2, pp. 176-184.

Campbell, MW.; Williams, J.; Hampton, A. & Wake, M. (2006). Maternal concern and perceptions of overweight in Australian preschool-aged children. *Med J Aust,* Vol.184, pp. 274-277.

Cardinal, RN.; Parkinson, JA.; Hall, J. & Everitt, BJ. (2002). Emotion and motivation: the role of the amygdala, ventral striatum, and prefrontal cortex. *Neurosci Biobehav Rev,* Vol.26, No.3, pp. 321-352.

Cecchini, M.; Sassi, F.; Lauer, JA.; Lee, YY.; Guajardo-Barron, V. & Chisholm, D. (2010). Tackling of unhealthy diets, physical inactivity, and obesity: health effects and cost-effectiveness. *Lancet,* Vol.376, pp. 1775-1784.

Chen, H.; Simar, D. & Morris, MJ. (2009). Hypothalamic neuroendocrine circuitry is programmed by maternal obesity: interaction with postnatal nutritional environment. *PLoS One,* Vol.4, pp. e6259.

Cheung, CY.; Tso, AW.; Cheung, BM.; Xu, A.; Ong, KL.; Fong, CH.; Wat, NM.; Janus, ED.; Sham, PC. & Lam, KS. (2010). Obesity susceptibility genetic variants identified from recent genome-wide association studies: implications in a Chinese population. *J Clin Endocrinol Metab,* Vol.95, No.3, pp. 1395-1403.

Cocores, JA. & Gold, MS. (2009). The Salted Food Addiction Hypothesis may explain overeating and the obesity epidemic. *Med Hypotheses,* Vol.73, No.6, pp. 892–899.

Colantuoni, C.; Rada, P.; McCarthy, J.; Patten, C.; Avena, NM.; Chadeayne, A. & Hoebel, BG. (2002). Evidence that intermittent, excessive sugar intake causes endogenous opioid dependence. *Obes Res,* Vol.10, No.6, pp. 478-488.

Colantuoni, C.; Schwenker, J.; McCarthy, J.; Rada, P.; Ladenheim, B.; Cadet, JL.; Schwartz, GJ.; Moran, TH. & Hoebel, BG. (2001). Excessive sugar intake alters binding to dopamine and mu-opioid receptors in the brain. *Neuroreport,* Vol.12, No.16, pp. 3549-3552.

Comings, DE.; Gade-Andavolu, R.; Gonzalez, N.; Wu, S.; Muhleman, D.; Chen, C.; Koh, P.; Farwell, K.; Blake, H.; Dietz, G.; MacMurray, JP.; Lesieur, HR.; Rugle, LJ. & Rosenthal, RJ. (2001). The additive effect of neurotransmitter genes in pathological gambling. *Clin Genet,* Vol.60, No.2, pp. 107-116.

Coon, KA.; Goldberg, J.; Rogers, BL. & Tucker, KL. (2001). Relationships between use of television during meals and children's food consumption patterns. *Pediatrics,* Vol.107, pp. E7.

Corsica, JA. & Pelchat, ML. (2010). Food addiction: true or false? *Curr Opin Gastroenterol,* Vol.26, pp. 165–169.

Cowley, MA.; Smart, JL.; Rubinstein, M.; Cerdan, MG.; Diano, S.; Horvath, TL.; Cone, RD. & Low, MJ. (2001). Leptin activates anorexigenic POMC neurons through a neural network in the arcuate nucleus. *Nature,* Vol.411, No.6836, pp. 480-484.

Dackis, C. & O'Brien, C. (2005). Neurobiology of addiction. *Nature Neuroscience,* Vol.8, pp. 1431-1436.

Dagher, A. & Robbins, TW. (2009). Personality, addiction, dopamine: insights from Parkinson's disease. *Neuron,* Vol.61, pp. 502–510.

Dagher, A. (2009). The neurobiology of appetite: hunger as addiction. *Int J Obes*, Vol.33, No.2, pp. S30–S33.

Davis, C. & Carter, JC. (2009). Compulsive overeating as an addiction disorder. A review of theory and evidence. *Appetite*, Vol.53, pp. 1–8.

Di Chiara, G. (1999). Drug addiction as dopamine-dependent associative learning disorder. *Eur J Pharmacol*, Vol.375, pp. 13–30.

De Castro, JM. (1997). How can energy balance be achieved by free-living human subjects? *Proc Nutr Soc*, Vol.56, No.1A, pp. 1-14.

Detar, DT. (2011). Understanding the disease of addiction. *Prim Care*. Vol.38, No.1, pp. 1-7.

Dietz, W. (2001). Childhood obesity. In: *Modern nutrition in health and disease* (9th Ed.) M. Shils, J. Olsen, M. Shike, et al. (Eds.), 1071–1080, Williams and Wilkins, Baltimore, MD, USA.

Ding, EL. & Malik, VS. (2008). Convergence of obesity and high glycemic diet on compounding diabetes and cardiovascular risks in modernizing China: an emerging public health dilemma. *Globalization and Health*, Vol.4, pp. 4.

Drucker, RR.; Hammer, LD.; Agras, WS. & Bryson, S. (1999). Can mothers influence their child's eating behavior. *J Dev Behav Pediatr*, Vol.20, pp. 88-92.

Ebbeling, CB.; Pawlak, DB. & Ludwig, DS. (2002). Childhood obesity: Public health crisis, common sense cure. *Lancet*, Vol.360, pp. 473–482.

Elliott, R.; Friston, KJ. & Dolan, RJ. (2000). Dissociable neural responses in human reward systems. *J Neurosci*, Vol.20, No.16, pp. 6159-6165.

Elmquist, JK.; Elias, CF. & Saper, CB. (1999). From lesions to leptin: hypothalamic control of food intake and body weight. *Neuron*, Vol.22, No.2, pp. 221-232.

Everitt, BJ.; Belin, D.; Economidou, D.; Pelloux, Y.; Dalley, JW. & Robbins, TW. (2008). Review. Neural mechanisms underlying the vulnerability to develop compulsive drug- seeking habits and addiction. *Philos Trans R Soc Lond B Biol Sci*, Vol.363, No.1507, pp.3125-3135.

Everitt, BJ. & Robbins, TW. (2005). Neural systems of reinforcement for drug addiction: from actions to habits to compulsion. *Nat Neurosci*, Vol.8, No.11, pp.1481-1489.

Fagerberg, B.; Hulten, LM. & Hulthe, J. (2003). Plasma ghrelin, body fat, insulin resistance, and smoking in clinically healthy men: the atherosclerosis and insulin resistance study. *Metabolism*, Vol.52, pp. 1460-1463.

Fan, Y.; Li, Y.; Liu, A.; Hu, X.; Ma, G. & Xu, G. (2010). Associations between body mass index, weight control concerns and behaviors, and eating disorder symptoms among non- clinical Chinese adolescents. *BMC Public Health*, Vol.10, pp. 314.

Farooqi, IS.; Bullmore, E.; Keogh, J.; Gillard, J.; O'Rahilly, S. & Fletcher, PC. (2007). Leptin regulates striatal regions and human eating behavior. *Science*, Vol.317, No.5843, pp. 1355.

File, SE.; Lippa, AS.; Beer, B. & Lippa, MT. (2004). Animal tests of anxiety. *Curr Protoc Neurosci*, Chapter 8, Unit 83.

Foster, GD.; Brownell, KD. & Fairburn, CG. (Eds). (2001). Non-dieting approaches. *Eating disorders and obesity: a comprehensive handbook*. Gulford, NY, USA.

Franklin, TR.; Acton, PD.; Maldjian, JA.; Gray, JD.; Croft, JR.; Dackis, CA.; O'Brien, CP. & Childress, AR. (2002). Decreased gray matter concentration in the insular, orbitofrontal, cingulate, and temporal cortices of cocaine patients. *Biol Psychiatry*, Vol.51, pp. 134–142.

Franklin, TR.; Wang, Z.; Wang, J.; Sciortino, N.; Harper, D.; Li, Y.; Ehrman, R.; Kampman, K.; O'Brien, CP.; Detre, JA. & Childress, AR. (2007). Limbic activation to cigarette smoking cues independent of nicotine withdrawal: a perfusion fMRI study. *Neuropsychopharmacology*, Vol.32, No.11, pp. 2301-2309.

Frayling, TM.; Timpson, NJ.; Weedon, MN.; Zeggini, E.; Freathy, RM.; Lindgren, CM.; Perry, JR.; Elliott, KS.; Lango, H.; Rayner, NW.; Shields, B.; Harries, LW.; Barrett, JC.; Ellard, S.; Groves, CJ.; Knight, B.; Patch, AM.; Ness, AR.; Ebrahim, S.; Lawlor, DA.; Ring, SM.; Ben-Shlomo, Y.; Jarvelin, MR.; Sovio, U.; Bennett, AJ.; Melzer, D.; Ferrucci, L.; Loos, RJ.; Barroso, I.; Wareham, NJ.; Karpe, F.; Owen, KR.; Cardon, LR.; Walker, M.; Hitman, GA.; Palmer, CN.; Doney, AS.; Morris, AD.; Smith, GD.; Hattersley, AT. & McCarthy, MI. (2007). A common variant in the FTO gene is associated with body mass index and predisposes to childhood and adult obesity. *Science*, Vol.316, pp. 889- 894.

Friedman, MA. & Brownell, KD. (1995). Psychological correlates of obesity: moving to the next research generation. *Psychol Bull*, Vol.117, No.1, pp. 3-20.

Fu, D.; Wang, J.; Chen, W. & Bi, Y. (2005). Disordered eating attitudes and behaviours and related mood states among female university students in Beijing. *Chin Ment Health J*, Vol.19, No.8, pp. 25-28.

Fu"hrer, D.; Zysset, S. & Stumvoll, M. (2008). Brain activity in hunger and satiety: an exploratory visually stimulated FMRI study. *Obesity (Silver Spring)*, Vol.16, No. 5, pp. 945-950.

Ge, K.; Weisell, R.; Guo, X.; Cheng, L.; Ma, H.; Zhai, F. & Popkin, BM. (1994). The body mass index of Chinese adults in the 1980s. *Eur J Clin Nutr*, Vol.48, No.3, pp. S148-154.

Gearhardt, AN.; Corbin, WR. & Brownell, KD. (2009a). Food addiction: an examination of the diagnostic criteria for dependence. *J Addict Med*, Vol.3, No.1, pp. 1-7.

Gearhardt, AN.; Corbin, WR. & Brownell, KD. (2009b). Preliminary validation of the Yale Food Addiction Scale. *Appetite*, Vol.52, No.2, pp. 430-436.

Gearhardt, AN.; Davis, C.; Kuschner, R. & Brownell, KD. (2011a). The addiction potential of hyperpalatable foods. *Curr Drug Abuse Rev*, Vol.4, No.3, pp. 140-145.

Gearhardt, AN.; Grilo, CM.; DiLeone, RJ.; Brownell, KD. & Potenza, MN. (2011b). Can food be addictive? Public health and policy implications. *Addiction*, Vol.106, No.7, pp. 1208- 1212.

Gearhardt, AN.; Yokum, S.; Orr, PT.; Stice, E.; Corbin, WR. & Brownell, KD. (2011c). Neural correlates of food addiction. *Arch Gen Psychiatry*, Vol.68, No.8, pp. 808-816.

Gerken, T.; Girard, CA.; Tung, YC.; Webby, CJ.; Saudek, V.; Hewitson, KS.; Yeo, GS.; McDonough, MA.; Cunliffe, S.; McNeill, LA.; Galvanovskis, J.; Rorsman, P.; Robins, P.; Prieur, X.; Coll, AP.; Ma, M.; Jovanovic, Z.; Farooqi, IS.; Sedgwick, B.; Barroso, I.; Lindahl, T.; Ponting, CP.; Ashcroft, FM.; O'Rahilly, S. & Schofield, CJ. (2007). The obesity-associated FTO gene encodes a 2-oxoglutarate-dependent nucleic acid demethylase. *Science*, Vol.318, No.5855, pp. 1469-1472.

Giovannucci, E. (2002). Modifiable risk factors for colon cancer. *Gastroenterol Clin North Am*, Vol.31, pp. 925-943.

Gold, MS. & Stembach, HA. (1984). Endorphins in obesity and in the regulation of appetite and weight. *Integrative Psychiatry*, Vol.2, No.6, pp. 1549-1555.

Gold, MS. (1999). Etiology and management of obesity. *Direction in Psychiatry*, Vol.19, No.20, pp. 1549-1555.

Goldstein, RZ. & Volkow, ND. (2002). Drug addiction and its underlying neurobiological basis: Neuroimaging evidence for the involvement of the frontal cortex. *American Journal of Psychiatry*, Vol.129, pp. 1642–1652.

Groschl, M.; Topf, HG.; Bohlender, J.; Zenk, J.; Klussmann, S.; Dötsch, J.; Rascher, W. & Rauh, M. (2005). Identification of ghrelin in human saliva: production by the salivary glands and potential role in proliferation of oral keratinocytes. *ClinChem*, Vol.51, pp. 997-1006.

Grundy, SM.; Brewer, B.; Cleeman, JI.; Smith, SC. & Lenfant, C. (2004). Definition of metabolic syndrome: Report of the national heart, lung, and blood institute/American heart association conference on scientific issues related to definition. *Circulation*, Vol.109, pp. 433-438.

Guldan, GS. (2010). Asian children's obesogenic diets—time to change this part of the energy balance equation? *Res Sports Med*, Vol.18, No.1, pp. 5-15.

Haddock, CK.; Dill, PL.; Poston, WSC. & Haddock, CK. (Eds.). (2000). *The effects of food on mood and behavior: implications for the addictions model of obesity and eating disorders. Food as a drug*, The Haworth Press, Inc., New York, NY.

Hodgkins, CC.; Cahill, KS.; Seraphine, AE.; Frost-Pineda, K. & Gold, MS. (2004). Adolescent drug addiction treatment and weight gain. *J Add Dis.*, Vol.23, No.3, pp. 55–66.

Hong, J. (1998). *The internationalization of television in China: an evolution of ideology, society, and media since the reform*, Praeger Publishers, Westport, CT.

Huang, JS.; Becerra, K. & Oda, T. (2007). Parental ability to discriminate the weight status of children: results of a survey. *Pediatrics*, Vol.120, pp. e112-119.

Hyman, SM.; Hong, KI.; Chaplin, TM.; Dabre, Z.; Comegys, AD.; Kimmerling, A. & Sinha, R. (2009). A stress-coping profile of opioid dependent individuals entering naltrexone treatment: a comparison with healthy controls. *Psychol Addict Behav*, Vol.23, No.4, pp. 613-619.

Ifland, JR.; Preuss, HG.; Marcus, MT.; Rourke, KM.; Taylor, WC.; Burau, K.; Jacobs, WS.; Kadish, W. & Manso, G. (2009). Refined food addiction: a classic substance use disorder. *Med Hypotheses*, Vol.72, No.5, pp. 518-526.

James, GA.; He, G.; Miller, AW.; Taeb, Y. & Liu, Y. (2002). MRI of hunger and insula activation during a fasting paradigm. *ISMRM*, Abstract.

James, GA.; Miller, JL.; Goldstone, AP.; Couch, JA.; He, G.; Driscoll, DJ. & Liu, Y. (2007). Enhanced activation of reward mediating prefrontal regions in response to food stimuli in Prader-Willi syndrome. *J Neurol Neurosurg Psychiatry*, Vol.78, No.6, pp. 615-619.

Jansen, A. (1998). A learning model of binge eating: cue reactivity and cue exposure. *Behav Res Ther*, Vol.36, No.3, pp. 257-272.

Jernigan, TL.; Butters, N.; DiTraglia, G.; Schafer, K.; Smith, T.; Irwin, M.; Grant, I.; Schuckit, M. & Cermak, LS. (1991). Reduced cerebral grey matter observed in alcoholics using magnetic resonance imaging. *Alcohol Clin Exp Res*, Vol.15, pp. 418-427.

Ji, MF. & McNeal, JU. (2001). How Chinese children's commercials differ from those of the United States: a content analysis. *J Advert*, Vol.30, pp. 79.

Jonas, JM. & Gold, MS. (1986). Cocaine abuse and eating disorders. *Lancet*, Vol.1, pp. 390-391.

Jones, N.; Furlanetto, DL.; Jackson, JA. & Kinn, S. (2007). An investigation of obese adults' views of the outcomes of dietary treatment. *J Human Nutr Diet*, Vol.20, pp. 486-494.

Joranby, L.; Pineda, K. & Gold, MS. (2005). Addiction to food and brain reward systems. *Sexual Addiction and Compulsivity*, Vol.12, No.2-3, pp. 201-217.

Jumabay, M.; Kawamura, H.; Mitsubayashi, H.; Ozawa, Y.; Izumi, Y.; Kasamaki, H.; Shimabukuro, Z.; Cheng, M.; Aisa & Wang, S. (2001). Urinary electrolytes and hypertension in elderly Kazakhs. *Clin Exp Nephrol*, Vol.5, pp. 217-221.

Kalra, PS. & Kalra, SP. (2002). Obesity and metabolic syndrome: long-term benefits of central leptin gene therapy. *Drugs Today (Barc)*, Vol.38, No.11, pp. 745-757.

Kalra, SP. & Kalra, PS. (1996). Nutritional infertility: the role of the interconnected hypothalamic neuropeptide Y-galanin-opioid network. *Front Neuroendocrinol*, Vol.17, No.4, pp. 371-401.

Kalra, SP. & Kalra, PS. (2004a). NPY and cohorts in regulating appetite, obesity and metabolic syndrome: beneficial effects of gene therapy. *Neuropeptides*, Vol.38, No.4, pp. 201-211.

Kalra, SP. & Kalra, PS. (2004b). Overlapping and interactive pathways regulating appetite and craving. *J Addict Dis*, Vol.23, No.3, pp. 5-21.

Kalra, SP.; Dube, MG.; Pu, S.; Xu, B.; Horvath, TL. & Kalra, PS. (1999). Interacting appetite-regulating pathways in the hypothalamic regulation of body weight. *Endocr Rev*, Vol.20, No.1, pp. 68-100.

Karatayev, O.; Gaysinskaya, V.; Chang, GQ. & Leibowitz, SF. (2009). Circulating triglycerides after a high-fat meal: predictor of increased caloric intake, orexigenic peptide expression, and dietary obesity. *Brain Res*, Vol.1298, pp. 111–122.

Kenny, PJ. (2011). 'Macrophage' cannabinoid receptor goes up in smoke. *Nat Neurosci*, Vol.14, No.9, pp. 1100-1102.

Kleiner, KD.; Gold, MS.; Frost-Pineda, K.; Lenz-Brunsman, B.; Perri, MG. & Jacobs, WS. (2004). Body mass index and alcohol use. *J Addict Dis*, Vol.23, No.3, pp. 105-118.

Ko, GT.; So, WY.; Chow, CC.; Wong, PT.; Tong, SD.; Hui, SS.; Kwok, R.; Chan, A.; Chan, CL.; Chan, JC. & BHBHK Research Committee. (2010). Risk associations of obesity with sugar-sweetened beverages and lifestyle factors in Chinese: the 'Better Health for Better Hong Kong' health promotion campaign. *Eur J Clin Nutrition*, Vol.64, pp. 1386-1392.

Kong, AP. & Chow, CC. (2010). Medical consequences of childhood obesity: a Hong Kong perspective. *Res Sports Med*, Vol.18, No.1, pp. 16-25.

Koob, GF.; Caine, B.; Markou, A.; Pulvirenti, L. & Weiss, F. (1994). Role for the mesocortical dopamine system in the motivating effects of cocaine. *NIDA Res Monogr*, Vol.145, pp. 1–18.

Koob, GF. & Le Moal, M. (2005). *Neurobiology of Addiction*. Academic Press, San Diego, CA.

Koob, GF. & Volkow, ND. (2010). Neurocircuitry of addiction. *Neuropsychopharmacology*, Vol.35, pp. 217–238.

Koob, GF. (2009). Dynamics of neuronal circuits in addiction: reward, antireward, and emotional memory. *Pharmacopsychiatry*, Vol.42, No.1, pp. S32–S41.

Kurihara, K. & Kashiwayanagi, M. (2000). Physiological studies on umami taste. *J Nutr*, Vol.130, No.4, pp. 931S-934S.

Levine, AS.; Kotz, CM. & Gosnell, BA. (2003). Sugars: hedonic aspects, neuroregulation, and energy balance. *Am J Clin Nutr*, Vol.78, pp. 834S–842S.

Li, HL.; Yu, YR.; Yu, HL.; Wang, C. & Zhang, XX. (2005). Relationship between peripheral insulin resistance and beta-cell function in obese subjects. *Sichuan Da Xue Xue Bao Yi Xue Ban*, Vol.36, pp. 378-381.

Li, X.; Song, F.; Jiang, H.; Zhang, M.; Lin, J.; Bao, W.; Yao, P.; Yang, X.; Hao, L. & Liu, L. (2010). A genetic variation in the fat mass-and obesity-associated gene is associated with obesity and newly diagnosed type 2 diabetes in a Chinese population. *Diabetes Metab Res Rev*, Vol.26, No.2, pp. 128-132.

Li, Y.; Zhai, F.; Yang, X.; Schouten, EG.; Hu, X.; He, Y.; Luan, D. & Ma, G. (2007). Determinants of childhood overweight and obesity in China. *British J Nutr*, Vol.97, pp. 210-215.

Liu, X.; Matochik, JA.; Cadet, JL. & London, ED. (1998). Smaller volume of pre-frontal lobe in polysubstance abusers: a magnetic resonance imaging study. *Neuropsychopharmacology*, Vol.18, pp. 243-252.

Liu, Y. & Gold, MS. (2003). Human functional magnetic resonance imaging of eating and satiety in eating disorders and obesity. *Psych Annals*, Vol.33, No.2, pp. 127-132.

Liu, Y.; Gao, JH.; Liu, HL. & Fox, PT. (2000). The temporal response of the brain after eating revealed by functional MRI. *Nature*, Vol.405, pp. 1058-1062.

Liu, Y.; von Deneen, KM.; Kobeissy, F. & Gold, MS. (2010). Food Addiction and obesity: Evidence from bench to bedside. *J of Psychoactive Drugs*, Vol.42, No.2, pp. 133-145.

Livingstone, S. (2002). *Young People and New Media*. Sage Publications, Thousand Oaks, CA.

Mark, GP.; Weinberg, JB.; Rada, PV. & Hoebel, BG. (1995). Extracellular acetylcholine is increased in the nucleus accumbens following the presentation of an aversively conditioned taste stimulus. *Brain Res*, Vol.688, No.1-2, pp. 184-188.

Martorell, R.; Stein, AD. & Schroeder, DG. (2001). Early nutrition and later adiposity. *J Nutr*, Vol.131, pp. 874S-880S.

Matsuda, M.; Liu, Y.; Mahankali, S.; Wang, J.; DeFronzo, RA.; Fox, PT. & Gao, JH. (1999). Altered hypothalamic response to oral glucose intake in obese humans. *Diabetes*, Vol.48, pp. 1801-1806.

Maynard, LM.; Galuska, DA.; Blanck, HM. & Serdula, MK. (2003). Maternal perceptions of weight status of children. *Pediatrics*, Vol.111, pp. 1226-1231.

McAuley, KA.; Williams, SM.; Mann, JI.; Walker, RJ.; Lewis-Barned, NJ.; Temple, LA. & Duncan, AW. (2001). Diagnosing insulin resistance in the general population. *Diabetes Care*, Vol.24, pp. 460-464.

McBride, D.; Barrett, SP.; Kelly, JT.; Aw, A. & Dagher, A. (2006). Effects of expectancy and abstinence on the neural response to smoking cues in cigarette smokers: an fMRI study. *Neuropsychopharmacology*, Vol.31, No.12, pp. 2728-2738.

McMillen, IC.; Rattanatray, L.; Duffield, JA.; Morrison, JL.; MacLaughlin, SM.; Gentili, S. & Muhlhausler, BS. (2009). The early origins of later obesity: pathways and mechanisms. *Advan Exp Med Biol*, Vol.646, pp. 71-81.

McNeal, JU. & Yeh, C. (1997). Development of consumer behavior patterns among Chinese children. *J Consum Market*, Vol.14, pp. 45-59.

Mi, J.; Cheng, H.; Zhao, XY.; Hou, DQ.; Chen, FF. & Zhang, KL. (2008). Developmental origin of metabolic syndrome: interaction of thinness at birth and overweight during adult life in Chinese population. *Obes Rev*, Vol.9, No.1, pp. 91-94.

Miller, EK. & Cohen, JD. (2001). An integrative theory of prefrontal cortex function. *Annu Rev Neurosci*, Vol.24, pp. 167-202.

Mogenson, GJ. (1982). Studies of the nucleus accumbens and its mesolimbic dopaminergic affects in relation to ingestive behaviors and reward. In: *The Neural Basis of Feeding and Reward*, GB. Hoebel & D. Novin (Eds.), Haer Institute, Brunswick, ME.

Mokdad, AH.; Marks, JS.; Stroup, DF. & Gerberding, JL. (2004). Actual causes of death in the United States, 2000. *JAMA*, Vol.291, No.10, pp. 1238-1245.

Morris, JS. & Dolan, RJ. (2001). Involvement of human amygdala and orbitofrontal cortex in hunger-enhanced memory for food stimuli. *J Neurosci*, Vol.21, pp. 5304–5310.

Murakami, K.; Sasaki, S.; Takahashi, Y.; Okubo, H.; Hosoi, Y.; Horiguchi, H.; Oguma, E. & Kayama, F. (2006). Dietary glycemic index and load in relation to metabolic risk factors in Japanese female farmers with traditional dietary habits. *Am J Clin Nutr*, Vol.83, pp. 1161-1169.

O'Doherty, J.; Rolls, ET.; Francis, S.; Bowtell, R.; McGlone, F.; Kobal, G.; Renner, B. & Ahne, G. (2000). Sensory-specific satiety-related olfactory activation of the human orbitofrontal cortex. *Neuroreport*, Vol.11, No.2, pp. 399-403.

O'Doherty, JP. (2004). Reward representations and reward-related learning in the human brain: insights from neuroimaging. *Curr Opin Neurobiol*, Vol.14, No.6, pp. 769-776.

Ogura, K.; Shinohara, M.; Ohno, K. & Mori, E. (2008). Frontal behavioral syndromes in Prader-Willi syndrome. *Brain Dev*, Vol.30, No.7, pp. 469-476.

Parvanta, SA.; Brown, JD.; Du, S.; Zimmer, CR.; Zhao, X. & Zhai, F. (2010). Television use and snacking behaviors among children and adolescents in China. *J Adolesc Health*, Vol.46, No.4, pp. 339-345.

Petry, NM. (2006). Should the scope of addictive behaviors be broadened to include pathological gambling? *Addiction*, Vol.101, No.1, pp. 152-160.

Pfefferbaum, A.; Sullivan, EV.; Mathalon, DH. & Lim, KO. (1997). Frontal lobe volume loss observed with magnetic resonance imaging in older chronic alcoholics. *Alcohol Clin Exp Res*, Vol.21, pp. 521–529.

Pi-Sunyer, FX. (2002). The medical risks of obesity. *Obesity Surg*, Vol., No.1, pp. 6S–11S.

Popkin, BM. (2001). The nutrition transition and obesity in the developing world. *J Nutr*, Vol.131, pp. 871S-873S.

Popkin, BM.; Paeratakul, S.; Zhai, F. & Ge, K. (1995). A review of dietary and environmental correlates of obesity with emphasis on developing countries. *Obes Res*, Vol.3, No.2, pp. 145s-53s.

Potenza, MN.; Hong, KI.; Lacadie, CM.; Fulbright, RK.; Tuit, KL. & Sinha, R. (2012). Neural correlates of stress-induced and cue-induced drug craving: influences of sex and cocaine dependence. *Am J Psychiatry*, [Epub ahead of print].

Rada, P. & Hoebel, BG. (2005). Acetylcholine in the accumbens is decreased by diazepam and increased by benzodiazepine withdrawal: a possible mechanism for dependency. *Eur J Pharmacol*, Vol.508, pp. 131–138.

Rada, P.; Avena, NM. & Hoebel, BG. (2005). Daily bingeing on sugar repeatedly releases dopamine in the accumbens shell. *Neuroscience*, Vol.134, No.3, pp. 737-744.

Raman, RP. (2002). Obesity and health risks. *Journal of the American College of Nutrition*, Vol.21, pp. 34S–139S.

Rhee, K. (2008). Childhood overweight and the relationship between parent behaviors, parenting style, and family functioning. *Annals Amer Acad Pol Soc Sci*, Vol.615, pp. 11-37.

Robbins, TW. & Everitt, BJ. (1999). Drug addiction: bad habits add up. *Nature*, Vol.398, No.6728, pp. 567-570.

Robinson, TE. & Berridge, KC. (1993). The neural basis of drug craving: an incentive-sensitization theory of addiction, *Brain Research Reviews*, Vol.18, pp. 247-291.

Rolls, ET. (2000). The orbitofrontal cortex and reward. *Cereb Cortex*, Vol.10, No.3, pp. 284-294.

Rosenbaum, M.; Sy, M.; Pavlovich, K.; Leibel, RL. & Hirsch, J. (2008). Leptin reverses weight loss-induced changes in regional neural activity responses to visual food stimuli. *J Clin Invest*, Vol.118, No.7, pp. 2583-2591.

Rosenkranz, JA. & Grace, AA. (2001). Dopamine attenuates prefrontal cortical suppression of sensory inputs to the basolateral amygdala of rats. *J Neurosci*, Vol.21, pp. 4090-4103.

Ross, HE. & Ivis, F. (1999). Binge eating and substance use among male and female adolescents. *International Journal of Eating Disorders*, Vol.26, pp. 245-260.

Ruiz, JR.; Labayen, I.; Ortega, FB.; Legry, V.; Moreno, LA.; Dallongeville, J.; Martínez-Gómez, D.; Bokor, S.; Manios, Y.; Ciarapica, D.; Gottrand, F.; De Henauw, S.; Molnár, D.; Sjöström, M.; Meirhaeghe, A. & HELENA Study Group. (2010). Attenuation of the effect of the FTO rs9939609 polymorphism on total and central body fat by physical activity in adolescents: the HELENA study. *Arch Pediatr Adolesc Med*, Vol.164, pp. 328-333.

Saad, MF.; Khan, A.; Sharma, A.; Michael, R.; Riad-Gabriel, MG.; Boyadjian, R.; Jinagouda, SD.; Steil, GM. & Kamdar, V. (1998). Physiological insulinemia acutely modulates plasma leptin. *Diabetes*, Vol. 47, No.4, pp. 544-549.

Sahu, A. & Kalra, SP. (1993). Neuropeptide regulation of feeding behavior: Neuropeptide Y. *TEM*, Vol.4, No.7, pp. 217-224.

Sato, Y.; Ito, T.; Udaka, N.; Kanisawa, M.; Noguchi, Y.; Cushman, SW. & Satoh, S. (1996). Immunohistochemical localization of facilitated-diffusion glucose transporters in rat pancreatic islets. *Tissue Cell*, Vol.28, No.6, pp. 637-643.

Schoenbaum, G. & Shaham, Y. (2008). The role of orbitofrontal cortex in drug addiction: a review of preclinical studies. *Biol Psychiatry*, Vol.63, No.3, pp. 256-262.

Schroeder, BE.; Binzak, JM. & Kelley, AE. (2001). A common profile of prefrontal cortical activation following exposure to nicotine- or chocolate associated contextual cues. *Neuroscience*, Vol.105, pp. 535-545.

Scuteri, A.; Sanna, S.; Chen, WM.; Uda, M.; Albai, G.; Strait, J.; Najjar, S.; Nagaraja, R.; Orrú, M.; Usala, G.; Dei, M.; Lai, S.; Maschio, A.; Busonero, F.; Mulas, A.; Ehret, GB.; Fink, AA.; Weder, AB.; Cooper, RS.; Galan, P.; Chakravarti, A.; Schlessinger, D.; Cao, A.; Lakatta, E. & Abecasis, GR. (2007). Genome-wide association scan shows genetic variants in the FTO gene are associated with obesity-related traits. *PLoS Genet*, Vol.3, No. e115.

Shapira, NA.; Liu, Y.; He, AG.; Bradley, MM.; Lessig, MC.; James, GA.; Stein, DJ.; Lang, PJ. & Goodman, WK. (2003). Brain activation by disgust-inducing pictures in obsessive- compulsive disorder. *Biol Psychiatry*, Vol.54, No.7, pp. 751-756.

Shi, Z.; Lien, N.; Kumar, BN. & Holmboe-Ottesen, G. (2005). Socio-demographic differences in food habits and preferences of school adolescents in Jiangsu Province, China. *Eur J Clin Nutr*, Vol.59, pp. 1439-1448.

Shi, Z.; Luscombe-Marsh, ND.; Wittert, GA.; Yuan, B.; Dai, Y.; Pan, X. & Taylor, AW. (2010). Monosodium glutamate is not associated with obesity or a greater prevalence of weight gain over 5 years: findings from the Jiangsu Nutrition Study of Chinese adults. *Br J Nutr*, Vol.104, pp. 457-463.

Shi, Z; Lien, N; Kumar, BN. & Holmboe-Ottesen, G. (2007). Perceptions of weight and associated factors of adolescents in Jiangsu Province, China. *Public Health Nutr*, Vol.10, pp. 298-305.

Simmons, WK.; Martin, A. & Barsalou, LW. (2005). Pictures of appetizing foods activate gustatory cortices for taste and reward. *Cerebral Cortex*, Vol.15, pp. 1602-1608.

Singh, NN.; Lancioni, GE.; Singh, AN.; Winton, AS.; Singh, J.; McAleavey, KM. & Adkins, AD. (2008). A mindfulness-based health wellness program for an adolescent with Prader- Willi syndrome. *Behav Modif*, Vol.32, No.2, pp. 167-181.

Small, DM.; Zatorre, RJ.; Dagher, A.; Evans, AC. & Jones-Gotman, M. (2001). Changes in brain activity related to eating chocolate: from pleasure to aversion. *Brain*, Vol.124, No.9, pp. 1720-1733.

Solinas, M. & Goldberg, SR. (2005). Motivational effects of cannabinoids and opioids of food reinforcement depend on simultaneous activation of cannabinoid and opioid systems. *Neuropscyhopharmacology*, Vol.30, No.11, pp. 2035-2045.

Spring, B.; Schneider, K.; Smith, M.; Kendzor, D.; Appelhans, B.; Hedeker, D. & Pagoto, S. (2008). Abuse potential of carbohydrates for overweight carbohydrate cravers. *Psychopharmacology (Berl)*, Vol.197, No.4, pp. 637-647.

Swanson, LW. & Petrovich, GD. (1998). What is the amygdala? *Trends Neurosci*, Vol.21, pp. 323-331.

Tartar, RE.; Ammerman, RT. & Ott, PJ. (1998). Handbook of substance abuse. *Neurobehavioral Pharmacology*. Premium Press, New York, NY.

Tataranni, PA. & DelParigi, A. (2003). Functional neuroimaging: a new generation of human brain studies in obesity research. *Obes Rev*, Vol.4, No.4, pp. 229-238.

Urban, NB. & Martinez, D. (2012). Neurobiology of addiction: insight from neurochemical imaging. *Psychiatr Clin North Am*, Vol.35, No.2, pp.:521-541.

Volkow, ND. & Fowler, JS. (2000). Addiction, a disease of compulsion and drive: involvement of the orbitofrontal cortex. *Cereb Cortex*, Vol. 10, No.3, pp. 318-325.

Volkow, ND. & Wise, RA. (2005). How can drug addiction help us understand obesity? *Nat Neurosci*, Vol.8, No.5, pp. 555-560.

Volkow, ND. & Li, TK. (2004). Science and society: drug addiction: the neurobiology of behaviour gone awry. *Nat. Rev. Neurosci*, Vol. 5, pp. 963–970.

Volkow, ND.; Fowler, JS. & Wang, GJ. (2004). The addicted human brain viewed in the light of imaging studies: brain circuits and treatment strategies. *Neuropharmacology*, Vol.47, No.1, pp. 3-13.

Volkow, ND.; Wang ,GJ.; Fowler, JS.; Logan, J.; Gatley, SJ.; Hitzemann, R.; Chen, AD.; Dewey, SL. & Pappas, N. (1997). Decreased striatal dopaminergic responsiveness in detoxified cocaine-dependent subjects. *Nature*, Vol.386, pp. 830–833.

Volkow, ND.; Wang, GJ.; Fowler, JS. & Telang, F. (2008). Overlapping neuronal circuits in addiction and obesity: evidence of systems pathology. *Philos Trans R Soc Lond B Biol Sci*. Vol.363, No.1507, pp. 3191-3200.

Volkow, ND.; Wang, GJ.; Fowler, JS.; Logan, J.; Jayne, M.; Franceschi, D.; Wong, C.; Gatley, SJ.; Gifford, AN.; Ding, Y-S. & Pappas, N. (2002). "Nonhedonic" food motivation in humans involves dopamine in the dorsal striatum and methylphenidate amplifies this effect. *Synapse*, Vol.44, No.3, pp. 175-180.

von Deneen, KM. & Liu, Y. (2011). Obesity as an addiction: Why do the obese eat more? *Maturitas*, Vol.68, No.4, pp. 342-345.

von Deneen, KM.; Gold, MS. & Liu, Y. (2009). Food addiction and cues in Prader-Willi Syndrome. *J Addict Med*, Vol.3, pp. 19-25.

von Deneen, KM.; Wei, Q.; Tian, J. & Liu, Y. (2011). Obesity in China. What are the causes? *Curr Pharm Des*, Vol.17, No.12, pp. 1132-1139.

Walther, K.; Birdsill, AC.; Glisky, EL. & Ryan, L. (2010). Structural brain differences and cognitive functioning related to body mass index in older females. *Hum Brain Mapp*, Vol.31, pp. 1052-1064.

Wang, GJ.; Volkow, ND.; Logan, J.; Rappas, NR.; Wong, CT.; Zhu, W.; Netusil, N. & Fowler JS. (2001). Brain dopamine and obesity. *Lancet*, Vol.357, No.9253, pp. 354-357.

Wang, GJ.; Volkow, ND.; Telang, F.; Jayne, M.; Ma, J; Rao, M.; Zhu, W.; Wong, CT.; Pappas, NR.; Geliebter, A. & Fowler, JS. (2004). Exposure to appetitive food stimuli markedly activates the human brain. *Neuroimage*, Vol.21, No.4, pp. 1790-1797.

Wang, GJ.; Volkow, ND.; Thanos, PK. & Fowler, JS. (2009). Imaging of brain dopamine pathways: implications for understanding obesity. *J Addict Med*, Vol.3, pp. 8-18.

Wang, K.; Ao, YT.; Zhao, L.; Guo, YY.; Shagedeke; Xu, YS.; Song, T.; Gerli & He, BX. (2006). Analysis on obesity and its risk factors among inhabitants of Bortala prefecture of Xinjiang autonomous region. *Chinese J Public Health*, Vol.22, No.9, pp. 1128-1130.

Wang, Y.; Beydoun, MA.; Liang, L.; Caballero, B. & Kumanyika, SK. (2008a). Will all Americans become overweight or obese? Estimating the progression and cost of the US obesity epidemic. *Obesity*, Vol.16, pp. 2323-2330.

Wang, Z.; Zhai, F.; Du, S. & Popkin, B. (2008b). Dynamic shifts in Chinese eating behaviors. *Asia Pac J Clin Nutr*, Vol.17, pp. 123-130.

Warren, MW. & Gold, MS. (2007). The relationship between obesity and drug use. *Am J Psychiatry*, Vol.164, No.8, pp. 1268-1269.

Wise, RA. (2006). Role of brain dopamine in food reward and reinforcement. *Philos Trans R Soc Lond B Biol Sci*, Vol.361,pp. 1149-1158.

Wurtman, RJ. & Wurtman, JJ. (1995). Brain serotonin, carbohydrate-craving, obesity and depression. *Obes Res*, Vol.3, No.4, pp. 477S-480S.

Xi, B. & Mi, J. (2009). FTO polymorphisms are associated with obesity but not with diabetes in East Asian populations: a meta-analysis. *Biomed Environ Sci*, Vol.22, No.6, pp. 449- 457.

Xu, H.; Song, Y.; You, NC.; Zhang, ZF.; Greenland, S.; Ford, ES.; He, L. & Liu, S. (2010). Prevalence and clustering of metabolic risk factors for type 2 diabetes among Chinese adults in Shanghai, China. *BMC Public Health*, Vol.10, pp. 683.

Zapata, A.; Chefer, VI.; Ator, R.; Shippenberg, TS. & Rocha, BA. (2003). Behavioural sensitization and enhanced dopamine response in the nucleus accumbens after intravenous cocaine self-administration in mice. *Eur J Neurosci*, Vol.17, No.3, pp. 590- 596.

Zemmet, P. (2000). Diabetes and obesity worldwide epidemics in full flight. *60th Scientific Sessions of the American Diabetes Association*, San Antonio, Texas.

Zhai, F.; Wang, H.; Du, S.; He, Y.; Wang, Z.; Ge, K. & Popkin, BM. (2009). Prospective study on nutrition transition in China. *Nutr Rev*, Vol.67, pp. S56-61.

Zhang, Y.; von Deneen, KM.; Tian, J.; Gold, MS. & Liu, Y. (2011). Food addiction and neuroimaging. *Curr Pharm Des*, Vol.17, No.12, pp. 1149-1157.

Zhang, YB. & Harwood, J. (2004). Modernization and tradition in an age of globalization: cultural values in Chinese television commercials. *J Commun*, Vol.54, pp. 156-172.

5

Addictive Drugs and Synaptic Plasticity

José Vicente Negrete-Díaz[1], Gonzalo Flores[1],
Talvinder S. Sihra[2] and Antonio Rodríguez-Moreno[3]
[1]Universidad Autonoma de Puebla, Puebla,
[2]University College London, London,
[3]Universidad Pablo de Olavide, Sevilla,
[1]México
[2]UK
[3]Spain

1. Introduction

The term addiction, derived from a Latin word meaning "bound to" or "enslaved by," was initially not linked to substance use. However, over the past several hundred years, addiction became associated with excessive alcohol and then drug use, such that by the late 1980s it was largely synonymous with compulsive drug use (O'Brien et al., 2006). The core features of addiction are manifest in the continued performance of the behavior despite adverse consequences, compulsive engagement or diminished control over the behavior, and an appetitive urge or craving state prior to the behavioral engagement representing core elements (Holden, 2010).

Addiction is a state of compulsive drug use; despite treatment and other attempts to control drug taking, addiction tends to persist. Hyman (2005) has summarized several studies where the authors have suggested that if the neurobiology is ultimately to contribute to the development of successful treatments for drug addiction, researchers must elucidate the molecular mechanisms by which drug-seeking behaviors are consolidated into compulsive use. Evidence at different levels of analysis suggest that addiction represents a pathological state of the neural mechanisms of learning and memory that, under normal circumstances, serve to shape survival behaviors related to the pursuit of rewards and the cues that predict them (Shultz et el., 1997; Montague et al., 2004; see Badiani et al., 2011 for review). The major substrates of persistent compulsive drug use are hypothesized to be molecular and cellular mechanisms that underlie long-term associative memories in several forebrain circuits (involving the ventral and dorsal striatum and prefrontal cortex) which receive inputs from midbrain dopamine neurons (see Hyman et al., 2006, for review). Also, the basolateral amygdala and nucleus accumbens core are key structures within limbic cortical-striatal circuitry where reconsolidation of a cue-drug memory occurs (Théberge et al., 2010). Vulnerability to stimulant addiction may depend on an impulsivity endophenotype. Impulsivity is the tendency to act prematurely without foresight, and is commonly associated with addiction to drugs, though its causal role in human addiction is unclear. Different groups (Dalley et al., 2007; Bezze et al., 2007 and Dalley et al., 2011) have characterized, in neurobehavioral and neurochemical terms, a rodent model of impulsivity based on premature responses in an attentional task. Evidence suggests that high impulsivity on this task precedes the subsequent escalation of cocaine self-administration behavior (Dalley et al., 2007, and also a tendency towards compulsive cocaine-seeking (Belin et al., 2008) and to relapse (Economidou et al., 2009). On the other hand, excessive consumption of palatable food can trigger neuroadaptive responses in brain reward circuitries similar to those produced by drugs of abuse. Thus, congruent genetic vulnerabilities in brain reward systems can increase predisposition to drug addiction and obesity. Kenny (2011) has recently advanced our understanding of the brain circuitries that regulate hedonic aspects of feeding behavior, with evidence suggesting that obesity and drug addiction may share common mechanisms.

Individuals take addictive drugs to elevate mood, but after repeated use these drugs produce serious unwanted effects, which include: tolerance to some drug effects, sensitization to others, and an adapted state–dependence, these setting the stage for withdrawal symptoms when drug use stops. The most serious consequence of repetitive drug taking is however addiction: a persistent state in which compulsive drug use escapes control, even when serious negative consequences ensue. Addiction is characterized by a long-lasting risk of relapse, which is often initiated by exposure to drug-related cues. Substantial progress has been made in understanding the molecular and cellular mechanisms of tolerance, dependence and withdrawal but, as yet, we understand little of the neural substrates of compulsive drug use and its remarkable persistence. Evidence exists for the possibility that compulsion and its persistence are based on a pathological usurpation of molecular mechanisms that are normally involved in memory (see Hyman and Malenka 2001 for review).

Genetic studies to date have been most successful at identifying factors that influence the transition from regular use to dependence. Numerous and large twin studies have indicated a significant genetic contribution to the process of conversion from eventual use to established use before development of dependence. The availability of large cohort samples for nicotine and alcohol dependence has resulted in significant progress being made in understanding at least some of the genetic contributions to these addictions (Tsuang et al., 1998, Kendler et al., 2003). Fewer studies have replicated specific genetic contributions to illicit drug use. Substance dependence can be thought of as a pharmacogenetic illness and, most likely, hundreds and more probably thousands of genetic variants will be required to fully explain the genetic input to this disease (see Bierut, 211 for review).

1.1 Neurobiology of addiction

Addictive drugs have in common the property that they are voluntarily self-administered by laboratory animals (usually avidly) (Di Chiara et al., 2004), and that they enhance the functioning of the reward circuitry of the brain (producing the 'high' that the drug user seeks). The core reward circuitry consists of an 'in-series' circuit linking the ventral tegmental area (VTA), nucleus accumbens (NAc) and ventral pallidum via the medial forebrain bundle. All addictive drugs have in common that they enhance (directly or indirectly or even transsynaptically) dopaminergic synaptic function in the NAc (Di Chiara et al., 2004), which is implicated in the reward process. Drug self-administration is regulated by NAc dopamine (DA) levels, which are retained within a specific elevated range (to maintain a desired hedonic level). The three classical sets of craving and relapse triggers are (a) reexposure to addictive drugs, (b) stress, and (c) reexposure to environmental cues (people, places, things) previously associated with drug-taking behavior. Knowledge of the neuroanatomy, neurophysiology, neurochemistry and neuropharmacology of addictive drug action in the brain is currently producing a variety of strategies for pharmacotherapeutic treatment of drug addiction, some of which appear promising (Gardner, 2011). Addictive drugs target the mesocorticolimbic dopamine (DA) system. This system originates in the VTA and projects mainly to the NAc and prefrontal cortex (PFC), affecting glutamatergic and GABAergic synaptic transmission in all three brain areas. These changes are refered to as drug-evoked synaptic plasticity, which outlasts the presence of the drug in the brain and contributes to the reorganization of neural circuits. While in most cases these early changes are not sufficient to induce the disease, with repetitive drug exposure, they may add up and contribute to addictive behavior (see Lüscher and Malenka, 2011 for review).

1.2 Learning and memory in addictive behavior

Two forms of cellular and synaptic plasticity, long-term potentiation (LTP) and long-term depression (LTD) remain the most extensively studied. They are considered the cellular and molecular basis of learning and memory (Kandel, 2004; Negrete-Díaz et al., 2007; Adermark et al., 2009; Abusch and Akirav, 2010; Collingridge et al., 2010; Huang et al., 2011, Figure 1).

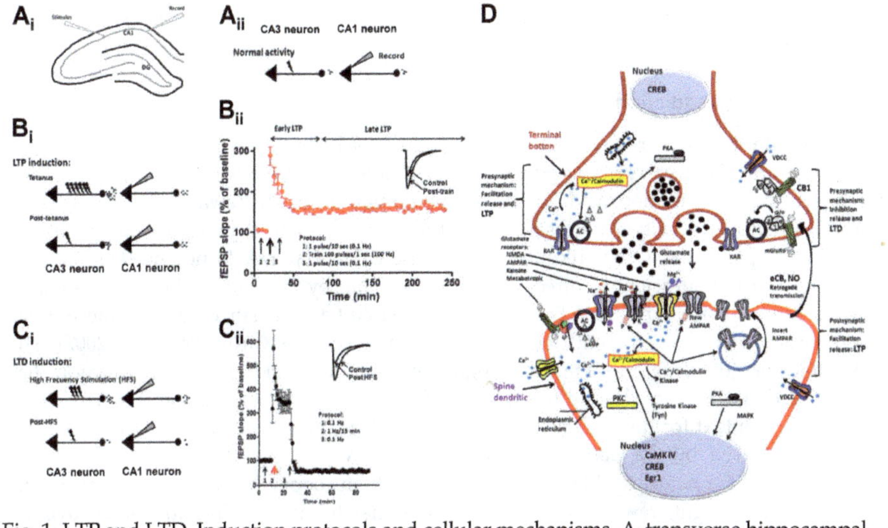

Fig. 1. LTP and LTD. Induction protocols and cellular mechanisms. A_i transverse hippocampal slice and estándar positioning of stimulating and recording electrodes. Hippocampus is the structure in which plasticity mechanisms have been more extensively estudied. A_{ii}, representation of presynaptic and postsynaptic neurons at synapse between CA3 and CA1 pyramidal cells. B_i, LTP protocol, tetanic (100 Hz, 1s) stimulation of presynaptic neurons induce and increase of the amplitude of excitatory postsynaptic potencial EPSP (B_{ii}) recorded from postsynaptic neurons. C_i, LTD protocol, stimulation at 1 Hz during 15 minutes induce a decrease of the amplitude of the EPSP (C_{ii}) recorded from postsynaptic neurons. D, schematic description of intracellular mechanisms involved in LTP and LTD

In addition, they can be used to demonstrate the repertoire of enduring modifications of individual synapses, circuits or neural networks. A classic triad arrangement of DA terminal varicosities, dendritic spines, and cortical inputs allows dopamine to enhance spike-time-dependent plasticity (STDP) at active cortico-striatal and cortico-cortical synapses. The induced LTP and LTD are candidate mechanisms for phasic DA signal to mediate behavioral learning. Thus, by affecting striatal and cortical plasticity, addictive drugs could lead to long-lasting changes of the motor, reward, and cognitive functions of these structures, striatum and PFC (Schultz, 2011). Conditioned stimuli (CSs) by Pavlovian association with reinforcing drugs (unconditioned stimuli; US) are thought to play an important role in the acquisition, maintenance and relapse of drug dependence. Bassareo et al. (2007) using microdialysis investigated the impact of pavlovian drug CSs on behaviour and on basal and drug-stimulated transmitter levels in three terminal DA areas: NAc shell and core, and the PFC. Drug CSs elicited incentive reactions and released DA; pre-exposure to CSs potentiated DA release to drug (Schultz, 2011). Théberge et al. (2010) demonstrated that the basolateral amygdala (BLA) and the NAc core are two structures importantly involved in the reconsolidation of a cocaine–CS memory. They show that, depending on the psychological processes involved, different neural substrates within limbic cortical-ventral striatal circuitry are required for the reconsolidation of a Pavlovian memory. Milton and Everitt, 2010, have shown with more detail the memory reconsolidation mechanisms underlying conditioned reinforcement and its relationship to drug addiction and the subsequent translation to the clinic of preclinical works.

1.3 Dopamine in addiction

DA's contribution appears to chiefly cause 'wanting' for hedonic rewards, more than 'liking' of or learning of those rewards (Schultz, 2011). However, the debate continues over the precise causal contribution made by mesolimbic DA systems to reward. Recent evidence indicates that DA is neither necessary nor sufficient to mediate changes in hedonic 'liking' for sensory pleasures. Other recent evidence indicates that DA is not needed for new learning, and not sufficient to directly mediate learning by causing teaching or prediction signals. Drugs of abuse promote DA signals, short circuit and sensitize dynamic mesolimbic mechanisms that evolved to attribute incentive salience to rewards (Berridge, 2007). The potential use of drugs to enhance cognition, emotion, and executive function has engendered controversy despite the fact that few such agents exist today. Hyman (2011) provided a context for discussions based on medical, regulatory, and ethical concerns that have been raised by the possibility that enhancers will emerge from current efforts to discover drugs for neuropsychiatric disorders. Addiction coopts the brain's neuronal circuits necessary for insight, reward, motivation, and social behaviors. This functional overlap results in addicted individuals making poor choices despite awareness of the negative consequences (Volkow et al., 2011). This explains why previously rewarding life situations and the threat of judicial punishment cannot stop drug taking and why a medical rather than a retributional approach is more effective in curtailing addiction.

We describe in this chapter the effects of cannabinoids, cocaine and amphetamines on the nervous system with particular emphasis on the effects of these compounds in plasticity processes. As the DA transporter is central to the effects of these drugs, we dedicate some special attention to the physiology of this type of transporter.

2. Cannabinoids (Table 1)

The use of marijuana for recreational and medicinal purposes has resulted in a large prevalence of chronic marijuana users (WHO, 2012). In the present decade, cannabis abuse has grown more rapidly than cocaine and opiate abuse. About 147 million people, 2.5% of the world population, consume cannabis (annual prevalence) compared with 0.2% consuming cocaine and 0.6% consuming amphetamine (WHO, 2012). The most rapid growth in cannabis abuse since the 1960s has been in developed countries in North America, Western Europe and Australia (WHO, 2012). Consequences of chronic cannabinoid administration include profound behavioral tolerance and withdrawal symptoms upon drug cessation. A marijuana withdrawal syndrome is only recently gaining acceptance as being clinically significant. Similarly, laboratory animals exhibit both tolerance and dependence following chronic administration of cannabinoids. These animal models are being used to evaluate the high degree of plasticity that occurs at the molecular level in various brain regions following chronic cannabinoid exposure (Lichtman and Martin, 2005).

2.1 The endocannabinoid (eCB) signaling system

The isolation and identification, in 1964 (Gaoni and Mechoulam, 1964), of delta-9-tetrahydrocannabinol (Δ9-THC), the primary psychoactive compound in cannabis, opened the door to a whole new field of medical research. The exploration of the therapeutic potential of THC and other natural and synthetic cannabinoid compounds was paralleled by the discovery of the endocannabinoid system, comprising cannabinoid receptors and their endogenous ligands, which offered exciting new insights into brain function (see Isbell et al., 1967 for review). Besides its well-known involvement in specific brain functions, such as control of movement (Di Marzo et al., 2000; Keeney et al., 2008; Fuss and Gass, 2010), memory (Deadwyler et al., 2007; Deadwyler and Hampson, 2008) and emotions (Paule et al., 2005; Tan et al., 2010), the endocannabinoid system plays an important role in fundamental developmental processes such as cell proliferation, migration and differentiation (Trezza et al., 2008, 2012). For this reason, changes in its activity during stages of high neuronal plasticity, such as the perinatal and the adolescent period, can have long-lasting neurobehavioral consequences (see Trezza et al., 2008 for review). Two subtypes of cannabinoid receptors (CBRs) have been identified to date, the CB1 receptor, essentially located in the CNS, but also in peripheral tissues, and the CB2 receptor, found only at the periphery. Many of the effects of cannabinoids, such as delta (9)-THC (Δ9-THC), the psychoactive principle of *cannabis sativa*, and endocannabinoids (eCBs) are mediated by these two metabotropic receptors, although additional receptors may be implicated. Both CB1 and CB2 are G-protein-coupled receptors (GPCRs), primarily operating through inhibitory G proteins, and are subject to the same pharmacological influences of other GPCRs (Chaperon and Thiébot, 1999; Basavarajappa et al., 2009). Freund et al. (2003) described a fine-grain anatomical distribution of the neuronal cannabinoid receptor CB1 in brain areas, emphasizing its general presynaptic localization and role in controlling neurotransmitter release, synaptic plasticity and network activity patterns. The eCBs as ligands for these CB1 and CB2 receptors are a family of lipidic mediators that signal through the same cell surface receptors that are targeted by Δ9-THC. Unlike neurotransmitter molecules that are typically held in vesicles before synaptic release, eCBs are liberated directly after synthesis and, once released, travel in a retrograde direction to suppress presynaptic neurotransmitter release through activation of CBRs (Basavarajappa, 2007).

Drug	Effect on brain plasticity and behaviour	Structures	Autor
Marijuana or CBR1 pharmacological manipulation	Presence of an 'amotivational' syndrome	Limbic system	Paule, 2005
	Regulation of ion channels, neurotransmitter release and synaptic plasticity	Multiples brain regions	Fisar, 2009
	Profound behavioral tolerance and withdrawal symptoms	Limbic system	Lichtman & Martin, 2005
	Activity of central reward pathways alterated	VTA	Lupica et al., 2004
	↑ Risk of developing psychotic disorders in adolescence Disturbs in glutamate and GABA release	PFC	Bossong & Niesink, 2010
	↑ Density of cannabinoid CB1R binding	Corticolimbic regions	Fernandez-Espejo et al., 2009
	↓ Hippocampal encoding and the ability to encode information into short-term memory	Hippocampus	Deadwyler et al., 2007; Deadwyler and Hampson, 2008.
	Impaired LTP Facilitated LTD	Schaffer collateral-CA1 projection	Abush & Akirav, 2010
	LTD blocked with CB1R antagonist	Glutamatergic and GABAergic synapses in the striatum	Adermark et al., 2009
	Impaired LTP Decrease in LTP prevented by pharmacological inhibition or deletion of the CB1R	Hippocampus	Fan et al., 2010
	Metaplastic effects on brain cortex	Motor cortex	Koch et al., 2009
	↑Response of mPFC neurons Modulate emotional memory formation	mPFC, BLA	Laviolette & Grace, 2006
	↓ Gray matter	Cerebral cortex	Stone et al., 2011
	Blocked LTP and acquisition of conditioned fear memories by CB1R antagonist	BLA-PLC pathway	Tan et al., 2010
	Changes in cell proliferation, migration and differentiation	Central nervous system, eCB system	Trezza et al., 2008

Table 1. Plastic changes on brain regions by chronic use of marijuana, Δ9-THC administration or CB1R pharmacological manipulation.
(Abbreviations: BLA: basolateral amygdale; CB1R: type 1 cannabinoid receptor; eCB: endocannabinoid; GABA: gamma aminobutyric acid; LTP: long-term potentiation; LTD: long-term depression; mPFC: medial prefrontal cortex; PLC: prelimbic cortex; PFC: prefrontal cortex).

Recent results have suggested that the eCB system may play an important role in early neuronal development having been detected from the earliest stages of embryogenesis and throughout pre- and postnatal development. Additionally, the eCB signaling system is being found to be involved in an increasing number of neuropathological conditions, with widespread roles being invoked in neurodegenerative disorders. The fact that eCB signaling is mostly inhibitory, imparts eCBs with the ability to modulate synaptic efficacy with a wide range of functional consequences and provides unique therapeutic possibilities in central nervous system (CNS) diseases, including alcoholism, Alzheimer's disease, Parkinson's disease, Huntington's disease, and multiple sclerosis (see Basavarajappa, 2007; Basavarajappa et al., 2009 for reviews).

Although CB1 receptors are distributed throughout the brain, they are found at very high levels in the cerebellum. Edwards and Skosnik (2007) have integrated two separate literatures. The first literature demonstrates that the eCB system mediates synaptic plasticity, specifically LTD of parallel fibers at the parallel fiber-Purkinje junction in the cerebellar cortex. The second literature suggests that LTD at this junction is necessary for the acquisition of the primary dependent variable in delay eyeblink conditioning. Also, they discuss recent evidence from CB1 knockout mice, human cannabis users, and schizophrenia patients, with the expectation that translational research on the cannabinoid system will be advanced. Wiskerke et al. (2008) summarize studies in which have been used CB1R knockout mice as well as CB1 antagonists to elucidate the role of this neurotransmitter system in psychostimulant addiction. CB1 receptors appear not to be involved in psychostimulant reward, nor in the development of dependence to such substances. In contrast, the eCB system appears to play a role in the persistence of psychostimulant addiction (see Wiskerke et al., 2008 for review). Interactions of the eCB system with afferent glutamatergic and possibly dopaminergic projections to the nucleus accumbens are most likely involved and CB1 receptors seem to modulate drug-related memories, in line with the hypothesized role of the eCB system in memory-related plasticity. Together, these findings suggest that modulators of the eCB system represent a promising novel type of therapy to treat drug addiction.

2.2 The reward system

The reward circuitry of the brain consists of neurons that synaptically connect a wide variety of nuclei. Of these brain regions, the VTA and the NAc play key roles in the processing of rewarding environmental stimuli and in drug addiction. The psychoactive properties of marijuana are produced by Δ9-THC, interacting primarily with CB1 receptors in a large number of brain areas. However, it is the activation of CB1 receptors located in reward circuits that is thought to be instrumental in sustaining the self-administration of marijuana in humans, and in mediating the anxiolytic and pleasurable effects of the drug. It has been suggested that, whereas Δ9-THC alters the activity of central reward pathways in a manner that is consistent with other abused drugs, the cellular mechanism through which this occurs is likely different, relying upon the combined regulation of several afferent pathways to the VTA (see Lupica et al., 2004 for review).

2.3 Cannabis, cannabinoids and neuronal plasticity

Changes in synaptic efficacy are thought to be crucial to experience-dependent modifications of neural function. eCB-mediated plasticity encompasses many forms of transient and long-lasting synaptic depression and is found at both excitatory and inhibitory synapses. Thus, the eCB system is emerging as a major player in synaptic plasticity and, given the wide distribution of CB1 receptors in the CNS, the list of brain structures and synapses expressing eCB-mediated plasticity is likely to expand (see Chevaleyre et al., 2006 for review). Glutamate is the principal excitatory neurotransmitter in CNS and altered glutamatergic transmission during critical periods (such as first postnatal weeks) may disturb circuitry in specific brain areas (including cortex and hippocampus), particularly in experience-dependent maturation. Recent hypotheses regarding disturbances in strengthening and pruning of synaptic connections in the PFC, and the link with latent psychotic disorders suggest that cannabis-induced schizophrenia is due to a distortion of normal late postnatal brain maturation (see Bossong and Niesink, 2010 for review). In this respect, cannabis use during adolescence increases the risk of developing psychotic disorders later in life. In animals, Bossong and Niesink (2010) postulated that adolescent exposure to Δ9-THC transiently disturbs physiological control of the eCB system over glutamate and GABA release. As a result, Δ9-THC may adversely affect adolescent experience-dependent maturation of neural circuitries within prefrontal cortical areas. Depending on dose, exact time window and duration of exposure, this may ultimately lead to the development of psychoses like schizophrenia.

There is substantial evidence that cannabis abuse is a risk factor for psychosis in genetically predisposed people, may lead to a worse outcome of the disease, or it can affect normal brain development during adolescence, increasing the risk for schizophrenia in adulthood. On the other hand, the eCB system is altered in schizophrenia (increased density of CB1 receptors binding in corticolimbic regions). Dysregulation of this system can interact with neurotransmitter systems in such a way that a "cannabinoid hypothesis" can be integrated in the neurobiological hypotheses of schizophrenia. Also, there is evidence that some genetic alterations of the CNR1 gene can act as a protectant factor against schizophrenia or can induce a better pharmacological response to atypical antipsychotics (see Fernandez-Espejo et al., 2009 for review). Awareness of cannabis dependence as a clinically relevant issue has grown in recent years. Clinical and laboratory studies demonstrate that chronic marijuana smokers can experience withdrawal symptoms upon cessation of marijuana smoking and have difficulty abstaining from marijuana use. The behavioral effects that directly contribute to the maintenance of chronic marijuana smoking are reward, subjective effects, and the positive and negative reinforcing effects of marijuana, Δ9-THC or synthetic cannabinoids (Cooper and Haney, 2008).

Studies using population codes derived from ensembles of hippocampal neurons have been assessed to determine whether eCBs were active when rats performed a short-term memory task in presence or absence of CB1 receptor antagonists or agonists. Results show that eCBs, like marijuana, reduced hippocampal encoding necessary to perform long-delay trials (Deadwyler et al., 2007). Also, CB1 receptor antagonism blocked an inherent hippocampal memory encoding bias used by all animals. These findings suggest a direct relationship between the actions of cannabinoids on hippocampal processes and the ability to encode information into short-term memory Deadwyler and Hampson, 2008. Considerable evidence demonstrates that cannabinoid receptor agonists impair, whereas cannabinoid receptor antagonists improve, memory and plasticity (Ademark et al., 2009; Fan et al., 2010). However, recent studies suggest that the effects of cannabinoids on learning do not necessarily follow these simple patterns, particularly when emotional memory processes are involved. Abush and Akirav (2010) have investigated the involvement of the CB system in hippocampal learning and plasticity using behavioral task and cellular models of learning and memory (LTP and LTD). They found that i.p. agonist administration impaired LTP in the Schaffer collateral-CA1 projection, whereas an inhibitor of eCB reuptake facilitated LTD. These findings suggest that the diverse effects of the cannabinoid system on CA1 memory and plasticity cannot be categorized simply into an impairing or an enhancing effect of cannabinoid activation and deactivation, respectively. Previous studies have indicated that eCB mobilization at excitatory synapses might be regulated by afferent activation. LTD at striatal synapses is mediated by postsynaptic eCB release and presynaptic CB1 receptor activation. Adermark et al. (2009) have examined changes in synaptic strength induced by activation of L-type calcium channels at glutamatergic and gamma-aminobutyric acid (GABA)ergic synapses in the striatum. They found that the basic mechanisms for eCB signaling are the same at glutamatergic and GABAergic synapses. LTD was blocked in slices treated with AM251, a CB1 receptor antagonist, but established depression was not reversed at either glutamatergic and GABAergic synapses. It is suggested that the level of neuronal firing regulates eCB signaling by modulating release from the postsynaptic cell, as well as interacting with presynaptic mechanisms to induce LTD at both glutamatergic and GABAergic synapses in the striatum.

Chronic use of marijuana impairs synaptic plasticity and cognitive function. Fan et al. (2010) found that repeated *in vivo* exposures to Δ9-THC for 7 consecutive days significantly impaired hippocampal LTP of excitatory glutamatergic synaptic transmission, and this decrease in LTP was prevented by pharmacological inhibition or deletion of the CB1 receptor. They showed that reduced expression and function of the GluR subunits and phosphorylation of cAMP response element-binding (CREB) may underlie the impaired long-term synaptic plasticity induced by repeated *in vivo* exposure to Δ9-THC. In animal models, the CB system has been convincingly implicated in the regulation of long-lasting synaptic plasticity. Both LTP and LTD can be induced in the human motor cortex by transcranial magnetic theta burst stimulation (TBS). Koch et al. (2009) explored the potential involvement of the CB system in TBS-induced synaptic plasticity in humans with multiple sclerosis. Continuous TBS induced the expected inhibition of motor-evoked potentials (MEPs) before cannabis-based preparation exposure (Sativex), whereas it caused a persisting enhancement of MEP amplitude 4 weeks after. The LTP-like phenomenon induced by intermittent TBS was conversely unaffected by preparation exposure. These results indicate that cannabis ingredients have metaplastic effects on the motor cortex. Laviolette and Grace (2006), using *in vivo* single-unit recordings in rats, found that a CB1 receptor agonist potentiated the response of medial prefrontal cortical (mPFC) neurons to olfactory cues paired previously with a footshock, whereas this associative responding was prevented by a CB1 receptor antagonist, providing the first demonstration that CB signaling in the mPFC can modulate the magnitude of neuronal emotional learning plasticity and memory formation through functional inputs from the basolateral amygdala (BLA, Laviolette and Grace, 2006).

Individuals with an "at risk mental state" (ARMS) are greatly more susceptible to developing a psychotic illness. There has been considerable interest in the interaction between psychosis risk and substance use. Cannabis at low to moderate intake may be associated with lower gray matter in both ARMS subjects and healthy volunteers, possibly representing low-level cortical damage or change in neural plasticity (Stone et al., 2011). The CB1 receptor system is functionally involved in the processing and encoding of emotionally salient sensory information, learning and memory. The CB1 receptor is found in high concentrations in brain structures that are critical for emotional processing, including the BLA and the mPFC. Synaptic plasticity in the form of LTP within the BLA-mPFC pathway is an established correlate of exposure to emotionally salient events (Laviolette and Grace, 2006). *In vivo* LTP studies showed that systemic pretreatment with AM-251, dose-dependently block LTP along the BLA-PLC pathway, and also the behavioral acquisition of conditioned fear memories (Tan et al., 2010). Experiments show that when CB1 receptor transmission within the BLA-PFC circuit was pharmacologically blocked, this prevented the acquisition of emotionally salient associative memory. These results indicate that coordinated CB1 receptor transmission within the BLA-PFC pathway is critically involved in the encoding of emotional fear memories and modulates neural plasticity related to the encoding of emotionally salient associative learning (Tan et al., 2010).

3. Cocaine (Table 2)

Behavioral sensitization is the augmented motor-stimulant response that occurs with repeated, intermittent exposure to most drugs of abuse, including cocaine. Sensitization, which is a long-lasting phenomenon, is thought to underlie drug craving and relapse to drug use (Steketee et al., 2003). The neural mechanisms of sensitization have focused on the NAc and VTA that comprise a part of the mesolimbic DA system. Cocaine sensitization results from a decrease in inhibitory modulation of excitatory transmission from the mPFC

Drug	Effect on brain plasticity and behaviour	Structures	Autor
Cocaine	Induced behavioural sensitization	mPFC, NAc, VTA	Steketee, 2003; 2005
	Induced conditioned place preference	mPFC, NAc shell, VTA	McBride et al., 1999
	↑ BDNF, ↓ mGluR5, LTD impared	NAc shell	Huang et al., 2011
	↑ DA transmission and induce CTA	NAc shell	Di Chiara et al., 2004
	Behavioral deficits at birth and/or during adulthood	Limbic system	Lidow, 2003
	Behavioral rigidity or lack of plasticity	PFC, limbic system	Paule, 2005
	Changes in Fos expression	Lateral hipotalamus	Aston-Jones et al., 2009
	Shift from impulsivity to compulsivity during the development of addictive behavior	PFC, ventral and dorsal striatum	Belin et al., 2008
	Increased MeCP2 expression and microRNA	Dorsal striatum	Welberg, 2010

Table 2. Plastic changes on brain regions by chronic use of cocaine.
(Abbreviations: BDNF: brain-derived neurotrophic factor; CTA: conditioned taste avoidance; DA: dopamine; LTD: long-term depression; MeCP2: methyl CpG binding protein 2; mGluR5: type 5 metabotropic glutamate receptor; mPFC: medial prefrontal cortex; NAc: nucleus accumbens; VTA: ventral tegmental area).

to the VTA and NAc. Repeated cocaine exposure alters DA, gamma-aminobutyric acid (GABA), and glutamate regulation of pyramidal cell activity (Di Chiara et al., 2004; Huang et al., 2011), with cocaine-induced alterations in cortical transmission occuring in two phases. During early withdrawal from repeated cocaine exposure, changes in neurotransmitter release are thought to underlie the decreased inhibitory modulation of pyramidal projection neurons. Following more prolonged withdrawal, the attenuation in inhibitory transmission appears to occur at the receptor level (Steketee, 2005).

3.1 Cocaine and dopaminergic system

Neuroadaptation in the NAc, a central component of the mesolimbic DA system, has been implicated in the development of cocaine-induced psychomotor sensitization and relapse to cocaine seeking (Zhang et al., 2001; Anderson et al., 2003; see Steketee, 2005 for review). Recent results suggest that withdrawal from repeated cocaine exposure may result in increased brain-derived neurotrophic factor (BDNF) levels in the NAc shell, which leads to a selective downregulation of mGluR5 and thereby impairs the induction of mGluR-dependent LTD (Huang et al., 2011). The effects of BDNF on cocaine-seeking are brain region-specific. Infusion of BDNF into subcortical structures, like the NAc and VTA, enhances cocaine-induced behavioral sensitization and cocaine-seeking. Conversely, repeated administration of BDNF antiserum into the NAc during chronic cocaine self-administration attenuates cocaine-induced reinstatement. Three weeks after BDNF antiserum infusion in animals with a cocaine self-administration history, suppressed basal levels of glutamate are normalized, and a cocaine prime-induced increase in extracellular glutamate levels in the NAc is prevented (McGinty et al., 2010). Although the development of behavioral sensitization to psychostimulants such as cocaine and amphetamine is confined mainly to one nucleus in the brain, the VTA, this process is nonetheless complex, involving an interplay between neurotransmitters, neuropeptides and trophic factors. Calcium-stimulated signalling molecules, including the calcium/calmodulin-dependent protein kinases, and the Ras/mitogen-activated protein kinases, represent the major biochemical pathways whereby converging extracellular signals are integrated and amplified, resulting in the biochemical and molecular changes in DA neurons in the VTA that represent the critical neuronal correlates of the development of behavioral sensitization to psychostimulants (see Licata and Pierce, 2003 for review).

Using a mouse model of behavioral sensitization, Huang et al. (2011) showed that animals withdrawn from repeated cocaine exposure have a selective deficit in the ability to elicit metabotropic glutamate receptor (mGluR)-dependent LTD in the shell of the NAc in response to bath application of the group I mGluR agonist DHPG. Experiments demonstrated that the impaired DHPG-LTD is likely attributable to a loss of mGluR5 function. Quantitative real-time reverse transcriptase-PCR and Western blot analysis revealed significant downregulation of mGluR5, but not mGluR1, mRNA or protein levels in the NAc shell. The inhibitory effect of repeated cocaine exposure on DHPG-LTD was selectively prevented when cocaine was coadministered with a selective D1 receptor antagonist. Furthermore, the levels of BDNF protein in the NAc shell increased progressively after cocaine withdrawal, and crucially, the impairment of DHPG-LTD in the NAc shell was not found in slices from BDNF-knock-out mice after cocaine withdrawal. Recent evidence suggests that CB1Rs may represent effective targets for therapeutic agents used to treat cocaine relapse. Li et al. (2008) determinated whether CBRs play a similar role in relapse to ketamine abuse. To establish a ketamine reinstatement model in the conditioned place preference paradigm, rats were trained to develop place preference conditioned by ketamine, which was subsequently extinguished through daily exposure to the test chambers in the absence of ketamine. The effects of rimonabant, a CB1Rs antagonist, were investigated on reinstatement of ketamine-induced place preference. While ketamine priming injections reinstated extinguished place preference, rimonabant administration significantly attenuated the reinstatement of ketamine-induced place preference in a dose-dependent manner. Importantly, rimonabant itself did not produce conditioned place preference or place aversion. Since the reinstatement effects of ketamine administration were inhibited by rimonabant, these findings suggest that a CB1 receptor antagonist may be useful in preventing relapse to ketamine abuse. VTA DA neurons play a pivotal role in processing reward-related information and are involved in drug addiction and mental illness in humans (Wise, 2004). Information is conveyed to the VTA in the large part by glutamatergic afferents that arise in various brain nuclei, including the pedunculopontine nucleus (PPN).

In rat brain slice preparations, Good and Lupica (2010) found that PPN stimulation activates afferents targeting GluR2-containing AMPA receptors (AMPAR) on VTA DA neurons, and these afferents did not exhibit long-term depression (LTD). In contrast, activation of glutamate afferents onto the same DA neurons via stimulation within the VTA evoked both, excitatory postsynaptic currents EPSCs mediated by GluR2-lacking AMPARs which showed LTD, and EPSCs mediated by GluR2-containing AMPA receptors that did not express LTD. Single cocaine injections increase GluR2-lacking AMPA receptors at all glutamate synapses on VTA dopamine neurons (and this permitted LTD expression in both pathways), whereas Δ9-THC selectively increased GluR2-lacking AMPA receptors at subcortical PPN synapses (and permitted LTD in the PPN pathway only), suggesting that different drugs of abuse may exert influence over distinct sets of glutamatergic afferents to VTA DA neurons, which may thereby be associated with different reinforcing or addictive properties of these drugs. Microdialysis studies in animals have shown that addictive drugs preferentially increase extracellular DA levels in the NAc rather than in the core. However, by acting directly on the brain, drugs bypass the adaptive mechanisms (habituation) that constrain the responsiveness of accumbens shell DA to food reward, abnormally facilitating Pavlovian incentive learning and promoting the acquisition of abnormal DA-releasing properties by drug conditioned stimuli (See Di Chiara & Bassareo, 2007 for review). Thus, whereas Pavlovian food conditioned stimuli release core but not shell DA, drug conditioned stimuli do the opposite, releasing shell but not core DA. This process, which results in the acquisition of excessive incentive-motivational properties by drug conditioned stimuli has been suggested to contribute to the initiation of the drug addiction process (Imperato and Di Chiara, 1986; Di Chiara and Bassareo, 2007).

Brain imaging studies, while extending these finding to humans, have shown a correlation between psychostimulant-induced increase of extracellular DA in the striatum and self-reported measures of liking and euphoria (Volkow et al., 2002a; 2002b). Although a correlate of drug reward, independent from associative learning and performance is difficult to obtain in animals, conditioned taste avoidance (CTA) might meet these requirements. Addictive drugs induce CTA to saccharin most likely as a result of anticipatory contrast of saccharin over drug reward. Consistently with a role of DA in drug reward, D2 or combined D1/D2 receptor blockade abolishes cocaine, amphetamine and nicotine CTA. Intracranial self-administration studies with mixtures of D1 and D2 receptor agonists point to the NAc shell as the critical site of DA reward (Di Chiara et al., 2004; Bassareo et al., 2007). NAc shell DA acting on D1 receptors is also involved in Pavlovian learning through pre-trial and post-trial consolidation mechanisms and in the utilization of spatial short-term memory for goal-directed behaviour (Volkow et al., 2011). Stimulation of NAc shell DA transmission by addictive drugs is shared by a natural reward like food, but lacks its adaptive properties (habituation and inhibition by predictive stimuli). These peculiarities of drug-induced stimulation of DA transmission in the NAc shell result in striking differences in the impact of drug-conditioned stimuli on DA transmission. It is speculated that drug addiction results from the impact exerted on behavior by the abnormal DA stimulant properties acquired by drug-conditioned stimuli as a result of their association with addictive drugs (Di Chiara et al., 2004; Everitt & Robbins, 2005). Di Chiara and Bassareo (2007) have summarized that addictive drugs share with palatable food, the property of increasing extracellular DA, preferentially in the NAc shell rather than in the core. However, by acting directly on the brain, drugs bypass the adaptive mechanisms (habituation) that constrain the responsiveness of NAc shell DA to food reward, abnormally facilitating Pavlovian incentive learning and promoting the acquisition of abnormal DA-releasing properties by drug conditioned stimuli. Thus, whereas Pavlovian foods conditioned stimuli release core but not NAc shell DA, drug conditioned stimuli do the opposite, releasing shell but not NAc core DA. Neuroadaptive processes related to the chronic influence of drugs on subcortical DA might secondarily impair the function of prefronto-striatal loops, resulting in impairments in impulse control and decision making that form the basis for the compulsive feature of drug seeking and its relapsing character (Belin and Everitt, 2010).

3.2 Prenatal cocaine exposure

The extent to which cocaine abuse by pregnant women can affect development of their offspring remains a matter of significant debate. In large part, this is due to difficulties in accurate determination of the type, dose, and pattern of cocaine administration by drug abusing women as well as to difficulties in controlling for a wide range of potentially confounding variables, such as other drugs used, race, socioeconomic status, and level of prenatal care. Examination of the effects of prenatal cocaine exposure in highly controlled nonhuman primate models represents an important complement to the human research. Data obtained in several different rhesus monkey models of cocaine exposure *in utero*, has demonstrated the potential of prenatal cocaine exposure to interfere with structural and biochemical development of the brain leading to behavioral deficits at birth and/or during adulthood. The differences in the outcomes between individual models also suggest that the specific types and severity of cocaine effects are likely dependent on the route, dose, gestational period, and daily pattern of administration (see Lidow, 2003 for review). Nonhuman primates (rhesus monkeys, Macaca mulatta) have been used to study the effects of chronic drug exposures on brain function during different stages of development. In the case of the marijuana studies, exposures occurred during the adolescent period; for the cocaine studies, exposures occurred *in utero*. A battery of behavioral tasks, designed to assess aspects of motivation, visual discrimination, time perception, short-term memory, and learning, was used to monitor treatment effects. Chronic marijuana smoke exposure resulted in an 'amotivational' syndrome. *In utero* cocaine exposure was shown to cause behavioral rigidity or lack of plasticity as evidenced by the difficulty of subjects to adjust to rules changes for some tasks. These effects were seen in adult subjects suggesting that the effects of gestational cocaine exposure are long-term or permanent (see Paul, 2005 for review).

3.3 Orexins in drug-seeking

Orexins (also known as hypocretins) are recently discovered neuropeptides, synthetised exclusively in hypothalamic neurons, which have been shown to be important in narcolepsy/cataplexy and arousal (Zhou et al., 2008). Aston-Jones et al. (2009) conducted behavioral, anatomical and neurophysiological studies that show that a subset of these cells, located specifically in lateral hypothalamus (LH), are involved in reward processing and addictive behaviors. They found that Fos expression in LH orexin neurons varied in proportion to preference for cocaine or food. Recently, using a self-administration paradigm, it was discovered that the Ox1 orexin receptor antagonist, SB-334867 (SB), blocks cocaine-seeking induced by discrete or contextual cues, but not by a priming injection of cocaine. Neurophysiological studies revealed that locally applied orexin often augmented responses of VTA DA neurons to activation of the mPFC, consistent with the view that orexin facilitates activation of VTA DA neurons by stimulus-reward associations. These findings are consistent with results from others showing that orexins facilitate glutamate-mediated responses, and are necessary for glutamate-dependent long-term potentiation, in VTA DA neurons (Anston-Jones et al., 2010). Boutrel et al., (2005) show that intracerebroventricular infusions of hypocretin-1 lead to a dose-related reinstatement of cocaine seeking without altering cocaine intake in rats and elevates intracranial self-stimulation threshold. The effect was prevented by blockade of noradrenergic and corticotrophin releasing factor systems, suggesting that hypocretin-1 reinstated drug seeking through induction of a stress-like state.

3.4 Regulation of cocaine intake

Recent studies have started to reveal the contribution of epigenetic regulation to addiction-related behaviours and neuroadaptation. Two studies focused on the role of the X-linked transcriptional repressor methyl CpG-binding protein 2 (MeCP2), wich contributes to the development and function of CNS synapses. They showed that drugs of abuse regulate the expression and/or activity of MeCP2 and that this contributes to behavioural and neural responses to the drug. MeCP2, known for its role in the neurodevelopmental disorder Rett syndrome, is emerging as an important regulator of neuroplasticity in postmitotic neurons.

Cocaine addiction is commonly viewed as a disorder of neuroplasticity (White, 1996; Everitt et al., 1999; Di Chiara, 1999). Heh-In et al. (2010) identified a key role for MeCP2 in the dorsal striatum in the escalating cocaine intake seen in rats with extended access to the drug, a process that resembles in some rats subjected to extended daily access to the drug, the increasingly uncontrolled cocaine use seen in addicted humans (See Badiani et al., 2011 for review). MeCP2 regulates cocaine intake through homeostatic interactions with microRNA-212 (miR-212) to control the effects of cocaine on striatal BDNF levels. They suggest that homeostatic interactions between MeCP2 and miR-212 in dorsal striatum may be important in regulating vulnerability to cocaine addiction. Deng et al. (2010) have shown that acute viral manipulation of MeCP2 expression in the NAc bidirectionally modulates amphetamine (AMPH)-induced conditioned place preference. *Mecp2* hypomorphic mutant mice have more NAc GABAergic synapses and show deficient AMPH-induced structural plasticity of NAc dendritic spines. Furthermore, these mice show deficient plasticity of striatal immediate early gene inducibility after repeated AMPH administration. Notably, psychostimulants induce phosphorylation of MeCP2 at Ser421, a site that regulates MeCP2's function as a repressor. Phosphorylation is selectively induced in GABAergic interneurons of the NAc, and its extent strongly predicts the degree of behavioral sensitization. These data reveal new roles for MeCP2, both, in mesolimbocortical circuit development, and in the regulation of psychostimulant-induced behaviors. Also, Im et al (2010) reported increased MeCP2 expression and miR-212 (as well as miR-132) levels in the dorsal striatum in rats that had extended access to cocaine. Knocking down striatal MeCP2 expression using small hairpin RNA (shRNA) promoted the cocaine-induced increase in miR-212 expression. It also prevented the escalation of cocaine intake that normally occurs with prolonged cocaine access, an effect that could be blocked by disruption of miR-212 signalling using an antisense oligonucleotide. Furthermore, overexpressing miR-212 in the dorsal striatum, a neurobiological locus of control of habitual (Belin and Everitt 2008; Belin et al., 2009, 2010, Zapata et al., 2010, Murray et al., 2012) and compulsive (Jonkman et al., 2012) cocaine seeking, using a lentiviral vector reduced MeCP2 levels and decreased cocaine intake in rats with extended access to the drug (Im et al., 2010). These findings indicate that miR-212 and MeCP2 homeostatically regulate one another in the dorsal striatum and suggest that this interaction has a role in controlling compulsive cocaine intake. Taken together, these results suggest a role for MeCP2 in the behavioural response to psychostimulant drugs, although many questions remain regarding the undoubtedly complex mechanisms involved in its interactions with microRNAs and its modulation of synaptic plasticity (Welberg, 2010).

4. Amphetamine (Table 3)

4.1 Dopaminergic system

The fundamental principle that unites addictive drugs appears to be that each enhances synaptic DA by means that dissociate it from normal behavioral control, so that they act to reinforce their own acquisition. This occurs via the modulation of synaptic mechanisms that can be involved in learning, including enhanced excitation or disinhibition of DA neuron activity, blockade of DA reuptake, and altering the state of the presynaptic terminal to enhance evoked over basal transmission. Amphetamines offer an exception to such modulation in that they combine multiple effects to produce nonexocytotic, stimulation-independent release of neurotransmitter, via reverse-transport, independent from normal presynaptic function (Sulzer, 2011). In addition, behavioral sensitization is accompanied by an increase in postsynaptic DA receptors; an increase in DA synthesis; an increase in DA utilization and/or release (Kalivas and Stewart, 1991; Flores et al., 2011). There is strong evidence to support the notion that behavioral sensitization is due to enhanced mesotelencephalic DA release, especially upon re-exposure to the drug (Robinson and Becker, 1986). The mesocorticolimbic dopamine system, which arises in the VTA and innervates the NAc, among numerous other regions, has been implicated in processes associated with drug addiction, including behavioral sensitization. The mPFC, defined as the cortical region that has a reciprocal innervation with the mediodorsal nucleus of the thalamus, is also a terminal region of the mesocorticolimbic DA system. The mPFC contains pyramidal glutamatergic neurons that serve as the primary output of this region and mPFC transmitter systems are involved in the development of behavioral sensitization to cocaine and amphetamine (Steketee, 2003).

Drug	Effect on brain plasticity and behaviour	Structures	Autor
Amphetamine	Behavioural sensitization	VTA	Licata & Pierce, 2003; Robinson & Becker, 1986
	↑ DA transmission and induce CTA	NAc shell	Di Chiara et al., 2004
	Induced conditioned place preference Enhancement of hippocampal CaMKII activity Altered structural plasticity of dendritic spines	Hippocampus, NAc	Tan, 2008; Deng et al., 2010
	↑ postsynaptic DAR ↑ DA synthesis ↑DA utilization and/or release Release of neurotransmitter via reverse transport	Mesotelencephalic system	Robinson & Becker, 1986
	Deficits in the passive avoidance and Y-maze tests LTP alterated Pleiotrophin expression regulated	Hippocampus Limbic system	del Olmo et al., 2009; Gramage et al., 2011
	↑ Learning of environmental stimuli ↑ mGluR-dependent facilitation ↑ Susceptible to LTP induction	VTA	Ahn et al., 2010
	↑ NMDA-dependent, AMPA-mediated LTP ↓ LTD	Dopamine neurons	Schultz, 2011
	↓ PFC thickness in control females ↑ Posterior striatum thickness in control males	PFC, Striatum	Muhammad et al., 2011a
	↑ Spine density in NAc and mPFC ↓ Spine density in the OFC	NAc, mPFC, OFC	Muhammad & Kolb, 2011b; 2011c
	Psychosis, similar to paranoid schizophrenia	Limbic system	Robinson & Becker, 1986
	↑ DAT at postpubertal age by prenatal exposure	NAc	Flores et al., 2011

Table 3. Plastic changes on brain regions by chronic use of amphetamine.

(Abbreviations: AMPA: α-amino-3-hydroxy-5-methyl-4-isoxazolepropionic acid; CaMKII: Ca2+/calmodulin-dependent protein kinase II CTA: conditioned taste avoidance; DA: dopamine; DAR: dopamine receptor eCB: endocannabinoid; LTP: long-term potentiation; LTD: long-term depression; mGluR: metabotropic glutamate receptor; mPFC: medial prefrontal cortex; NAc: nucleus accumbens; NMDA: N-Methyl-D-aspartic acid; OFC: orbital frontal cortex; PFC: prefrontal cortex; VTA: ventral tegmental area).

Intracranial self-administration (ICSA) and intracranial place conditioning (ICPC) methodologies have been mainly used to study drug reward mechanisms, but they have also been applied toward examining brain reward mechanisms (McBride et al., 1999; Di Chiara et al., 2004). ICSA studies in rodents have established that the VTA is a site supporting reinforcement. The NAc also appears to have a major role in brain reward mechanisms. Rodents will self-infuse a variety of drugs of abuse (amphetamine and cocaine) into the NAc, and this occurs primarily in the shell region. ICPC studies also indicate that injection of amphetamine into the shell portion of the NAc produces conditioned place preference (CPP). Activation of the DA system within the shell subregion of the NAc appears to play a key role in brain reward mechanisms. The PFC supports the ICSA of cocaine and phencyclidine. The DA system also seems to play a role in this behavior since cocaine self-infusion into the PFC can be blocked by co-infusing a D2 antagonist. Among other regions, ICPC findings suggest that cocaine and amphetamine are rewarding in the rostral ventral pallidum (VP). Finally, substance P-mediated systems within the caudal VP (nucleus basalis magnocellularis) and serotonin systems of the dorsal and median raphe nuclei may also be important anatomical components involved in brain reward mechanisms. Overall, the ICSA and ICPC studies indicate that there are a number discrete CNS sites involved in brain reward mechanisms (McBride et al., 1999).

4.2 Amphetamine alters learning, LTP and LTD

Recent studies suggest LTP expression in locally activated glutamate synapses onto DA neurons (local Glu-DA synapses) of the midbrain VTA following a single or chronic exposure to many drugs of abuse, whereas a single exposure to cannabinoid did not significantly affect synaptic plasticity at these synapses. It is unknown whether chronic exposure of cannabis (marijuana or cannabinoids), the most commonly used illicit drug worldwide, induce LTP or LTD at these synapses. Pleiotrophin (PTN) is a cytokine with important roles in the modulation of synaptic plasticity, which levels of expression are significantly regulated by amphetamine administration. Gramage et al. (2011), have reported that amphetamine during adolescence causes long-term cognitive deficits in rats. Periadolescent amphetamine treatment daily during 10 days in normal and in PTN genetically deficient mice result in significant deficits in the passive avoidance and Y-maze tests (two tasks related to learning and memory abilities), only observed in amphetamine-pretreated PTN mutant mice. However, 13 and 26 days after the last administration, they did not find significant differences in Y-maze between amphetamine- and saline-pretreated PTN-/- mice. A significantly enhanced LTP in CA1 hippocampal slices from saline-pretreated PTN-/- mice compared with saline-pretreated PTN+/+ mice was observed. Interestingly, amphetamine pre-treatment during adolescence significantly enhanced LTP in adult PTN+/+ mice but did not cause any effect in PTN-/- mice, suggesting LTP mechanisms saturation in naïve PTN-/- mice. The data demonstrate that periadolescent amphetamine treatment causes transient cognitive deficits and long-term alterations of hippocampal LTP depending on the endogenous expression of PTN. Pleiotrophin (PTN) is a growth factor that has been shown to be involved in hippocampal synaptic plasticity and learning. Del Olmo et al. (2009), using *in vitro* electrophysiological recordings in PTN-stimulated CA1 from rat hippocampal slices, found that PTN inhibited hippocampal LTP induced by high-frequency stimulation (HFS). Also, they observed significant differences in recognition memory between PTN genetically deficient (PTN-/-) mice and wild type (WT) mice using the Y-maze test, whereas WT mice showed disruption of recognition memory,

PTN -/- mice maintained the recognition memory. The data demonstrate that PTN inhibits hippocampal LTP *in vitro* and might play a role in memory processes *in vivo*.

Synaptic plasticity in the mesolimbic DA system is critically involved in reward-based conditioning and the development of drug addiction (Schultz et al., 1998; Wise, 2004). Ca^{2+} signals triggered by postsynaptic action potentials (APs) drive the induction of synaptic plasticity in the CNS. Ahn et al. (2010) have recently proposed that enhancement of mGluR-dependent n-methyl-d-aspartate receptor (NMDAR) plasticity in the VTA may promote the learning of environmental stimuli repeatedly associated with amphetamine experience. In this study, using brain slices prepared from male rats, it was shown that repeated *in vivo* exposure to the psychostimulant amphetamine upregulates mGluR-dependent facilitation of burst-evoked Ca^{2+} signals in DA neurons of the VTA. Protein kinase A (PKA)-induced sensitization of IP_3 receptors mediates this upregulation of mGluR action. As a consequence, NMDAR-mediated transmission becomes more susceptible to LTP induction after repeated amphetamine exposure. It was also found that the magnitude of amphetamine-conditioned place preference (CPP) in behaving rats correlates with the magnitude of mGluR-dependent Ca^{2+} signal facilitation measured in VTA slices prepared from these rats.

Major drugs of abuse such as cocaine, amphetamine, morphine, heroine, nicotine, and ethanol act on glutamatergic synapses on midbrain DA neurons and lead to NMDA-dependent, AMPA-mediated long-term potentiation in DA neurons. Thus, excitatory influences on these neurons become enhanced; in particular NMDA-dependent burst firing. Amphetamine also leads to reduction of LTD in DA neurons (Swope et al., 1999; Ahn et al., 2010; Liu et al., 2010, Good and Lupica, 2010). Thus, subthreshold fluctuations of excitatory inputs to DA neurons would increase or even generate action potentials in the absence of reward, generating a false reward signal (Schultz, 2011). There are glutamatergic projections from the hippocampus to the NAc, which regulate DA transmission in this structure. Ventral hippocampal (VH) glutamatergic neurons project to the NAc shell region, whereas the dorsal hippocampus (DH) sends glutamatergic projections to the NAc core region. Tan (2008) investigated the roles of hippocampal NMDA receptors and NAc D1 receptor in AMPH-produced conditioned place preference (AMPH-CPP) in rats. It was shown that AMPH-CPP results in the enhancement of hippocampal CaMKII activity which can be impaired by NMDA antagonist (AP5). Inactivation of hippocampal area (dorsal hippocampus or ventral hippocampus) impaired AMPH-CPP, but its effect was diminished by the activation of D1 receptors in NAc core or NAc shell. It was concluded that if the deterioration of AMPH-CPP expression resembles the formation of new learning, then this active process might have been facilitated by the hippocampal NMDA receptor activations during testing.

4.3 Amphetamine sensitization

Muhammad et al. (2011a) studied the effect of postnatal tactile stimulation (TS) on juvenile behavior, adult amphetamine (AMPH) sensitization, and the interaction of TS and AMPH on prefrontal cortical (PFC) thickness and striatum size. AMPH administration resulted in gradual increase in behavioral sensitization that persisted at least for 2 weeks. However, TS rats exhibited attenuated AMPH sensitization compared to sex-matched controls. Neuroanatomically, AMPH reduced the PFC thickness in control females but enlarged the posterior striatum in control males. It was suggested that TS during development modulated the response to novel objects and altered social behaviors and attenuated AMPH-induced behavioral sensitization by preventing drug-induced structural alteration in the PFC and the striatum, brain regions implicated in drug abuse. Subsequently, these same investigators studied the effect of prenatal stress (PS) on juvenile behavior and adult AMPH sensitization, as well as the effect of the interaction between experience and drug on cortical thickness and neuronal morphology in corticolimbic regions in rats. PS did not influence AMPH-induced behavioral sensitization in either male or female rats. Moreover, PS increased the spine density in the NAc and decreased it in the mPFC without any alteration in the orbital frontal cortex (OFC). Similarly, AMPH administration increased spine density in the NAc and mPFC, whereas a decrease was observed in the OFC. However, PS prevented the drug-induced alterations in the spine density observed in controls. In sum, PS modulated juvenile behavior and altered brain morphology without influencing AMPH-induced behavioral sensitization substantially (Muhammad and Kolb, 2011b). Also, more recently Muhammad and Kolb (2011c) studied the long-term influence of maternal separation (MS) on periadolescent behavior, adult amphetamine (AMPH) sensitization, and structural plasticity in the corticolimbic regions in rats. Male and female pups, separated daily for 3h from the dam during postnatal day 3-21, were tested for periadolescent exploratory, emotional, cognitive, and social behaviors. The results showed that MS enhanced anxiety-like behavior in males. Repeated AMPH administration increased the spine density in the NAc and the mPFC, and decreased it in the OFC. MS blocked the drug-induced alteration in these regions. MS during development influenced periadolescent behavior in males, and structurally reorganized cortical and subcortical brain regions without affecting AMPH-induced behavioral sensitization.

4.4 Amphetamine and mental disorders

Individuals who repeatedly use stimulant drugs, such as AMPH, develop an AMPH-induced psychosis that is similar to paranoid schizophrenia. There has been, therefore, considerable interest in characterizing the effects of chronic stimulant drug treatment on brain and behavior in non-human animals (Robinson and Becker, 1986).

5. Dopamine transporter and neural plasticity

Dopamine (DA) is one of the most important neurotransmitters affecting fine brain processes. Dysfunction of dopaminergic neurotransmission precipitates diseases such as Parkinson's disease (PD), schizophrenia, attention-deficit hyperactivity disorder (ADHD), and drug addiction (see Zhang et al., 2010 for review). DA synthesis occurs within the DA neurons. Tyrosine is transported into the cell via amino acid carriers in the blood–brain barrier and cell membranes. Once in the intracellular space, tyrosine is hydroxylated to L-3,4-dihydroxyphenylalanine (L-DOPA) by tyrosine hydroxylase (TH). L-DOPA is then decarboxylated by aromatic acid decarboxylase (AADC) to DA (for review see Miyake et al., 2011). Extracellular DA concentration and lifetime after release is regulated by diffusion, dilution as well as reuptake (for review see Rice and Cragge, 2008). Reuptake of synaptic DA by the dopamine transporter (DAT) is the principal mechanism regulating dopamine neurotransmission, and is often used as a marker for presynaptic DA function (for review see Zhang et al., 2010). In addition DA itself can regulate DAT via its interaction with the transporter or presynaptic autoreceptors (Williams and Galli, 2006). Interestingly, a recent report has found that unmedicated bipolar disorder (BPD) subjects had significantly lower DAT availability relative to healthy controls in bilateral dorsal caudate (Anand et al., 2011), thus the authors suggest that DAT availability may be related to the neuropathology of BPD.

The DAT is a target for the development of pharmacotherapies for a number of central disorders including PD, Alzheimer's disease, schizophrenia, Tourette's syndrome, Lesch-Nyhan disease, ADHD, obesity, depression, and stimulant abuse, as well as normal aging (for review see Runyon and Carroll, 2006). DAT is located on the presynaptic membrane of DA terminals and regulates phasic DA transmission at the synapse by rapidly removing DA from the synaptic cleft through reuptake (for review see Rice and Cragge, 2008). Interestingly, this protein is expressed exclusively by DA neurons and is found extrasynaptically on DA axons in CPu and NAc (for review see Rice and Cragge, 2008). In addition, DA receptors are also predominantly extrasynaptic (Sesack et al., 1994; Yung et al., 1995; Hersch et al., 1995; Khan et al., 1998). Interestingly, several recent reports suggest that synuclein proteins have a critical role in monoamine neurotransmitter homeostasis. In addition, the physical interactions between synuclein proteins and monoamine transporters (DA, serotonin (5HT) and norepinephrine (NE) transporters) indicate an important role for the synucleins in regulating transporter function, trafficking and distribution at the DA, 5HT and NE synapses (for review see Oaks and Sidhu, 2011).

The synuclein family of proteins includes α-synuclein (α-Syn), β-synuclein (β-Syn), and γ-synuclein (γ-Syn). The genes cloned from multiple species demonstrate that synucleins, a group of prevalent pre-synaptic proteins, are highly conserved, but unique to vertebrate organisms (Surguchov, 2008). In addition, these proteins participate in numerous interactions with other proteins, lipid membranes, and nucleic acids, suggesting a possible role in the chaperoning or trafficking of biomolecules (Surguchov, 2008). Two-hybrid and immunoprecipitation experiments have identified a physical interaction between α-Syn and the carboxy terminal of DAT (Lee et al., 2001). In addition, release of DA synthesized by DA neurons in the brain requires packaging of the neurotransmitter into vesicles by the vesicular monoamine transporter 2 (VMAT2). VMAT2 co-localizes with α-Syn in the Lewy bodies of PD (Yamamoto, 2006), and overexpression of α-Syn can disrupt VMAT2 function (Surguchov, 2008). However, the influence of β-Syn and γ-Syn upon VMAT2 expression and activity are not known. Recent reports suggest that psychostimulants such as amphetamines and cocaine induced overexpression of α-synuclein (Fornai et al., 2005; Mauceli et al., 2006; Ajjimaporn et al., 2007; Klongpanichapak et al., 2008; Mukda et al., 2011, Sae-Ung et al., 2011). Interestingly, recent reports suggest that low levels of the γ-synuclein in the NAc results to an increased self-administration of cocaine in the rat (Boyer et al., 2011). In addition, cocaine induced a 1.9-fold increase in locomotor activity after overexpression of α-synuclein in the NAc (Boyer and Dreyer, 2007). It is noteworthy that the neurotoxicity induced by the psychostimulants such as amphetamine are mediated by enhanced oxidative stress and these effects are abolished by melatonin (Govitrapong et al., 2010), a main secretory product of pineal gland. Interestingly, a recent report suggested that this melatonin effect is mediated by the reduction of the overexpression of α-synuclein induced by amphetamine (Sae-Ung et al., 2011).

Amphetamines and cocaine are psychostimulants with a target in the monoaminergic system. These drugs reverse the action of monoamine transporters and enhance the release of DA as well as norepinephrine and 5-hydroxytriptamine (5-HT, serotonin) into the synaptic cleft, increasing their availability to act upon post-synaptic receptors. Reuptake blocking and decreased degradation of these neurotransmitters increases their concentrations in the synaptic cleft.

Locomotor activity induced by psychostimulants such as amphetamine is the result of increases in synaptic DA, by blocking or reversing the direction of DAT (Sulzer et al., 1995; Sulzer et al., 2005), which in turn acts on postsynaptic receptors. Interestingly, mice lacking DAT exhibit spontaneous hyperlocomotion and are unresponsive to amphetamine (Giros et al., 1996). Recent reports suggest that DAT, but not the serotonin transport (SERT), is critical in mediating the reinforcing effects of cocaine. In addition, mice lacking DAT generally failed to acquire and maintain cocaine self-administration (Thompson et al., 2009) compared to wild-type or SERT-/- mice. Therefore, DAT may play a role in mediating the long-lasting neural changes associated with drug addiction (Martin et al., 2011; Schmitt and Reith 2010).

Drug addiction involves several molecules such as CART (Cocaine-and amphetamine-regulated transcript) peptide. This peptide is a neurotransmitter believed to play a homeostatic role in psychostimulant reward and reinforcement, as well as in other processes (Jaworski and Jones, 2006; Rogge et al., 2008). CART has also been proved to attenuate locomotion induced by direct intraaccumbal injections of DA (Jaworski et al., 2003). Recently, it has been documented that the role of CART peptide in the NAc is to homeostatically regulate the activity of the DA system (Rogge et al., 2008). Moreover CART mRNA and CART peptide are found abundantly in the NAc (Douglass et al., 1995; Koylu et al., 1998). CART peptide (CART55-1029) has been shown to have minor psychostimulant-like properties when injected into the VTA, inducing locomotor activity and producing a slightly conditioned place preference (Kimmel et al., 2000, 2002). In this sense, a new study supports the idea that CART peptide reduces the effects of psychostimulants by modulating the simultaneous activation of both D1 and D2 receptors, rather than by affecting the action of any individual DA receptor (Moffett et al., 2011). In addition, our recent report suggests that prenatal amphetamine exposure produced, at postpubertal age, an enhanced DAT in the NAc (Flores et al., 2011, Figures 2, 3, 4) and children with prenatal psychostimulant exposure have greater risk of addictions (McKenna, 2011).

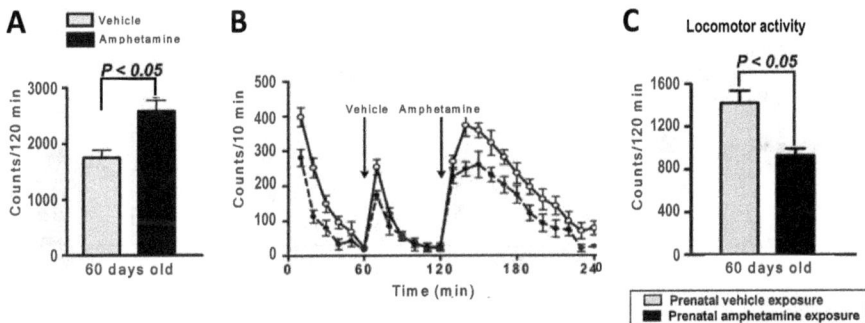

Fig. 2. Effect of amphetamine on locomotor behavior in a novel environment. A) Analysis of total activity scores revealed that the rats at PD60 were more active after amphetamine injection than their corresponding control group. B) Temporal profile of locomotor activity at PD60. C) Rats with prenatal amphetamine exposure were less active than control animals. Modified from Flores et al., 2011.

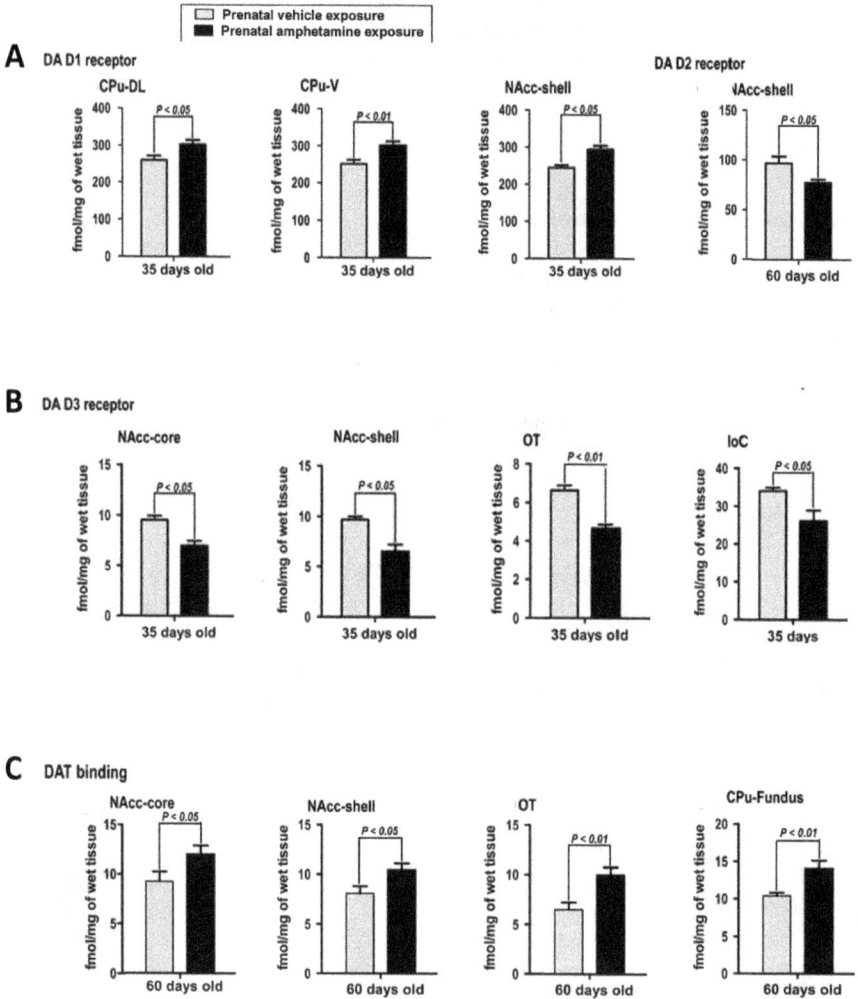

Fig. 3. Quantitative autoradiographic analysis of [3H]- SCH-23390/dopamine D1-like receptor binding, [3H]-spiperone/dopamine D2-like receptor binding, [3H]7-OHDPAT/dopamine D3 receptor binding and [3H] WIN-35428/dopamine transporter binding in prenatal amphetamine exposure (PAE)- and prenatal vehicle exposure (PVE)-rats Dopamine (DA), Postnatal (PD), nucleus accumbens (NAcc), caudate–putamen (CPu), olfactory tubercle (OT) and the island of Calleja. (Modified from Flores et al., 2011).

NAc core

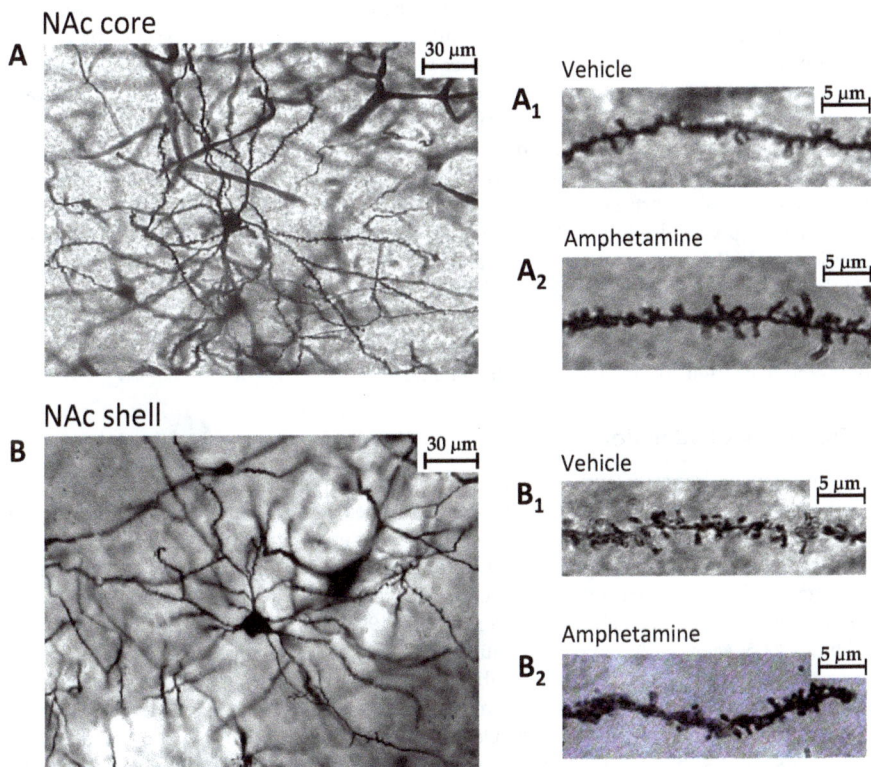

NAc shell

Fig. 4. Photomicrograph showing representative Golgi-Cox-impregnated medium spiny neurons and spines dendritic from the nucleus accumbens. Neurons in the nucleus accumbens core (A) and shell (B). The spine density is higher at PD60 in the dendritic segments from the core (A2) and shell (B2) subregions of the NAc of rats prenatally exposed to amphetamine compared to their corresponding vehicle group.

Cocaine and amphetamine may induce neural changes, including an increase in the density of spines on neuron dendrites in the NAc and PFC (Robinson and Kolb, 2004) associated with locomotor sensitization (Manev and Uz, 2009). More recently it has been suggested that cocaine-induced dendritic spine changes are correlated with the presence of DAT, because mice lacking DAT did not show an increase in dendritic spine density in the NAc (Martin et al., 211). In addition, the stereotypy induced by cocaine is also absent in this transgenic mice (Tilley and Gu, 2008). However, amphetamine and cocaine, although similar in many respects, do not produce identical patterns of structural plasticity when given to rats at different ages. In adult rats, several reports have demonstrated that cocaine increases spine density on the basilar dendrites of pyramidal neurons in the PFC, while amphetamine has either no effect or a weak effect on these dendrites. In contrast, in juvenile (P22–P34) rats, amphetamine increases spine density on the basilar dendrites of PFC (for review see Robinson and Kolb, 2011).

In conclusion, DAT is one of the principal mechanisms regulating DA neurotransmission via reuptake of synaptic DA. The psychostimulants amphetamine and cocaine alter DAT function and alter the lifetime of the DA after release. Exposure to amphetamine or cocaine produced persistent changes in the structure of dendrites and dendritic spines in brain regions such as the NAc and PFC, limbic structures related with the addictions. This structural plasticity associated with the use of the drugs of abuse results in a reorganization of synaptic connectivity in these neural systems, which may associate with addiction symptoms. Several reports suggest that cocaine abusers have an increase in DAT levels with a decrease in gray and white matter density (Gould et al., 2011), however, abstainers have significantly higher gray matter density and lower DAT levels than current cocaine users (Hanlon et al., 2011; Gould et al., 2011). Therefore, both, DAT levels and gray matter density in cocaine users reverse after prolonged abstinence (Volkow et al., 2001; Beverigde et al., 2009; Hanlon et al., 2011). Interestingly, cocaine abstainers perform better cognitive test compared to current cocaine users (Hanlon et al., 2011).

6. Treatment of addiction

Despite intensive research and significant advances, drug addictions remain a substantial public health problem. Drug addictions have a high economical cost annually and impact not only the addicted individuals, but also their spouses, children, employers, and others. Thus, the development of improved prevention and treatment strategies is of importance (Potenza et al., 2011). Learning processes have been shown to play a major role in the maintenance of addictive behaviour (Everitt et al., 1999; Robbins & Everitt, 2002; Everitt & Robbins, 2005; Moreira & Lutz, 2008; Liu et al., 2010). Humans and animals rapidly learn cues and contexts that predict the availability of addictive drugs. Once learned, these cues and contexts initiate drug seeking, craving and relapse in both animal models and clinical studies (Von der Goltz & Kiefer, 2009; De Vries & Schoffelmeer, 2005; Micale et al., 2007). Evidence suggests that several types of neuroadaptation occur, including synapse-specific adaptations of the type thought to underlie specific long-term associative memory. Thus, understanding learning and memory processes in the addicted is an important key for understanding the persistence of addiction, and it is reasonable to hypothesize that the disruption of drug-related memories may help to prevent relapses (von der Goltz & Kiefer, 2009). The study of structure-activity relationships of molecules which influence the cannabinoid system in the brain and body is crucial in the search of medical preparations with the therapeutic effects of the phytocannabinoids without the negative effects on cognitive function attributed to cannabis (see Fisar, 2009 for review).

As discussed before, cannabinoid CB1Rs are novel targets for a new class of therapeutic agents used to treat drug addiction. Blockade of the CB1 receptor is particularly effective in reducing cue-induced reinstatement of drug seeking, an animal analogue of cue-induced relapse in human addicts (See Gardner, 2002, 2005, 2011 for review). These relapse-preventing properties are observed with different classes of abused drug (i.e. psychostimulants, opiates, nicotine and alcohol). In addition, recent evidence indicates a more general role of CB1 receptors in reward-related memories, which is consistent with the proposed role of endocannabinoids in memory-related plasticity. Relapse-preventing actions and inhibitory effects on weight gain were confirmed recently in clinical trials with the CB1 antagonist rimonabant (De Vries and Schoffelmeer, 2005). Preclinical results provide support for the suggestion that targeting the endocannabinoid system may aid in the treatment of disorders associated with impaired extinction-like processes, such as post-traumatic stress disorder (Abush and Akirav, 2010). Liu et al. (2010) provided evidence that NMDA receptor-dependent synaptic depression at VTA dopamine circuitry requires GluR2 endocytosis, also suggest an essential contribution of such synaptic depression to cannabinoid-associated addictive learning, in addition to pointing to novel pharmacological strategies for the treatment of cannabis addiction. They found in rats that chronic cannabinoid exposure activates VTA CB1 receptors to induce transient neurotransmission depression at VTA local Glu-DA synapses through activation of NMDA receptors and subsequent endocytosis of AMPA receptor GluR2 subunits. A GluR2-derived peptide blocks cannabinoid-induced VTA synaptic depression and conditioned place preference, i.e., learning to associate drug exposure with environmental cues.

6.1 Pharmacological treatments and targets

Multiple pharmacological targets have been identified for the treatment of addictive disorders. "Classic" approaches tend to target the drug "reward" system, such as normalization of function through agonist approaches and negative reinforcement strategies. Agonist medications have their main impact on the same types of neurotransmitter receptors as those stimulated by abused substances. Most notably, dextroamphetamine has reduced drug use in short-term clinical trials in cocaine and methamphetamine users. The long-term safety and abuse liability of amphetamines as a treatment for cocaine addiction remains to be determined. Another example of an agonist approach for cocaine dependence is modafinil, a weak DAT inhibitor and increases synaptic DA levels, which has stimulant-like effects. On other hand, antagonists block the effects of drugs by either pharmacological or pharmacokinetic mechanisms. More recently, immunotherapies have been developed for the treatment of cocaine and methamphetamine addictions. The antibodies produced by immunotherapies sequester the drug in the circulation and reduce the amount of drug and the speed at which it reaches the brain. A potentially promising target for agonist and antagonist treatment of cocaine addiction is the D3 dopamine receptor. D3 partial agonists can act like agonists and stimulate DA receptors when endogenous levels of dopamine are low, as in cocaine withdrawal. An important limitation of vaccines is that the antibodies produced are specific for a given drug of abuse, a characteristic that will limit their clinical efficacy in polydrug abusers.

Drug addiction is associated with adaptive changes in multiple neurotransmitter systems in the brain. These adaptive changes are thought to underlie the negative reinforcing effects of abstinence from drug use that are clinically observed as withdrawal symptoms, craving for drug use, and negative mood states like anhedonia and anxiety (Hasin et al., 2007; Treadway and Zald, 2011). Examples of medications targeting negative reinforcement of drugs include methadone or buprenorphine, drugs that relieve opioid withdrawal symptoms. Cocaine users with more severe withdrawal symptoms respond more favorably to propranolol, a beta-adrenergic antagonist (Kampman et al., 2006). Several agents targeting glutamate system are also under investigation as potential treatment medications. Memantine, a noncompetitive NMDA glutamate receptor antagonist, may be efficacious and operate by reducing cognitive measures of compulsivity (Grant et al., 2010). However, clinical trials with an NMDA receptor antagonist have demonstrated negative findings for cocaine dependence (Bisaga et al., 2010).

Activation of cannabinoid receptors on synaptic terminals results in regulation of ion channels, neurotransmitter release and synaptic plasticity. Neuromodulation of synapses by the cannabinoids is proving to have a wide range of functional effects, making them potential targets as medical preparations in a variety of illnesses, including some mental disorders and neurodegenerative illnesses (see Fisar, 2009 for review).

In conclusion, the review of existing evidences indicates that addictive drugs induce synaptic plasticity at DA system and produce changes in DA at different target structures of the brain, affecting glutamateric, GABAergic transmission and LTP and LTD processes (Figure 5). New research will without doubt shed light onto the mechanisms of addiction induction and better design of drug-addiction treatments.

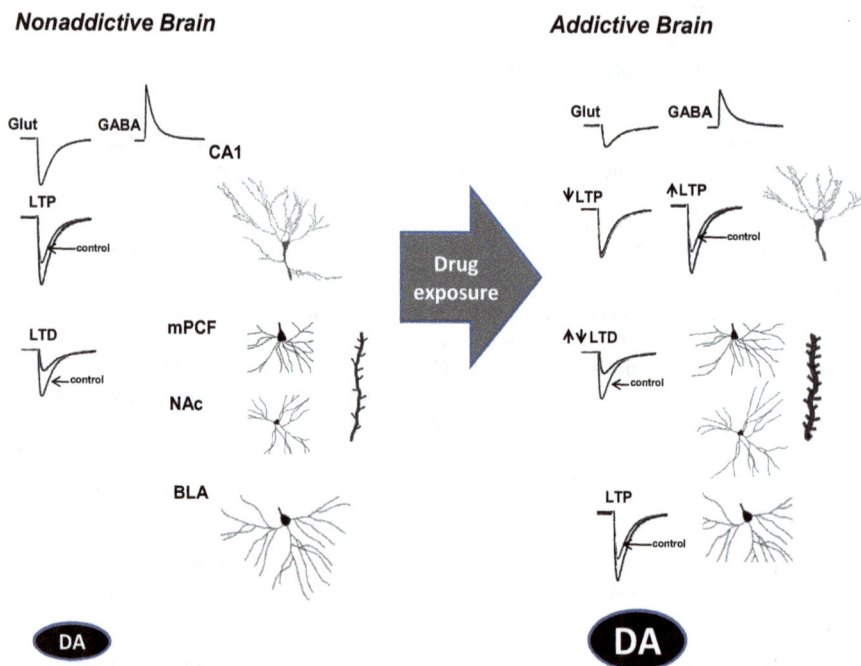

Fig. 5. Addictive drug affects DA levels, glutamatergic and GABAergic transmission and LTP and LTD processes at different brain structures. DA: dopamine; CA1: CA1 region of the hippocampus; PFC, prefrontal cortex; NAc: accumbens nucleus; BLA: basolateral amygdala.

7. References

Abush, H. & Akirav, I. (2010). Cannabinoids modulate hippocampal memory and plasticity. *Hippocampus*, Vol.20, No.10, pp. 1126-1138.

Adermark, L.; Talani, G. & Lovinger, D.M. (2009). Endocannabinoid-dependent plasticity at GABAergic and glutamatergic synapses in the striatum is regulated by synaptic activity. *Eur J Neurosci.*, Vol.29, No.1, pp. 32-41.

Ahn K.C.; Bernier, B.E.; Harnett, M.T. & Morikawa, H. (2010). IP3 receptor sensitization during in vivo amphetamine experience enhances NMDA receptor plasticity in dopamine neurons of the ventral tegmental area. *J Neurosci.*, Vol.30, No.19, pp. 6689-6699.

Ajjimaporn, A.; Phansuwan-Pujito, P.; Ebadi M. & Govitrapong, P. (2007). Zinc protects SK-N-SH cells from methamphetamine-induced alpha-synuclein expression. *Neurosci Lett.*, No.419, pp. 59-63.

Anand, A.; Barkay, G.; Dzemidzic, M.; Albrecht, D.; Karne, H.; Zheng, Q.H,; Hutchins, G.D.; Normandin, M.D. & Yoder, K.K. (2011). Striatal dopamine transporter availability in unmedicated bipolar disorder. *Bipolar Disord.*, No.13, pp. 406-413.

Anderson, S.M.; Bari, A.A. & Pierce, R.C. (2003). Administration of the D1-like dopamine receptor antagonist SCH-23390 into the medial nucleus accumbens shell attenuates cocaine priming-induced reinstatement of drug-seeking behavior in rats. *Psychopharmacology*, No. 168, pp.132-138.

Aston-Jones, G.; Smith, R.J.; Moorman, D.E. & Richardson, K.A. (2009). Role of lateral hypothalamic orexin neurons in reward processing and addiction. *Neuropharmacol.*, No.56, Suppl 1, pp. 112-121.

Aston-Jones, G.; Smith, R.J.; Sartor, G.C.; Moorman, D.E.; Massi, L.; Tahsili-Fahadan, P. & Richardson, K.A. (2010). Lateral hypothalamic orexin/hypocretin neurons: A role in reward-seeking and addiction. *Brain Res.*, Vol.16, No.1314, pp. 74-90.

Badiani, A.; Belin, D.; Epstein, D.; Calu, D. & Shaham, Y. (2011). Opiate versus psychostimulant addiction: the differences do matter. *Nat Rev Neurosci.*, Vol. 12, No. 11, pp. 685-70.

Basavarajappa, B.S. (2007). Neuropharmacology of the endocannabinoid signaling system-molecular mechanisms, biological actions and synaptic plasticity. *Curr Neuropharmacol.*, Vol.5, No.2, pp. 81-97.

Basavarajappa, B.S.; Nixon, R.A. & Arancio, O. (2009). Endocannabinoid system: emerging role from neurodevelopment to neurodegeneration. *Mini Rev Med Chem.*, Vol.9, No.4, pp. 448-462.

Bassareo, V.; De Luca, M.A. & Di Chiara, G. (2007). Differential impact of pavlovian drug conditioned stimuli on in vivo dopamine transmission in the rat accumbens shell and core and in the prefrontal cortex. *Psychopharmacol. (Berl)*, Vol.191, No.3, pp. 689-703.

Belin, D.; Mar, A.C.; Dalley, J.W.; Robbins, T.W. & Everitt, B.J. (2008). High impulsivity predicts the switch to compulsive cocaine-taking. *Science.* Vol. 320, No. 5881, pp. 1352-5.

Belin, D.; Jonkman, S.; Dickinson, A., Robbins, T. & Everitt, B. (2009) Parallel and interactive learning processes within the basal ganglia: Relevance for the understanding of addiction. *Behav. Brain Res.* No. 199, Vol. 11, pp. 89–102.

Belin, D. & Everitt, B.J. (2010). Drug Addiction: The Neural and Psychological Basis of a Compulsive Incentive Habit. In: *Handbook of Basal ganglia. Structure and Function.* Steiner, H. & Tseng, K. Eds. Academic Press.

Berridge, K.C. (2007). The debate over dopamine's role in reward: the case for incentive salience. *Psychopharmacol. (Berl)*, Vol.191, No.3, pp. 391-431.

Beveridge, T.J.; Smith, H.R.; Nader, M.A. & Porrino, L.J. (2009). Abstinence from chronic cocaine self-administration alters striatal dopamine systems in rhesus monkeys. Neuropsychopharmacol., Vol. 34, No. 5, pp. 1162-1171.

Bierut, L.J. (2011). Genetic Vulnerability and Susceptibility to Substance Dependence. Neuron, Vol.69, No.4, pp. 618-627.

Bossong, M.G. & Niesink, R.J. (2010). Adolescent brain maturation, the endogenous cannabinoid system and the neurobiology of cannabis-induced schizophrenia. Prog Neurobiol., Vol.92, No.3, pp. 370-385.

Boutrel B, Kenny PJ, Specio SE, Martin-Fardon R, Markou A, Koob GF, de Lecea L. (2005). Role for hypocretin in mediating stress-induced reinstatement of cocaine-seeking behavior. Proc Natl Acad Sci., No. 102, Vol. 52, pp. 19168-19173.

Boyer, F.; Balado, E.; Piazza, P.V.; Dreyer, J.L. & Deroche-Gamonet, V. (2011). A decrease in gamma-synuclein expression within the nucleus accumbens increases cocaine intravenous self-administration in the rat. Addict Biol., No.16, pp. 120-123.

Boyer, F. & Dreyer, J.L. (2007). Alpha-synuclein in the nucleus accumbens induces changes in cocaine behaviour in rats. Eur J Neurosci., No.26, pp. 2764-2776.

Chaperon, F. & Thiébot, M.H. (1999). Behavioral effects of cannabinoid agents in animals. Crit Rev Neurobiol., Vol.13, No.3, pp. 243-281.

Chevaleyre, V.; Takahashi, K.A. & Castillo, P.E. (2006). Endocannabinoid-mediated synaptic plasticity in the CNS. Annu Rev Neurosci., No.29, pp. 37-76.

Cooper, Z.D. & Haney, M. (2008). Cannabis reinforcement and dependence: role of the cannabinoid CB1 receptor. Addict Biol., Vol.13, No.2, pp. 188-195.

Dalley, J.W.; Fryer, T.D.; Brichard, L.; Robinson, E.S.; Theobald, D.E.; Lääne, K.; Peña, Y.; Murphy, E.R.; Shah, Y.; Probst, K.; Abakumova, I.; Aigbirhio, F.I.; Richards, H.K.; Hong, Y.; Baron, J.C.; Everitt, B.J. & Robbins, T.W. (2007). Nucleus accumbens D2/3 receptors predict trait impulsivity and cocaine reinforcement. Science, Vol. 15, No. 5816, pp. 1267-70.

Dalley, J.W.; Everitt, B.J. & Robbins, T.W. (2011). Impulsivity, Compulsivity, and Top-Down Cognitive Control. Neuron Vol.69, No.4, pp. 680-694.

Deadwyler, S.A.; Goonawardena, A.V. & Hampson, R.E. (2007). Short-term memory is modulated by the spontaneous release of endocannabinoids: evidence from hippocampal population codes. Behav Pharmacol., Vol.18, No.5-6, pp. 571-80.

Deadwyler, S.A. & Hampson, R.E. (2008). Endocannabinoids modulate encoding of sequential memory in the rat hippocampus. Psychopharmacol (Berl)., Vol.198, No.4, pp. 577-586.

Del Olmo, N.; Gramage, E.; Alguacil, L.F.; Pérez-Pinera, P.; Deuel, T.F. & Herradón, G. (2009). Pleiotrophin inhibits hippocampal long-term potentiation: a role of pleiotrophin in learning and memory. Growth Factors, Vol.27, No.3, pp. 189-194.

Deng, J.V.; Rodriguiz, R.M.; Hutchinson, A.N.; Kim, I.K.; Wetsel, W.C. & West, A.E. (2010). MeCP2 in the nucleus accumbens contributes to neural and behavioral responses to psychostimulants. Nature Neurosci., No.13, pp, 1128-1136.

De Vries, T.J. & Schoffelmeer, A.N. (2005). Cannabinoid CB1 receptors control conditioned drug seeking. Trends Pharmacol Sci., Vol.26, No.8, pp. 420-426.

Di Chiara, G. (1999). Drug addiction as dopamine-dependent associative learning disorder. Eur J Pharmacol., No. 375, pp. 13–30.

Di Chiara, G.; Bassareo, V.; Fenu, S.; De Luca, M.A.; Spina, L.; Cadoni, C.; Acquas, E.; Carboni, E.; Valentini, V. & Lecca, D. (2004). Dopamine and drug addiction: the nucleus accumbens shell connection. *Neuropharmacol.*, No.47, Suppl 1, pp. 227-241.

Di Chiara, G. & Bassareo, V. (2007). Reward system and addiction: what dopamine does and doesn't do. *Curr Opin Pharmacol.*, Vol.7, No.1, pp. 69-76.

Di Marzo, V.; Hill M.P.; Bisogno, T.; Crossman, A.R. & Brotchie, J.M. (2000). Enhanced levels of endogenous cannabinoids in the globus pallidus are associated with a reduction in movement in an animal model of Parkinson's disease. *FASEB J.*, Vol. 14, No. 10, pp.1432-1438.

Economidou, D.; Pelloux, Y., Robbins, T.W.; Dalley, J.W. & Everitt, B.J. (2009) High impulsivity predicts relapse to cocaine-seeking after punishment-induced abstinence. Biol Psychiatry. Vol. 65, No. 10, pp. 851-6.

Edwards, C.R. & Skosnik, P.D. (2007). Cerebellar-dependent learning as a neurobehavioral index of the cannabinoid system. *Crit Rev Neurobiol.*, Vol.19, No.1, pp. 29-57.

Everitt, B. J.; Parkinson, J.A.; Olmstead, M.C.; Arroyo, M.; Robledo, P. & Robbins, T.W. (1999). Associative processes in addiction and reward. The role of amygdala-ventral striatal subsystems. *Ann. NY Acad. Sci.*, No. 877, pp. 412–438.

Everit, B.J. & Robbins, T.W. (2005). Neural systems of reinforcement for drug addiction: from actions to habits to compulsion. Nat Neurosci., Vol. 7, No. 8, pp.1481-1489.

Fan, N.; Yang, H.; Zhang, J. & Chen, C. (2010). Reduced expression of glutamate receptors and phosphorylation of CREB are responsible for in vivo Delta9-THC exposure-impaired hippocampal synaptic plasticity. *J Neurochem.*, Vol.112, No.3, pp. 691-702.

Fernandez-Espejo, E.; Viveros, M.P.; Núñez, L.; Ellenbroek, B.A. & Rodriguez de Fonseca, F. (2009). Role of cannabis and endocannabinoids in the genesis of schizophrenia. *Psychopharmacol (Berl).*, Vol.206, No.4, pp. 531-549.

Fisar, Z. (2009). Phytocannabinoids and endocannabinoids. *Curr Drug Abuse Rev.*, Vol.2, No.1, pp. 51-75.

Flores, G.; de Jesús, Gómez-Villalobos M. & Rodríguez-Sosa, L. (2011). Prenatal amphetamine exposure effects on dopaminergic receptors and transporter in postnatal rats. *Neurochem Res.*, No.36, pp. 1740-1749.

Fornai, F.; Lenzi, P.; Ferrucci, M.; Lazzeri, G.; di Poggio, A.B.; Natale, G.; Busceti, C.L.; Biagioni, F.; Giusiani, M.; Ruggieri, S. & Paparelli, A. (2005). Occurrence of neuronal inclusions combined with increased nigral expression of alpha-synuclein within dopaminergic neurons following treatment with amphetamine derivatives in mice. *Brain Res Bull.*, No.65, pp. 405-413.

Freund, T.F.; Katona, I. & Piomelli, D. (2003). Role of endogenous cannabinoids in synaptic signaling. *Physiol Rev.*, Vol.83, No.3, pp. 1017-1066.

Fuss, J. & Gass, P. (2010). Endocannabinoids and voluntary activity in mice: runner's high and long-term consequences in emotional behaviors. *Exp Neurol.* Vol. 224, No. 1, pp. 103-105.

Gaoni, Y. & Mechoulam, R. (1964). Isolation, structure and partial synthesis of an active constituent of hashish. J Am Chem Soc., No. 86, p.1646.

Gardner, E.L. (2002). Addictive potential of cannabinoids: the underlying neurobiology. *Chem Phys Lipids.*, Vol. 121, No. 1-2, pp. 267-290.

Gardner, E.L. (2005). Endocannabinoid signaling system and brain reward: emphasis on dopamine. *Pharmacol Biochem Behav.*, Vol. 81, No. 2, pp. 263-284.

Gardner, E.L. (2011). Addiction and brain reward and antireward pathways. *Adv Psychosom Med.*, No.30, pp. 22-60.

Giros, B.; Jaber, M.; Jones, S.R.; Wightman, R.M. & Caron, M.G. (1996). Hyperlocomotion and indifference to cocaine and amphetamine in mice lacking the dopamine transporter. *Nature*, No.379, pp. 606-612.

Govitrapong, P.; Boontem, P.; Kooncumchoo, P.; Pinweha, S.; Namyen, J.; Sanvarinda, Y. & Vatanatunyakum, S. (2010). Increased blood oxidative stress in amphetamine users. *Addict Biol.*, Vol.15, No.1, pp. 100-102.

Good, CH. & Lupica, C.R. (2010). Afferent-specific AMPA receptor subunit composition and regulation of synaptic plasticity in midbrain dopamine neurons by abused drugs. *J Neurosci.*, Vol.30, No.23, pp. 7900-7909.

Gould, R.W.; Porrino, L.J. & Nader, M.A. (2011). Nonhuman Primate Models of Addiction and PET Imaging: Dopamine System Dysregulation. Curr Top Behav Neurosci. DIO: 10.1007/7854.

Gramage, E.; Del Olmo, N.; Fole, A.; Martín, Y.B. & Herradón, G. (2011). Periadolescent amphetamine treatment causes transient cognitive disruptions and long-term changes in hippocampal LTP depending on the endogenous expression of pleiotrophin. *Addict Biol.* 2011, August 4, doi: 10.1111/j.1369-1600.2011.00362.x.

Hasin, D.S.; Stinson, F.S.; Ogburn, E. & Grant, B.F. (2007). Prevalence, correlates, disability, and comorbidity of DSM-IV alcohol abuse and dependence in the United States: Results from the National Epidemiologic Survey on Alcohol and Related Conditions. *Arch. Gen. Psychiatry*, No. 64, pp. 830–842.

Hersch, S.M.; Ciliax, B.J.; Gutekunst, C.A.; Rees, H.D.; Heilman, C.J.; Yung, K.K.; Bolam, J.P.; Ince, E.; Yi, H. & Levey, A.I. (2005). Electron microscopic analysis of D1 and D2 dopamine receptor proteins in the dorsal striatum and their synaptic relationships with motor corticostriatal afferents. *J Neurosci.*, No.15, pp. 5222-5237.

Huang, C.C.; Yeh, C.M.; Wu, M.Y.; Chang, A.Y.; Chan, J.Y.; Chan, S.H. & Hsu, K.S. (2011). Cocaine withdrawal impairs metabotropic glutamate receptor-dependent long-term depression in the nucleus accumbens. *J Neurosci.*, Vol.31, No.11, pp. 4194-4203.

Hyman, S.E. & Malenka, R.C. (2001). Addiction and the brain: the neurobiology of compulsion and its persistence. *Nat Rev Neurosci.*, Vol.2, No.10, pp. 695-703.

Hyman, S.E. (2005). Addiction: A Disease of Learning and Memory. *Am J Psychiatry*, No.162, pp. 1414-1422.

Hyman, S.E.; Malenka, R.C. & Nestler, E.J. (2006). Neural mechanisms of addiction: the role of reward-related learning and memory. *Annu Rev Neurosci.*, No.29, pp. 565-598.

Hyman, S.E. (2011). Cognitive enhancement: promises and perils. *Neuron*, Vol.69, No.4, pp. 595-598.

Holden, C. (2010). Psychiatry. Behavioral addictions debut in proposed DSM-V. *Science*, No. 327, pp. 935.

Im, H.I.; Hollander, J.A.; Bali, P. & Kenny, P.J. (2010). MeCP2 controls BDNF expression and cocaine intake through homeostatic interactions with microRNA-212. *Nature Neurosci.* No.13, pp. 1120–1127.

Imperato, A. & Di Chiara, G. (1986). Preferential stimulation of dopamine release in the nucleus accumbens of freely moving rats by ethanol. *J Pharmacol Exp Ther.*, No. 239, pp. 219–228.

Isbell, H.; Gorodetzsky, C.W.; Jasinski, D., Claussen, U.; Spulak, F.V. & Korte, F. (1967). Effects of (-)Delta (9)-Trans-Tetrahydrocannabinol in Man. *Psychopharmacologia (Berl.)*, No. 11, pp. 184-188.

Jaworski, J.N.; Kozel, M.A.; Philpot, K.B. & Kuhar, M.J. (2003). Intra-accumbal injection of CART (cocaine-amphetamine regulated transcript) peptide reduces cocaine-induced locomotor activity. *J Pharmacol Exp Ther.*, No.307, pp. 1038-1044.

Jaworski, J.N. & Jones, D.C. (2004). The role of CART in the reward/reinforcing properties of psychostimulants. *Peptides*, No.27, pp. 1993-2004.

Jonkman, S.; Pelloux, Y. & Everitt, B.J. (2012) Differential roles of the dorsolateral and midlateral striatum in punished cocaine seeking. *J Neurosci.*, No. 32, pp. 4645–4650.

Kalivas, P.W. & Stewart, J. (1991) Dopamine transmission in the initiation and expression of drug- and stress-induced sensitization of motor activity. *Brain Res Rev.*, No. 16, pp. 223–244.

Kandel, E.R. (2004). The Molecular Biology of Memory Storage: A Dialogue Between Genes and Synapses. *Science*, No. 294, pp. 1030-1038.

Kendler, K.S., Prescott C.A., J. Myers, J. & Neale, M.C. (2003). The structure of genetic and environmental risk factors for common psychiatric and substance use disorders in men and women. *Arch. Gen. Psychiatry*, 60, pp. 929–937.

Keeney, B.K.; Raichlen, D.A.; Meek, T.H.; Wijeratne, R.S.; Middleton, K.M.; Gerdeman, G.L. & Garland, T. Jr. (2008). Differential response to a selective cannabinoid receptor antagonist (SR141716: rimonabant) in female mice from lines selectively bred for high voluntary wheel-running behaviour. *Behav Pharmacol.*, Vol. 19, No. 8, pp. 812-20.

Kenny, P.J. (2011). Reward Mechanisms in Obesity: New Insights and Future Directions. *Neuron*, Vol.69, No.4, pp. 664-679.

Khan, Z.U.; Gutiérrez, A.; Martín, R.; Peñafiel, A.; Rivera, A. & De La Calle, A. (1998). Differential regional and cellular distribution of dopamine D2-like receptors: an immunocytochemical study of subtype-specific antibodies in rat and human brain. *J Comp Neurol.*, No.402, pp. 353-371.

Kimmel, H.L.; Gong, W.; Vechia, S.D.; Hunter, R.G. & Kuhar, M.J. (2000). Intra-ventral tegmental area injection of rat cocaine and amphetamine-regulated transcript peptide 55-102 induces locomotor activity and promotes conditioned place preference. *J Pharmacol Exp Ther.*, No.294, pp. 784-792.

Kimmel, H.L.; Thim, L. & Kuhar, M.J. (2002). Activity of various CART peptides in changing locomotor activity in the rat. *Neuropeptides*, No.36, pp. 9-12.

Klongpanichapak, S.; Phansuwan-Pujito, P.; Ebadi, M. & Govitrapong, P. (2011). Melatonin inhibits amphetamine-induced increase in alpha-synuclein and decrease in phosphorylated tyrosine hydroxylase in SK-N-SH cells. *Neurosci Lett.*, No. 436, pp. 309-313.

Koch, G.; Mori, F.; Codecà, C.; Kusayanagi, H.; Monteleone, F.; Buttari, F.; Fiore, S.; Bernardi, G. & Centonze, D. (2009). Cannabis-based treatment induces polarity-reversing plasticity assessed by theta burst stimulation in humans. *Brain Stimul.*, Vol.2, No.4, pp. 229-233.

Laviolette, S.R. & Grace, A.A. (2006). Cannabinoids Potentiate Emotional Learning Plasticity in Neurons of the Medial Prefrontal Cortex through Basolateral Amygdala Inputs. *J Neurosci.*, Vol.26, No.24, pp. 6458-6468.

Lee, F.J.; Liu, F.; Pristupa, Z.B. & Niznik, H.B. (2001). Direct binding and functional coupling of alpha-synuclein to the dopamine transporters accelerate dopamine-induced apoptosis. *FASEB J.*, No.15, pp. 916-926.

Licata, S.C. & Pierce, R.C. (2003). The roles of calcium/calmodulin-dependent and Ras/mitogen-activated protein kinases in the development of psychostimulant-induced behavioral sensitization. *J Neurochem.*, Vol.85, No.1, pp. 14-22.

Lichtman, A.H. & Martin, B.R. (2005). Cannabinoid tolerance and dependence. *Handb Exp Pharmacol.*, No.168, pp. 691-717.

Lidow, M.S. (2003). Consequences of prenatal cocaine exposure in nonhuman primates. *Brain Res Dev Brain Res.*, Vol.147, No.1-2, pp. 23-36.

Li, F; Fang, Q.; Liu, Y.; Zhao, M.; Li, D.; Wang, J. & Lu, L. (2008). Cannabinoid CB(1) receptor antagonist rimonabant attenuates reinstatement of ketamine conditioned place preference in rats. *Eur J Pharmacol.*, Vol.589, No.1-3:122-126.

Liu, Z.; Han, J.; Jia, L.; Maillet, J.C.; Bai, G.; Xu, L.; Jia, Z.; Zheng, Q.; Zhang, W.; Monette, R.; Merali, Z.; Zhu, Z.; Wang, W.; Ren, W. & Zhang, X. (2010). Synaptic neurotransmission depression in ventral tegmental dopamine neurons and cannabinoid-associated addictive learning. *PLoS One*, Vol.5, No.12, e15634.

Lupica, C.R.; Riegel, A.C. & Hoffman, A.F. (2004). Marijuana and cannabinoid regulation of brain reward circuits. *Br J Pharmacol.*, Vol.143, No.2, pp. 227-234.

Lüscher, C. & Malenka, R.C. (2011). Drug-Evoked Synaptic Plasticity in Addiction: From Molecular Changes to Circuit Remodeling. *Neuron*, Vol.69, No.4, pp. 650-663.

Manev, H. & Uz, T. (2009). Dosing time-dependent actions of psychostimulants. *Int Rev Neurobiol.*, No.88, pp. 25-41.

Martin, B.J.; Naughton, B.J.; Thirtamara-Rajamani, K.; Yoon, D.J.; Han, D.D.; Devries, A.C. & Gu, H.H. (2011). Dopamine transporter inhibition is necessary for cocaine-induced increases in dendritic spine density in the nucleus accumbens. *Synapse*, No.65, pp. 490-496.

Mauceli, G.; Busceti, C.I.; Pellegrini, A.; Soldani, P.; Lenzi, P.; Paparelli, A. & Fornai, F. (2006). Overexpression of alpha-synuclein following methamphetamine: is it good or bad? *Ann N Y Acad Sci.*, No.1074, pp. 191-197.

McBride, W.J.; Murphy, J.M. & Ikemoto, S. (1999). Localization of brain reinforcement mechanisms: intracranial self-administration and intracranial place-conditioning studies. *Behav Brain Res.*, Vol.101, No.2, 129-152.

McGinty, J.F.; Whitfield, T.W. Jr & Berglind, W.J. (2010). Brain-derived neurotrophic factor and cocaine addiction. *Brain Res.*, No.1314, pp. 183-93.

McKenna, S.A. (2011). Reproducing Hegemony: The Culture of Enhancement and Discourses on Amphetamines in Popular Fiction. *Cult Med Psychiatry*, Vol. 35, No.1, pp. 90-97.

Micale, V.; Mazzola, C. & Drago, F. (2007). Endocannabinoids and neurodegenerative diseases. *Pharmacol Res.*, Vol. 56, No. 5, pp. 382-392.

Milton, A.L. & Everitt, B.J. (2010). The psychological and neurochemical mechanisms of drug memory reconsolidation: implications for the treatment of addiction. *Eur J Neurosci.* Vol. 31, No.12, pp. 2308-19.

Miyake, N.; Thompson, J.; Skinbjerg, M. & Abi-Dargham, A. (2011). Presynaptic dopamine in schizophrenia. *CNS Neurosci Ther.*, No.17, pp. 104-109.

Moffett, M.C.; Song, J. & Kuhar, M.J. (2011). CART peptide inhibits locomotor activity induced by simultaneous stimulation of D1 and D2 receptors, but not by stimulation of individual dopamine receptors. *Synapse*, No.65, pp. 1-7.

Montague, P.R.; Hyman, S.E. & Cohen J.D. (2004). Computational roles for dopamine in behavioural control. *Nature*, No. 431, pp. 760-767.

Moreira, F.A. & Lutz, B. (2008). The endocannabinoid system: emotion, learning and addiction. *Addict Biol.*, Vol.13, No. 2, pp.196-212.

Muhammad, A.; Hossain, S.; Pellis, S.M. & Kolb, B. (2011a). Tactile stimulation during development attenuates amphetamine sensitization and structurally reorganizes prefrontal cortex and striatum in a sex-dependent manner. *Behav Neurosci*, Vol.125, No.2, pp. 161-74.

Muhammad, A. & Kolb, B. (2011b). Mild Prenatal Stress-Modulated Behavior and Neuronal Spine Density without Affecting Amphetamine Sensitization. *Dev Neurosci.* 2011, May 12, (DOI: 10.1159/000324744), [Epub ahead of print].

Muhammad, A. & Kolb, B. (2011c). Maternal separation altered behavior and neuronal spine density without influencing amphetamine sensitization. *Behav Brain Res.*, Vol.223, No.1, pp. 7-16.

Mukda, S.; Vimolratana, O. & Govitrapong, P. (2011). Melatonin attenuates the amphetamine-induced decrease in vesicular monoamine transporter-2 expression in postnatal rat striatum. *Neurosci Lett.*, No.488, pp. 154-157.

Murray, J.; Belin, D. & Everitt, B.J. (2012) Double dissociation of the dorsomedial and dorsolateral striatum control over the acquisition and performance of cocaine seeking. *Neuropsychopharmacology*, In Press.

Oaks, A.W. & Sidhu, A. (2011). Synuclein modulation of monoamine transporters. *FEBS Lett.*, No.585, pp. 1001-1006.

O'Brien, C.P.; Volkow, N. & Li, T.K. (2006). What's in a word? Addiction versus dependence in DSM-V. *Am J Psychiatry*, No. 163, pp. 764–765.

Paule, M.G. (2005). Chronic drug exposures during development in nonhuman primates: models of brain dysfunction in humans. *Front Biosci.*, No.10, pp. 2240-2249.

Pezze, M.A.; Dalley, J.W. & Robbins, T.W. (2007). Differential roles of dopamine D1 and D2 receptors in the nucleus accumbens in attentional performance on the five-choice serial reaction time task. *Neuropsychopharmacol.* Vol. 32, No.2, pp. 273-83.

Potenza, M.N.; Sofuoglu, M.; Carroll, K.M. & Rounsaville, B.J. (2011). Neuroscience of Behavioral and Pharmacological Treatments for Addictions. *Neuron*, Vol.69, No.4, pp. 695-712.

Rice, M.E. & Cragg, S.J. (2008). Dopamine spillover after quantal release: rethinking dopamine transmission in the nigrostriatal pathway. *Brain Res Rev.*, No.58, pp. 303-313.

Robbins, T.W. & Everitt, B.J. (2002). Limbic-striatal memory systems and drug addiction. *Neurobiol Learn Mem.*, Vol.78, No.3, pp. 625-636.

Robinson, T.E. & Becker, J.B. (1986). Enduring changes in brain and behavior produced by chronic amphetamine administration: a review and evaluation of animal models of amphetamine psychosis. *Brain Res.*, Vol.396, No.2, pp. 157-198.

Robinson, T.E. & Kolb, B. (2004). Structural plasticity associated with exposure to drugs of abuse. *Neuropharmacology*, No.47, pp. 33-46.

Robinson, T.E. & Kolb, B. (2011). Structural plasticity associated with exposure to drugs of abuse. *Neuropharmacology* 2004, No.47, Suppl 1, pp. 33-46.

Rogge, G.; Jones, D.; Hubert, G.W.; Lin, Y. & Kuhar, M.J. (2008). CART peptides: regulators of body weight, reward and other functions. *Nat Rev Neurosci.*, No.9, pp. 747-758.

Runyon, S.P. & Carroll, F.I. (2006). Dopamine transporter ligands: recent developments and therapeutic potential. *Curr Top Med Chem.*, No.6, pp. 1825-1843.

Sae-Ung, K.; Uéda, K.; Govitrapong, P. & Phansuwan-Pujito, P. (2012). Melatonin reduces the expression of alpha-synuclein in the dopamine containing neuronal regions of amphetamine-treated postnatal rats. *J Pineal Res.*, Vol. 52, No. 1, pp. 128-137.

Schmitt, K.C. & Reith, M.E. (2010). Regulation of the dopamine transporter: aspects relevant to psychostimulant drugs of abuse. *Ann N Y Acad Sci.*, No.1187, pp. 316-340.

Schultz, W.; Dayan, P. & Montague, P.R. (1997). A neural substrate of prediction and reward. *Science*, No. 275, pp. 1593-1599.

Schultz, W. (1998). Predictive reward signal of dopamine neurons. *J Neurophysiol.*, No. 80, pp.1-27.

Schultz, W. (2011). Potential vulnerabilities of neuronal reward, risk, and decision mechanisms to addictive drugs. *Neuron*, Vol.69, No.4, pp. 603-617.

Sesack, S.R.; Aoki, C. & Pickel, V.M. (1994). Ultrastructural localization of D2 receptor-like immunoreactivity in midbrain dopamine neurons and their striatal targets. *J Neurosci.*, No.14, pp. 88-106.

Steketee, J.D. (2003). Neurotransmitter systems of the medial prefrontal cortex: potential role in sensitization to psychostimulants. *Brain Res Brain Res Rev.*, Vol.41, No.2-3, pp. 203-228.

Steketee, J.D. (2005). Cortical mechanisms of cocaine sensitization. *Crit Rev Neurobiol.*, Vol.17, No.2, pp. 69-86.

Sulzer, D.; Chen, T.K.; Lau, Y.Y.; Kristensen, H.; Rayport, S. & Ewing, A. (1995). Amphetamine redistributes dopamine from synaptic vesicles to the cytosol and promotes reverse transport. *J Neurosci.*, No.15, pp. 4102-4108.

Sulzer, D.; Sonders, M.S.; Poulsen, N.W. & Galli, A. (2005). Mechanisms of neurotransmitter release by amphetamines: a review. *Prog Neurobiol.*, No.75, pp. 406-433.

Sulzer, D. (2011). How Addictive Drugs Disrupt Presynaptic Dopamine Neurotransmission. *Neuron*, Vol.69, No.4, pp. 628-649.

Surguchov, A. (2008). Molecular and cellular biology of synucleins. *Int. Rev. Cell Mol. Biol.*, No.270, pp. 225-317.

Stone, J.M.; Bhattacharyya, S.; Barker, G.J. & McGuire, P.K. (2011). Substance use and regional gray matter volume in individuals at high risk of psychosis. *Eur Neuropsychopharmacol.* Vol. 22, No. 2, pp. 114-122.

Swope, S.L.; Moss, S.J.; Raymond, L.A. & Huganir, R.L. (1999). Regulation of ligand-gated ion channels by protein phosphorylation. *Adv Second Messenger Phosphoprotein Res.* No. 33, pp. 49-78.

Tan, H.; Lauzon, N.M.; Bishop, S.F.; Bechard, M.A. & Laviolette, S.R. (2010). Integrated cannabinoid CB1 receptor transmission within the amygdala-prefrontal cortical pathway modulates neuronal plasticity and emotional memory encoding. *Cereb Cortex*, Vol.20, No.6, pp. 1486-1496.

Tan, S.E. (2008). Roles of hippocampal NMDA receptors and nucleus accumbens D1 receptors in the amphetamine-produced conditioned place preference in rats. *Brain Res Bull.*, Vol.77, No.6, pp. 412-419.

Théberge, F.R.; Milton, A.L.; Belin, D.; Lee J.L. & Everitt B.J. (2010). The basolateral amygdala and nucleus accumbens core mediate dissociable aspects of drug memory reconsolidation. *Learn Mem.* Vol. 17, No.9, pp. 444-53.

Thompson, B.L.; Levitt, P. & Stanwood, G.D. (2009). Prenatal exposure to drugs: effects on brain development and implications for policy and education. *Nat Rev Neurosci.*, No.10, pp. 303-312.

Tilley, M.R. & Gu, H.H. (2008). Dopamine transporter inhibition is required for cocaine-induced stereotypy. *Neuroreport*, No.19, pp. 1137-1140.

Tsuang, M.T., Lyons, M.J., Meyer, J.M., Doyle, T., Eisen, S.A, Goldberg, J., True, W., Lin, N., Toomey, R. & Eaves, L. (1998). Co-occurrence of abuse of different drugs in men: The role of drug-specific and shared vulnerabilities. *Arch. Gen. Psychiatry*, 55, pp. 967-972.

Treadway, M.T. and Zald, D.H. (2011). Reconsidering anhedonia in depression: Lessons from translational neuroscience. *Neurosci Biobehav Rev.*, No. 35, pp. 537-555.

Trezza, V.; Cuomo, V. & Vanderschuren, L.J. (2008). Cannabis and the developing brain: insights from behavior. *Eur J Pharmacol.*, Vol.585, No.2-3, pp. 441-452.

Trezza, V.; Campolongo, P.; Manduca, A.; Morena, M.; Palmery, M.; Vanderschuren, L.J. & Cuomo V. (2012). Altering endocannabinoid neurotransmission at critical developmental ages: impact on rodent emotionality and cognitive performance. *Front Behav Neurosci.*, Vol. 6, No. 2, pp. 1-12.

White, N. M. (1996). Addictive drugs as reinforcers: multiple partial actions on memory systems. *Addiction Vol.* 91, No. 7, pp. 921-949.

Volkow, N.D.; Fowler, J.S. & Wang, G.J. (2002a). Role of dopamine in drug reinforcement and addiction in humans:results from imaging studies. *Behav Pharmacol.* No. 13, pp. 355-366.

Volkow, N.D; Wang, G.J.; Fowler, J.S.; Thanos, P.P.; Logan, J.; Gatley, S.J.; Gifford, A.; Ding, Y.S.; Wong, C.; Pappas, N. & Thanos, P. (2002b). Brain DA D2 receptors predict reinforcing effects of stimulants in humans:replication study. *Synapse*, No. 46, pp. 79-82.

Volkow, N.D.; Baler, R.D. & Goldstein, R.Z. (2011). Addiction: pulling at the neural threads of social behaviors. *Neuron*, Vol.69, No.4, pp. 599-602.

Von der Goltz, C. & Kiefer, F. (2009). Learning and memory in the aetiopathogenesis of addiction: future implications for therapy? *Eur Arch Psychiatry Clin Neurosci.*, No.259, Suppl 2, pp. S183-S187.

Welberg, L. (2010). Addiction: Cracking the code of addiction. *Nat Rev Neurosci.*, Vol.11, No.10, p. 668.

WHO (2012). Cannabis. In *"Management of substance abuse"*. January 6, 2012. Available from: http://www.who.int/substance_abuse/facts/cannabis/en/

Wise, R.A. (2004). Dopamine, learning and motivation. *Nat Rev Neurosci.*, Vol.5, No. 6, pp.483-494.

Wiskerke, J.; Pattij, T.; Schoffelmeer, A.N. & De Vries T.J. (2008). The role of CB1 receptors in psychostimulant addiction. *Addict Biol.*, Vol.13, No.2, pp. 225-238.

Williams, J.M. & Galli, A. (2006). The dopamine transporter: a vigilant border control for psychostimulant action. *Handb Exp Pharmacol.*, No.175, pp. 215-232.

Yamamoto, S.; Fukae, J.; Mori, H.; Mizuno, Y. & Hattori, N. (2006). Positive immunoreactivity for vesicular monoamine transporter 2 in Lewy bodies and Lewy neurites in substantia nigra. *Neurosci. Lett.*, Vol.396, No.3, pp. 187–191.

Yung, K.K.; Bolam, J.P.; Smith, A.D.; Hersch, S.M.; Ciliax, B.J. & Levey, A.I. (1995). Immunocytochemical localization of D1 and D2 dopamine receptors in the basal ganglia of the rat: light and electron microscopy. *Neuroscience*, No.65, pp. 709-730.

Zapata, A.; Minney, V.L. & Shippenberg, T.S. (2010). Shift from goal-directed to habitual cocaine seeking after prolonged experience in rats. *J Neurosci.*, No. 30, pp.15457–15463.

Zhang, J.; Liu, X.; Lei, X.; Wang, L.; Guo, L.; Zhao, G. & Lin, G. (2010). Discovery and synthesis of novel luteolin derivatives as DAT agonists. Bioorg Med Chem., No.18, pp. 7842-7848.

Zhou, Y.; Cui, C.L.; Schlussman, S.D.; Choi, J.C.; Ho, A.; Han, J.S. & Kreek, M.J. (2008). Effects of cocaine place conditioning, chronic escalating-dose "binge" pattern cocaine administration and acute withdrawal on orexin/hypocretin and preprodynorphin gene expressions in lateral hypothalamus of Fischer and Sprague-Dawley rats. *Neuroscience*, Vol. 153, No. 4, pp.1225-1234.

6

Cocaine Addiction: Changes in Excitatory and Inhibitory Neurotransmission

Edgar Antonio Reyes-Montaño and Edwin Alfredo Reyes-Guzmán
Protein Research Group (Grupo de Investigación en Proteínas, GRIP)
Universidad Nacional de Colombia, Sede Bogotá
Colombia

1. Introduction

The principal routes of cocaine administration are oral, intranasal, intravenous, and inhalation. The slang terms for these routes are, respectively, "chewing," "snorting," "mainlining," "injecting," and "smoking" (including freebase and crack cocaine). Cocaine use ranges from occasional use to repeated or compulsive use, with a variety of patterns between these extremes. There is no safe way to use cocaine. Any route of administration can lead to absorption of toxic amounts of cocaine, allowing to acute cardiovascular or cerebrovascular emergencies that could result in sudden death. Repeated cocaine use by any route of administration can produce addiction and other adverse health consequences. Those who snort or sniff cocaine through their noses suffer damage to their nasal and sinus passages. These include nasal crusting, nosebleeds, nasal congestion, irritation, facial pain caused by sinusitis and hoarseness.

Cocaine addiction changes the responsiveness of the brain to various neurotransmitters or chemicals. The development of drug addiction involves persistent cellular and molecular changes in the Central Nervous System. The brain dopamine, GABA and glutamate systems play key roles in mediating drug-induced neuroadaptation. We show some physiological changes that can occur in some key pathways in which glutamate, dopamine and GABA receptors are involved. These chemical changes cause different effects in users, including: anxiety, confusion, dizziness, psychosis, headaches and nausea.

Cocaine use and addiction affects the sympathetic nervous system (which controls automatic functions such as breathing, heartbeat, etc.). This system secretes adrenaline which raises ones heart rate, narrows blood vessels and significantly increases blood pressure. Chest pain, heart attacks and strokes are common side effects of cocaine use.

The most widely studied neurobiological characteristic of cocaine addiction is the role played by dopamine transmission. It is clear that enhanced dopamine transmission in neurons projecting from the ventral mesencephalon to the limbic forebrain, including the medial prefrontal cortex (mPFC) and nucleus accumbens (NAc), is the pharmacological target for cocaine-induced reinforcement and locomotor stimulation (O' Brien., 2001) However, persistence of the behavioral characteristics of cocaine addiction, such as paranoia (sensitization) and the propensity to relapse years after the acute rewarding effects of the drug have disappeared, indicates that there must also be neuronal substrates undergoing long-term neuroplastic changes. Although studies have endeavored to identify enduring changes in dopamine transmission that might underlie behavioral sensitization and the reinstatement of drug-seeking (relapse), the results have not been entirely consistent with an obligatory role for dopamine.

Addiction can be viewed as a form of drug-induced neural plasticity. One of the best-established molecular mechanisms of addiction is up-regulation of the cAMP second messenger pathway, which occurs in many neuronal cell types in response to chronic administration of opiates or other drugs of abuse. This up-regulation and the resulting activation of the transcription factor CREB appear to mediate aspects of tolerance and dependence. In contrast, induction of another transcription factor, termed 1FosB, exerts the opposite effect and may contribute to sensitized responses to drug exposure. Knowledge of these mechanisms could lead to more effective treatments for addictive disorders.

2. The neurobiology of cocaine addiction

Dopamine acts as a modulator for many nerve cells throughout the brain. Dopamine is responsible for keeping those cells operating at the appropriate levels of activity to accomplish our needs and aims (Nestler., 2005). Whenever we need to mobilize our muscles or mind to work harder or faster, dopamine drives some of the involved brain cells to step up to the challenge (Nestler., 2005). The targets in brain and other organs are shown in figure 1.

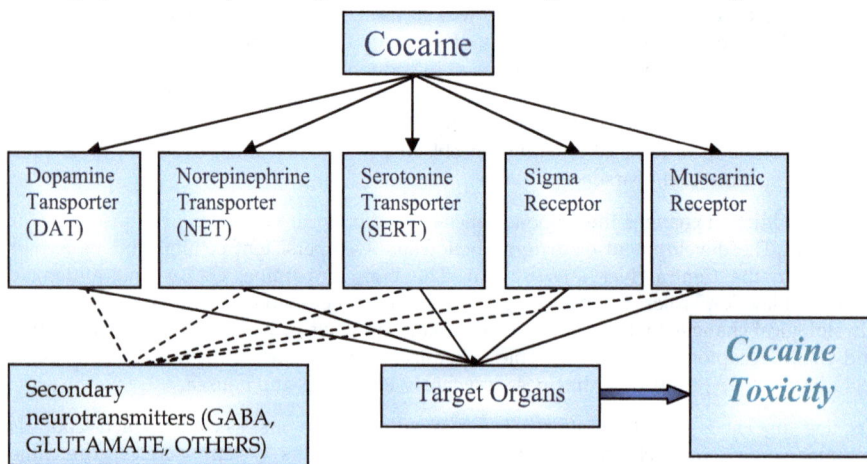

Fig. 1. Cocaine and receptors associated with its toxicity. Continuous lines show the main target organs affected; dashed lines represent the secondary neurotransmitters associated. (Adapted from Nestler., 2005)

Dopamine is originated in dopaminergic neurons and launch them into their surroundings. Some of the free-floating dopamine molecules latch onto receptor proteins on neighboring cells. Once attached, dopamine stimulates the receptors to alter electrical impulses in the receiving cells and thereby alter the cells' function. To keep the receiving cells in each brain region functioning at appropriate intensities for current demands the dopaminergic cells continually increase and decrease the number of dopamine molecules they launch. They further regulate the amount of dopamine available to stimulate the receptors by pulling some previously released dopamine molecules back into themselves (Nestler., 2005).

One of the most addictive drugs is cocaine. Cocaine can act mainly on the mesoaccumbens dopamine (DA) pathway of the midbrain, extending from the ventral tegmental area (VTA) to the nucleus accumbens (NAc). This pathway is also known as the reward pathway as it is the area of the brain that is activated when someone has a pleasurable experience such as eating, sex, or receiving praise. Cocaine interferes with the dopamine control mechanism: It ties up the dopamine transporter. As a result, with cocaine on board, dopamine molecules that otherwise would be picked up remain in action. Dopamine builds up and overactivates the receiving cells. However, DA is not the only system affected by cocaine. Glutamate and neurotransmission mediated for this aminoacid is also modified and has an importantt role in the mechanism of this drug addiction.

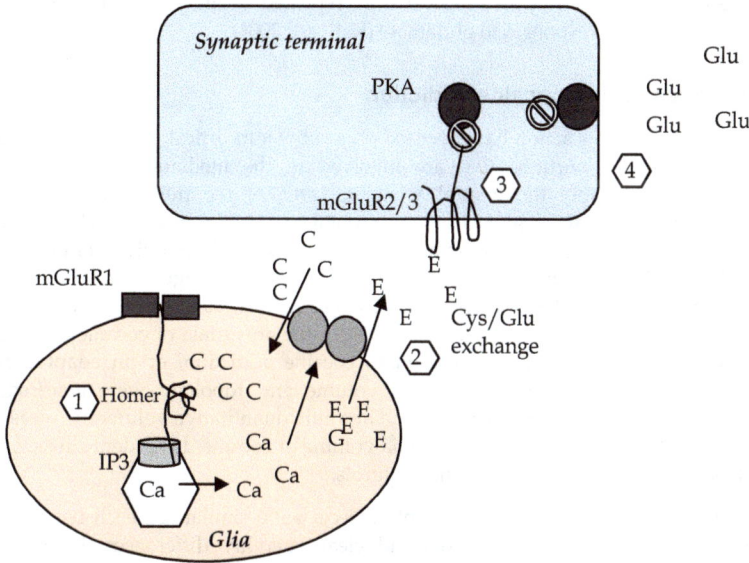

Fig. 2. The potential mechanisms regulating glutamatergic transmission in the NAc that are involved in the reinstatement of drug-seeking behavior. The cocaine-induced changes in extrasynaptic glutamate release outlined below are postulated to increase the signal-to-noise ratio of synaptically released glutamate, thereby facilitating drug-seeking. 1. Homer protein is reduced in the nucleus accumbens, causing a reduction in signaling via mGluR1 receptors through inositol trisphosphate (IP3) receptor regulation of internal calcium (Ca) stores. 2. Because glutamate release stimulated by mGluR1 receptors results from activation of the cystine/glutamate exchanger, it is proposed that down regulated mGluR1 signaling may mediate the reduced activity of the cystine/glutamate exchanger produced by chronic cocaine administration. 3. The reduced heteroexchange of extracellular cystine (C) for intracellular glutamate (E) in glia results in reduced basal extracellular glutamate and reduced tone on mGluR2/3 presynaptic autoreceptors. 4. This reduced tone, accompanied by mGluR2/3 residing in a more phosphorylated (desensitized) state, results in reduced inhibitory regulation of synaptically released glutamate (Glu) (Adapted from Kalivas., 2004)

The way in which this sequence of adaptations could synergize to dysregulate presynaptic glutamate transmission in cocaine addiction is illustrated in Figure 2. This hypothetical model describes how reduced Homer1bc could account for reduced activity of the cystine-glutamate exchanger and the accompanying reduced basal levels of extracellular glutamate. The reduced levels of glutamate, combined with desensitization of the mGluR2/3 receptor, results in a loss of regulatory feedback on synaptic glutamate release. Thus, lower basal levels of glutamate, combined with increased release of synaptic glutamate in response to activation of prefrontal cortical afferents to the NAc, results in an amplified signal and behavioral drive to engage drug seeking (e.g. to relapse). In addition to adaptations in presynaptic and possibly glial release of glutamate that regulate the expression of sensitization and/or reinstatement   a variety of changes in postsynaptic glutamate transmission have been documented in the NAc. Interestingly, although presynaptic release of glutamate was augmented by withdrawal from repeated cocaine, most data indicate a reduction in postsynaptic responses to glutamate (Kalivas., 2004).

3. Brain changes during cocaine addiction

Animal studies of cocaine´s action have focused on a set of subcortical gray matter of some structures as paralimbic cortices, that are involved in the mediation of reward and reinforcement, most notably the ventral tegmental area of the midbrain, the nucleus accumbens, the amygdala, and regions of the prefrontal cortex (Makris et al., 2004). Existing studies of brain structure in cocaine users have reported abnormalities only in brain regions connected to the amygdala, such as the orbitofrontal and anterior cingulate cortex (Franklin et al., 2002; Matochik et al., 2003). Markis et al., (2004) sought to evaluate the hypothesis that topological and volumetric abnormalities may exist in the amygdala of cocaine-dependent subjects that may represent a predisposition to cocaine addiction, or an adaptation to protracted exposure to the drug. Amygdala volume and topology were assessed by segmentation-based morphometric analysis, and absolute quantitative volumetric measures were performed. It was observed that amygdala volume of cocaine-dependent subjects was significantly smaller than the one of matched controls.

The amygdala volumes of cocaine-dependent subjects were similar for each hemisphere, whereas those of their matched controls had clear laterality differences. In addition, amygdala volume in addicts did not correlate with (1) measures of anxiety or depression, (2) any measure of the amount of cocaine use, or (3) age at which cocaine use began (Makris et al., 2004)

Barrós-Loscertales et al., (2011) reported reduced gray matter (GM) volume in the striatum and in the supramarginal gyrus. Likewise, another set of cortical and subcortical structures, such as the amygdala, the insula and dorsolateral prefrontal cortex, were seen to have volume reductions related to years of cocaine exposure (Barrós-Loscertales et al., 2011). All these structural changes associated with cocaine addiction seem to merge in the striato-cortico-limbic circuitry linked not only to addiction, but also to the wider set of disinhibitory disorders (Barrós-Loscertales et al., 2011). Although causal relationships are very difficult to determine in human studies, the significant relationship between years of use and reduced GM volumes are consistent with these volumetric effects arising from the cumulative exposure to cocaine or the concomitant lifestyle (e.g., stress) that accompanies prolonged drug use (Yücel et al., 2008).

In other aspects, Ersche et al., (2011) found some differences between healthy and cocaine users, specially in the gray matter abundance in some regions of the brain. There was widespread significant loss of grey matter in orbitofrontal cortex bilaterally in the cocaine user group. Grey matter volume was also abnormally reduced in the insula, the medial frontal and anterior cingulate cortex, temporoparietal cortex and the cerebellum. In contrast to this extensive system of decreased cortical grey matter volume, cocaine users also showed a significant increase of grey matter volume mainly localized to basal ganglia structures (including putamen, caudate nucleus and pallidum), and cerebellum (figure 3).

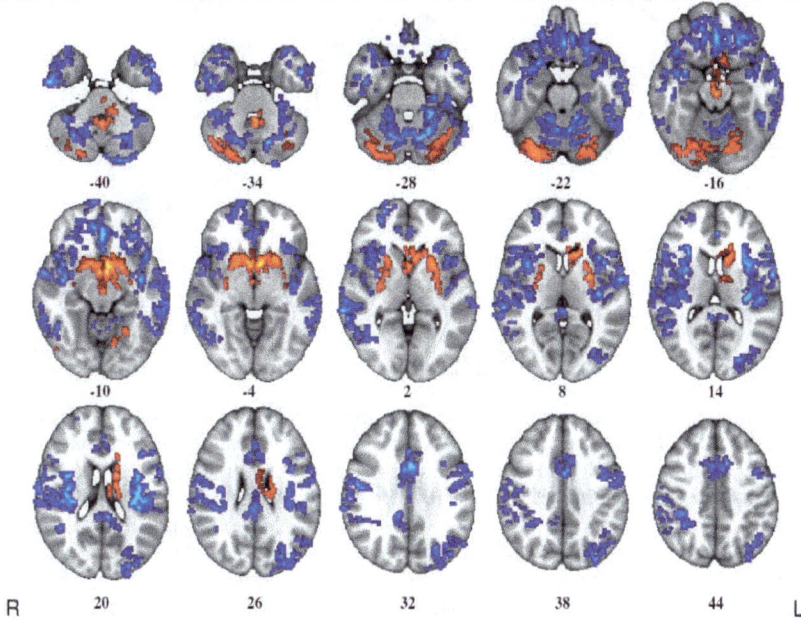

Fig. 3. Whole-brain maps of significant differences in grey matter volume between healthy volunteers and cocaine users. Voxels coloured blue indicate brain areas in which cocaine users have reduced grey matter volume compared with healthy volunteers, and voxels coloured red indicate brain areas in which cocaine users have abnormally increased grey matter volume. These results were generated by permutation testing of voxel cluster statistics with cluster-wise P50.001, at which level we expect less than one false positive cluster per map. The statistical results are overlaid on the FSL MNI152 standard T1 image and the numbers beneath each section of the image refer to its position (mm) relative to the intercommissural plane in standard stereotactic space. L = left; R = right. (Ersche et al., 2011)

In addition, it has been found that the caudate enlargement in cocaine users was associated with significant attentional impairments, whereas the reduction in grey matter in the orbitofrontal cortex was associated with cocaine-related compulsivity. The abnormal changes in grey matter in the striatum and in the orbitofrontal cortex were both related to the duration of cocaine abuse (Ersche et al., 2011).

In another interesting description, Ersche et al., (2011) showed some maps of brain regions demonstrating significant association between grey matter volume and measures of duration of cocaine use, compulsivity and impulsivity in the group of cocaine users (figure 4). This study allow see that is possible find some positive and negative correlations between grey matter and duration of cocaine use, or compulsive cocaine taking or impulsivity in cocaine users.

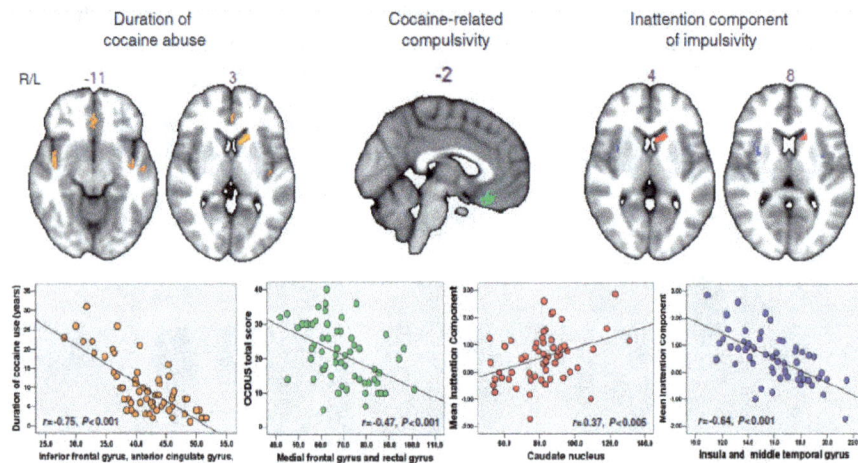

Fig. 4. Maps of brain regions. Regions where grey matter volume correlated significantly with the duration of cocaine use in drug users are indicated in orange. Regions that correlated significantly with compulsive cocaine-taking are coloured in green. Regions where grey matter volume correlated significantly with the inattention component of impulsivity in cocaine users are indicated in red (if the correlation was positive) and blue (if the correlation was negative). The scatter plots beneath each section of the brain image show the correlation between these measures and the total grey matter volume for each drug user. The numbers above each section of the image refer to its plane position (mm) relative to the origin in MNI stereotactic space. L = left; R = right (Ersche et al., 2011).

In addition, there are differences between the cocaine-dependent and healthy groups. For example, the cocaine users had higher depressive scores than the healthy people, and fewer years in formal education (11.5 compared to 12.3 years). Most of the cocaine users also had nicotine dependence (83%), some also had alcohol dependence (27%), cannabis dependence (18%) and heroin dependence (7%). These factors may also have been related to the brain differences seen, rather than just the cocaine use. Morever, Ersche et al., (2011), noted that impulsivity is a complex trait and that the measures they used would not have captured all aspects of it.

4. The signaling pathways involved in cocaine addiction

The drugs of abuse differ greatly in their chemical structure, they act on their own unique target that are mostly proteins involved in synaptic transmission, although different drugs affect different neurotransmitter systems (Nestler, E., 2004).

All addictive drugs facilitate dopamine transmission. The dopamine projection to the prefrontal cortex (PFC), nucleus accumbens (NAc) and amygdala is a primary site of pharmacological action by cocaine, as well as a site where addictive behaviors such as relapse and sensitization can be initiated (Berridge and Robinson., 1998). The regions of the prefrontal cortex most clearly tied to addiction in both neuroimaging studies in addicts and lesion/pharmacological studies in animal models of addiction (rats) are the anterior cingulate/prelimbic cortex and the ventral orbital cortex (Neisewander et al., 2000; Goldstein and Volkow., 2002; Kalivas., 2004).

The NAc is composed of two compartments termed the core and the shell (Zahm and Brog., 1992) and, although the shell is more clearly associated with dopamine-dependent reward, the core has been linked to the enduring cellular changes elicited by repeated use of addictive drugs (Di Ciano and Everitt., 2001; Kalivas and McFarland., 2003). The projections from the amygdala and prefrontal cortex to the nucleus accumbens are glutamatergic, as are the reciprocal connections between the basolateral amygdala and prefrontal cortex (figure 5). The prefrontal cortex also sends glutamatergic efferents to the dopamine cell body region in the ventral tegmental area (VTA). This circuit has primary output through co-localized γ-amino butyric acid (GABA)ergic and peptidergic neurons in the NAc that project to the ventral pallidum (PV) and ventral tegmental area (Kalivas., 2004).

The changes in the NAc, influenced by activation of dopamine receptors, are critically involved in behavioral adaptations (Marinelli and White., 2000). Natural rewards, but also drugs of abuse, increase VTA release of dopamine in downstream structures such as the NAc (Di Chiara, 2002; Schultz., 2002). However, an essential difference between natural rewards and drugs of abuse is that, over time, the dopamine response to the natural rewards, but not drugs of abuse, diminishes (Kalivas and O'Brien., 2008). Additionally, the amount of dopamine released following administration of a drug of abuse, particularly cocaine, typically exceeds what occurs following exposure to a natural reward. Thus, the repeated large release of dopamine is believed to be critical in the development of addiction, as it alters and modifies structures and their connections (Uys and LaLumiere,. 2008).

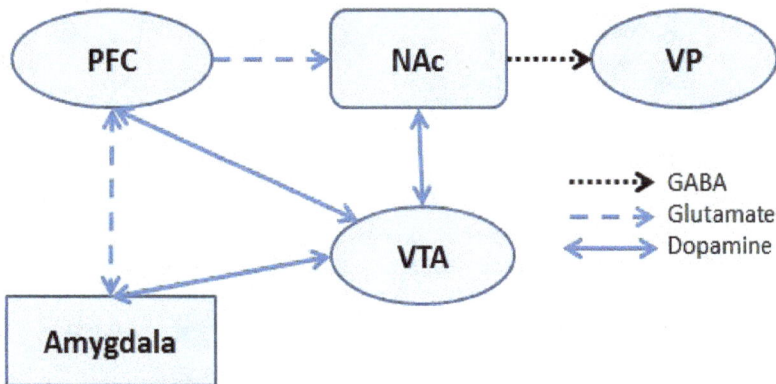

Fig. 5. The schematic diagram identify the critical structures involved in drug reward and relapse to cocaine seeking. VTA, Ventral tegmental area; PFC, Prefrontal cortex; NAc, Nucleus accumbens; VP, Ventral pallidum.

The VTA–NAc, so called mesolimbic, pathway seems to be a site where virtually all drugs of abuse converge to produce their acute reward signals. Two major mechanisms are involved: first, all drugs of abuse increase dopamine-mediated transmission in the NAc, although by very different mechanisms; second, some drugs also act directly on NAc neurons by dopamine-independent mechanisms (Everitt and Wolf., 2002).

An interesting point is the intracellular event precipitated by stimulation of dopamine receptors as a result of repeated use of cocaine. In dopamine D1 receptor stimulation of cAMP-dependent protein kinase (or PKA) and subsequent changes in protein function and gene expression in the NAc and VTA appear critical to establishing sensitization (Nestler., 2001). The most well-characterized effect of increased cAMP-dependent protein kinase activity is the induction of cAMP response element and the subsequent change in ΔFosB and cyclin-dependent kinase 5 (Nestler et al., 2001; Lu et al., 2003). In addition to the immediate consequences of dopamine receptor signaling, calcium/calmodulin and ras/mitogen-activated protein kinase activity in the ventral tegmental area are critical for the development of sensitization (figure 6). The dopamine D1 receptor stimulation–dependent activation of L-type Ca^{2+} channels and CaMKII facilitates the reinstatement of cocaine seeking by promoting the transport of GluA1-containing AMPA receptors in the NAc shell to the plasma membrane. The CaMKII activity in the NAc shell may be an essential link between dopamine and glutamate systems involved in the neuronal plasticity underlying cocaine craving and relapse (figure 6). (Wolf et al., 2004; Boehm and Malinow., 2005; Schmidt and Pierce., 2010).

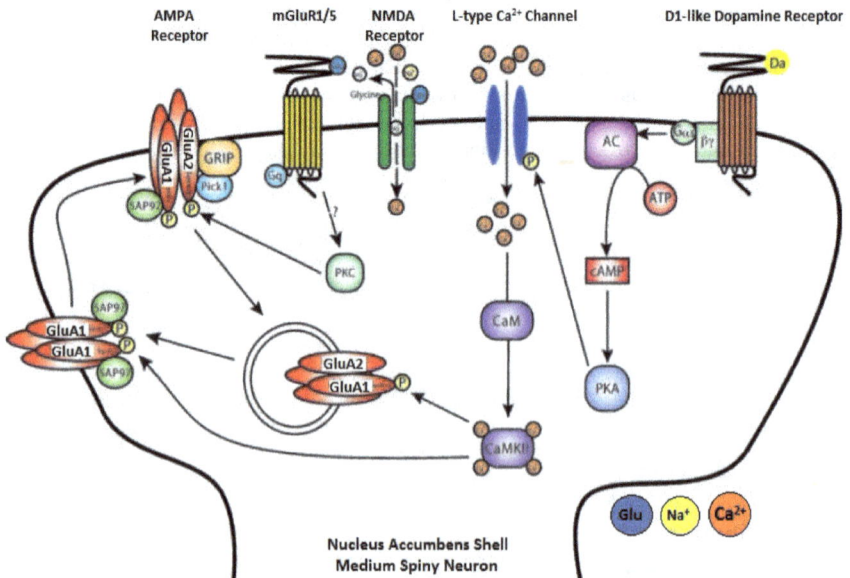

Fig. 6. Pathway between NAc shell dopamine and glutamate systems, via L-type Ca^{2+} channels and Ca^{2+}/calmodulin kinase II (CaMKII), which is proposed to underlie the reinstatement of cocaine seeking. (Adapted from Schmidt and Pierce., 2010).

In contrast to dopamine, glutamate transmission appears to be a primary contributor in the majority of examples of enduring neuroplasticity in the brain, and the development and expression of cocaine addiction is no exception (Winder et al., 2002). The activation of glutamatergic efferents from the amygdala and prefrontal cortex is critical in the expression of addictive behaviors.

Cocaine indirectly influences glutamate transmission in the limbic system, including the NAc, producing persistent changes in neuronal function that can alter the behavioral effects that generate this drug. (Gass and Olive., 2008; Uys and LaLumiere., 2008; Thomas et al., 2008). Thus, maladaptive forms of neuroplasticity in the NAc contribute to cocaine-seeking behavior, and reversing these cocaine-induced neuroadaptations in glutamatergic transmission may prevent relapse of cocaine taking.

The interaction between glutamate and dopamine in VTA and NAc is rather complex, but in simplified terms, glutamatergic input to the VTA increases the activity of dopaminergic cells and enhances dopamine release in the NAc (Tzschentke., 2001). At the level of the NAc, glutamate also facilitates dopaminergic transmission, presumably by presynaptically influencing dopamine release (Floresco et al., 1998; Tzschentke and Schmidt., 2003).

5. The role of glutamate, and GABA receptors in cocaine addiction

The glutamate as neurotransmitter interacts with specific ionotropic glutamate receptors (iGluR) or metabotropic glutamate receptors (mGluR) (Dingledine et al., 1999; Cull-Candy et al., 2001). The ionotropic family of glutamate receptors consists of three subfamilies of tetrameric receptors; N-methyl-D-aspartate (NMDA) receptors, α-amino-3-hydroxy-5-methylisoxazole-4-propionic acid receptors (AMPAR), and kainate receptors. Agonist binding induces a conformation change in NMDA, AMPA, and kainate receptors that increases the probability of channel opening. Different subunit compositions of ionotropic glutamate receptors produce functionally diverse NMDA, AMPA, and kainate receptors that are expressed differently throughout the brain (Dingledine et al., 1999).

The latter are the G protein-coupled receptor. Through various G proteins, they connect to multiple second messenger systems. There are three functional groups of mGluRs (group I–III) classified from eight subtypes (mGluR1–8) (Conn and Pin., 1997). Group I mGluRs (mGluR1/5 subtypes) are positively coupled to phospholipase Cβ1 through Gαq proteins. Activation of mGluR1/5 increases phosphoinositol hydrolysis, resulting in intracellular Ca^{2+} release and protein kinase C (PKC) activation (Conn and Pin, 1997). Both group II (mGluR2/3) and group III (mGluR4/6/7/8) receptors are negatively coupled to adenylyl cyclase through Gαi/o proteins. Their activation reduces cAMP formation and inhibits protein kinase A (PKA).

Group I mGlu receptors can also couple Homer proteins through a Homer-phosphatidyl-inositol 3-kinase enhancer (PIKE) adaptor complex (Szumlinski et al., 2008). This is particularly important for mGlu receptor trafficking into and out of the synapse and also to functionally connect mGlu to iGlu receptors.

5.1 Ionotropic receptors and cocaine

The glutamate neurotransmission in the NAc core is necessary for cocaine-induced behaviors, which are regulated by AMPA receptors (Pierce et al., 1996). In addition, chronic cocaine treatment changes iGluR's in both the PFC and NAc. In cocaine sensitized rats, there is an increase in GluN2B receptors in the NAc shell and decreased Tyr1472 phosphorylation in the NAc core with an increase in GluA1 Ser845 phosphorylation in the PFC, NAc shell and core (Zhang et al., 2007). Interestingly, glutamate receptor trafficking may be highly relevant for cocaine-induced neuroplasticity (Lau and Zukin., 2007).

Dopamine D1 receptor stimulation of rat PFC cortical neurons increases surface expression of GluA1-containing AMPA receptors through a protein kinase A-dependent mechanism (Sun et al., 2005). Cocaine self-administration increases synaptic GluA2-lacking AMPA receptors in the NAc after withdrawal (Conrad et al., 2008). Likewise when sensitized animals are re-exposed to cocaine after 10–14 days of withdrawal, both AMPAR surface expression and AMPA/NMDA ratio were shown to be decreased 24 h later (Boudreau et al., 2007; Ferrario et al., 2010; Kourrich et al., 2007; Thomas et al., 2001). GluA2-lacking AMPA receptors may therefore be a novel target for treating cocaine addiction.

The effect of repeated cocaine exposure on the cellular distribution of AMPARs is of functional significance because it has been shown that drug seeking requires AMPAR transmission in the NAc (Cornish and Kalivas, 2000; Di Ciano and Everitt, 2001) and that enhanced AMPAR transmission in the NAc is associated with enhanced drug seeking (Anderson et al., 2008; Conrad et al., 2008; Suto et al., 2004; Wolf and Ferrario, 2010).

Carrie et al., (2011) showed effects of a single cocaine exposure in rats and the difference from those previously reported after repeated cocaine administration. They further suggested that cocaine exerts these effects by influencing neuronal circuits rather than simply stimulating NAc DA transmission.

Cocaine injection administered to rats pretreated with repeated cocaine injections results in increased glutamate release in the NAc core (McFarland et al., 2003; Pierce et al., 1996; Hotsenpiller et al., 2001). There are different neuroadaptations in the accumbens core and the accumbens shell. When cocaine is injected during withdrawal from repeated cocaine exposure, occurs that cocaine decreased presynaptic glutamate immunoreactivity in the accumbens core, but not the accumbens shell (Kozell et al., 2003, 2004). Similarly, cocaine–induced reinstatement of drug seeking was associated with increased glutamate release in the core of the nucleus accumbens, an effect that is attenuated by pharmacological inactivation of the medial prefrontal cortex (mPFC) (McFarland et al., 2003). Then, the administration of an AMPA receptor antagonist into the NAc blocked the reinstatement of cocaine seeking induced by administration of cocaine directly into the mPFC (Park et al., 2002). The activation of the glutamatergic projection from the mPFC to the NAc promotes cocaine seeking (Park et al., 2002)., a finding supported by brain imaging studies of human cocaine addicts, which demonstrate that cocaine craving is associated with metabolic activation of the mPFC (Volkow et al., 2005). These findings also demonstrate that stimulation of AMPA glutamate receptors in the NAc plays a critical role in cocaine seeking (Schmidt and Pierce., 2010).

Has been established an association (correlation) between AMPAR phosphorylation and enduring behavioral plasticity (behavioral sensitization and more significantly drug-seeking behavior), although a causal link between them remains to be proven experimentally (Mao et al., 2011). S845/S831 phosphorylation is likely to be up-regulated to increase surface AMPAR expression   thereby enhancing AMPAR transmission related to behavioral plasticity (Boudreau and Wolf, 2005; Conrad et al., 2008). However, self-administration of cocaine induced lesser S845 phosphorylation in the striatum as compared to acute cocaine injection, establishing a tolerance of S845 phosphorylation in response to chronic cocaine (Edwards et al., 2007). This tolerance may reflect a down-regulated GluA1 function in accumbens neurons and may contribute to cocaine sensitization and cocaine-seeking behavior (Sutton et al., 2003; Bachtell et al., 2008). These imply a phosphorylation-dependent mechanism for AMPAR plasticity and drug-seeking (Mao et al., 2011).

In terms of NMDA receptors there is evidence that links post-translational modifications of glutamate receptors to excitatory synaptic plasticity and drug-seeking behavior (Di Ciano, Everitt, 2001). Generally, modification processes of striatal glutamate receptors are sensitive to addictive drugs such as cocaine.

Dopamine D2 receptors are involved in the regulation of NMDA receptor phosphorylation (Liu et al., 2006). A single dose of cocaine induced a heteroreceptor complex formation between D2 receptors and GluN2B-containing NMDA receptor in D2 receptor-bearing striatopallidal neurons. The interaction of D2 receptors with GluN2B disrupted the association of CaMKII with GluN2B, thereby reducing phosphorylation at the CaMKII-sensitive site S1303 and inhibiting NMDA receptor currents. Behaviorally, this phosphorylation, involving D2–GluN2B interaction, suppressed the inhibitory indirect pathway to promote a full motor response to cocaine. Chronic cocaine reduced GluN1 S896 phosphorylation in the rat frontal cortex at 24 h, although not 14 days after of withdrawal (Loftis and Janowsky, 2002). However, acute, repeated, and self-administration of cocaine increased GluN1 S897 phosphorylation in the rat striatum (Edwards et al., 2007). Then the fact that S897 is a sensitive site modified by cocaine can show the importance of post-translational modifications in NMDA receptor plasticity and drug craving (Mao et al., 2011; Hemby et al., 2005).

5.2 Metabotropic receptors and cocaine

An acute injection of cocaine did not alter the total accumbal expression of mGluR5 protein but was enough to reduce surface expression of mGluR5 in the nucleus accumbens, suggesting that trafficking of mGluRs plays a critical role in cocaine-induced synaptic plasticity (Fourgeaud et al., 2004). There is evidence that indicates that mGluR2/3 and mGluR5 proteins are redistributed to the synaptosomal membrane fraction after a period of extended, but not acute, forced abstinence (Ghasemzadeh et al., 2009).

In fact, mGluR2/3s have already been demonstrated to play a key role in the excessive glutamate release believed to promote drug-seeking (Kalivas, 2004). Acute and chronic cocaine treatment alter the normal function, expression or traficking of group I metabotropic receptors in the NAc of rats (Mitrano et al., 2008). A single injection of cocaine decreases the proportion of plasma membrane-bound mGluR1a in the NAc shell dendrites 45 minutes after the injection, while chronic cocaine treatment decreased mGluR1a in the NAc core dendrites. This is in contrast to acute and chronic cocaine treatment having no effect on the localization of mGluR5 receptors (Mitrano et al., 2008). Another study found a decrease in mGluR1a in the NAc shell of chronic cocaine treated rats (Ary and Szumlinski., 2007; Uys and LaLumiere., 2008). Mice lacking mGluR5 receptors do not self-administer cocaine or show an increase in locomotor activity after cocaine treatment, despite having a similar increase in dopamine levels in the NAc as compared to wild-type mice (Chiamulera et al., 2001). Activation of the perisynaptic group II mGluR receptors, mGluR2/3, decreases presynaptic glutamate release in the NAc (Xi et al., 2002; Moran et al., 2005)

Likewise the cocaine-induced plasticity in excitatory synapses within the NAc initiates adaptive changes in neuronal ensembles that lead to drug-seeking behavior and alters subsequent physiological responses to cocaine, including increased trafficking and surface expression of AMPA receptors, during protracted withdrawal (Schmidt and Pierce., 2010).

Glutamate receptors antagonists produce undesirable side effects on neurological functions. Therefore, modulation, rather than blockade, of glutamatergic transmission would be more advantageous. Accordingly, glutamate transmission-modulating agents have emerged as possible therapeutic compounds in preclinical and clinical studies (Kalivas, 2004).

5.3 GABA in cocaine addiction

GABA is an inhibitory neurotransmitter that is found primarily in the brain. As mentioned previously, the VTA plays a role in the reinforcing effects of most drugs of abuse, including cocaine, and consists of both dopaminergic and GABAergic cell bodies along with afferent terminals containing a variety of neurotransmitters. Then GABA acts as the primary inhibitory neurotransmitter in the VTA, and the GABAergic environment in the VTA has been understudied in the realm of cocaine abuse. High GABA levels result in low levels of dopamine. However cocaine diminishes transmission through of type a GABA-A receptor on dopaminergic cells in the VTA, and stimulation of other GABA-B receptor, instead, can counteract the reinforcing properties of cocaine.

The activation of GABA-A and GABA-B receptors inhibit VTA neurons, reduce dopamine release, and reduce cocaine-induced increases in extracellular dopamine (Klitenick et al., 1992; Fadda et al., 2003). GABA-A receptors are also located on GABAergic interneurons presynaptic to dopaminergic VTA neurons, and activation of these receptors would be predicted to inhibit GABAergic interneurons, disinhibit VTA neurons, enhance dopamine release, and enhance cocaine-induced increases in extracellular dopamine (Klitenick et al., 1992; Xi and Stein, 1998). Now, given the interactions between GABA and dopaminergic systems, GABAergic ligands may be useful for modifying some of the abuse-related effects of cocaine. Then the use of an among mechanistically diverse GABA agonists, high-efficacy GABA-A modulators may be the most effective for modifying the abuse-related effects of cocaine (Barrett et al., 2005).

On the other hand, acute cocaine toxicity is frequently associated with seizures. The mechanisms underlying the convulsant effect of cocaine are not well understood. Previously, studies have shown that cocaine depresses whole-cell current evoked by gamma-aminobutyric acid (GABA) in hippocampal neurons freshly isolated from rats. Cocaine's effect was voltage-independent and concentration-dependent. Ye and Ren, (2006), suggest that cocaine induces an increase from intracellular calcium [Ca]i, which stimulates phosphatase activity and thus leads to dephosphorylation of GABA receptors. This dephosphorylation-mediated disinhibitory action may play a role in cocaine-induced convulsant states.

6. Therapeutical targets for cocaine addiction

Studying the pathways involved in cocaine addiction, it is possible to know that pharmaceutical industries are hardly working on pharmacotherapies to treat this addiction and that must be directed toward the molecular transductors of abnormalities found in cocaine users. In the present section, we'll show some of the most used pharmacotherapies and the usual targets that are regulated for them. In general, we can say that most of those therapies have been used firstly in other pathologies and assayed in cocaine addiction according to their action mode or target.

Topiramate: is a sulphamatefructopyranose derivative, thought to antagonize a drug's rewarding effects by inhibiting mesocorticolimbic dopamine release via the gamma aminobutyric acid (GABA) activity and inhibition of glutamate function after drug intake. Through this activity, topiramate may decrease extracellular release of dopamine in the VTA projecting to the nucleus accumbens. This action may mediate drug-seeking behaviors and craving by reducing the rewarding effects associated with drug use (Johnson et al., 2004).

Disulfiram: inhibits plasma and microsomal carboxylesterases and plasma cholinesterase that inactivate cocaine systemically thereby increasing blood levels of cocaine without any cardiovascular toxicity. Another important role is that disulfiram chelates copper, and since copper is essential in the function of the dopamine beta-hydroxylase enzyme, disulfiram inhibits the conversion of dopamine to norepinephrine. Dopamine betahydroxylase inhibition by disulfiram leads to decreases in peripheral and central norepinephrine and increases in dopamine levels. This effect is believed to contribute to disulfiram's efficacy in treating cocaine addiction (McCance-Katz et al., 1998)

Ondansetron: Post-synaptic 5-HT3 receptors are located densely on the terminals of corticomesolimbic dopamine containing neurons, where they promote DA release. A primary effect of ondansetron a 5-HT3 antagonist is to decrease dopamine release, especially under suprabasal conditions in these regions (Haile et al., 2009)

Baclofen: is a GABA B receptor agonist used to reduce muscle spasticity in different neurological diseases. It is believed to modulate cocaine-induced dopamine release in the nucleus accumbens. In animal studies baclofen was found to reduce cocaine self-administration, reinstatement, and cocaine seeking behaviors in rats suggesting its potential utility as a medication for treatment of cocaine addiction. In humans, an open label study found that baclofen 20 taken three times daily significantly reduced cocaine craving in cocaine-dependent subjects. However, this trial had a sample size of 10 and did not have a placebo arm. An analysis of the same data found that baclofen significantly reduced cocaine use in the subgroup of patients with the heaviest cocaine use only (Fadda et al., 2003)

Modafinil: a functional stimulant, is FDA approved for the treatment of narcolepsy and idiopathic hypersomnia. The mechanisms underlying modafinil's therapeutic actions remain unknown. It is believed to occupy both the dopamine and norepinephrine transporters consistent with a stimulant like effect. In addition, modafinil appears to increase release of the excitatory neurotransmitter glutamate, and decrease the inhibitory neurotransmitter GABA. Modafinil is usually well tolerated, although up to 3% of patients on modafinil experienced cardiovascular side-effects such as hypertension, tachycardia, and palpitations. Because of its stimulant-like activity, modafinil was suggested and later tested as a treatment for cocaine dependence. It was believed to diminish not only the symptoms of cocaine withdrawal, but also act as a "substitution treatment" for cocaine (Ballon and Feifel., 2006).

Naltrexone: (NTX) has long been available as an orally available antagonist at opioid receptors, with a relative selectivity for the μ-opioid receptor at lower doses. It was originally studied as a potential treatment for opiate dependence, where it seems to be effective in special cases, but not across the broad range of patients. NTX taps into known EtOH actions in a seemingly logical manner. EtOH administration leads to release of endogenous opioid peptides, and one of the downstream effects of this is to activate mesolimbic dopamine (DA) release. This in turn contributes to acute positive reinforcing properties of drugs of abuse (Kreek et al., 2002). Consistant with this chain of events, μ-receptor null-mutant mice do not self-administer EtOH (Roberts et al., 2000; Heilis and Egli., 2006).

Other medications that interact with GABA- or glutamate-mediated neuronal systems have been tried as potential treatment for cocaine dependence. While there is preclinical evidence that acamprosate can inhibit conditioned place preference to cocaine and attenuates both drug and cue-induced reinstatement of cocaine-seeking behavior there is to date, no clinical trial testing its utility in treating humans with cocaine dependence. Gabapentin is another gabanergic drug used to treat both epilepsy and neuropathic pain. Its exact pharmacological mechanism remains unclear. Gabapentin has showed some promising results in an open-label study and case series suggesting that it might have utility in the treatment of cocaine dependence. There are encouraging preclinical data that support the utility of vigabatrin as a treatment agent for cocaine dependence. Vigabatrin is another anticonvulsant that increases GABA neurotransmission but this time by inhibiting GABA transaminase. It is a drug with great potentials but needs to be tested in adequately powered placebo controlled randomized studies. Tiagabine is yet another anticonvulsant that increases GABA neurotransmission by blocking the presynaptic reuptake of GABA. In 2 randomized clinical trials involving cocaine dependent patients who were maintained on methadone, tiagabine (12-24 mg/day) was found to decrease cocaine use compared with placebo (Bowers et al., 2007; Gonzalez et al., 2003) .

Finally, the use of stimulants has been tried for the treatment of cocaine dependence under the premise of a drug substitution for a drug with slower onset formulation and less abuse liability. Methylphenidate, a dopamine and nerepinephrine reuptake inhibitor used to treat attention deficit hyperactivity disorders (ADHD) was found to be no better than placebo in the treatment of cocaine dependent patients without comorbid ADHD. However when used in a population with dual diagnosis of cocaine dependence and ADHD, results from clinical trials were mixed. While a controlled clinical trial using immediate release methylphenidate (90 mg/day) found no difference between the active drug and placebo groups, another trial using sustained release methylphenidate (60 mg/day), found significant improvement in ADHAD symptoms that were associated with decrease in cocaine use compared with placebo. Though medications such as those that facilitate gabaergic function, modulate dopaminergic function or act as an agonist replacement therapy show promise in treating cocaine dependence, there are certain drawbacks (Levin et al., 2007).

Other authors (Heilis and Egli., 2006) have organized medication used in cocaine addiction in three different groups. The medications described in past paragraphs are classified in the "first wave: currently available treatments" and "second wave: the near future". Those medications have been used in mixes between them and have shown interesting results.

Table 1 summarizes some aspects related to treatment and targets of first, and second wave medications.

Medication	Group (wave)	Target, mechanism	References
Disulfiram	First	Blocking aldehyde dehydrogenase (alcohol treatment), and dopamine beta-hydroxylase (cocaine dependence)	Carroll et al., 2004
Naltrexone (NTX)	First	Antagonist at opioid receptors	Kirchmayer et al., 2000
Acamprosate (ACM)	First	Glutamate antagonist, attenuates NMDA signaling through spermidine site and actions at metabotropic glutamate receptors	Spanagel & Zieglgansberger, 1997; Harris et al., 2002.
NTX and ACM mixed	First	Opioid receptors, NMDA receptors and metabotropic receptors	Rist et al., 2005; Spanagel & Mann, 2005.
Ondansetron	Second	Serotonin receptors	Higgins et al., 1992; Meert, 1993; Tomkins et al., 1995.
Baclofen	Second	Agonist at GABA-B receptor. Treatment when in detected additional alcohol dependence	Stromberg, 2004.
Topiramate	Second	Proposed effects: blockade of voltage dependent sodium channels, antagonism of kainite receptors and potentiation of GABA signaling through increased GABA availability	Zona et al., 1997; Gryder & Rogawski, 2003; Kaminski et al., 2004, White et al.,1997

Table 1. Medications used in cocaine dependence, showing its classification and possible mechanism (or target) of action. The main use of those medications is in alcohol dependence treatment but they have shown good results in other dependences as cocaine addiction (adapted from Heilis and Egli., 2006)

The third wave medications in cocaine addiction have been used with promising results. The development of pharmacotherapy for cocaine addiction is based on previous strategies designed to alleviate other chemical dependencies such as alcoholism and opiate addiction, focusing on the neurobiological and the behavioral bases of addiction. To date, however, no pharmacotherapy has been approved by the U.S. Food and Drug Administration for cocaine dependence, but two major classes of medications have been investigated: (1) dopaminergic agents and (2) antidepressants. Studies have been relatively brief for both types of agents and have focused on abstinence initiation rather than on relapse prevention. In addition to dopaminergic agents and antidepressants, other compounds such as calcium channel blockers, have been examined as potential treatments of cocaine dependence (figure 7) (Carrera et al., 2004)

In the first group, some dopaminergic agents have been used based on the theory that chronic cocaine use reduces the efficiency of central DA neurotransmission, several dopaminergic compounds, including amantadine, bromocriptine, mazindol, and methylphenidate, have been examined as treatments for cocaine abuse. Investigators hoped that these dopaminergic agents, which have a fast onset of action, would correct the DA dysregulation and alleviate the withdrawal symptoms that often follow cessation of stimulant use.

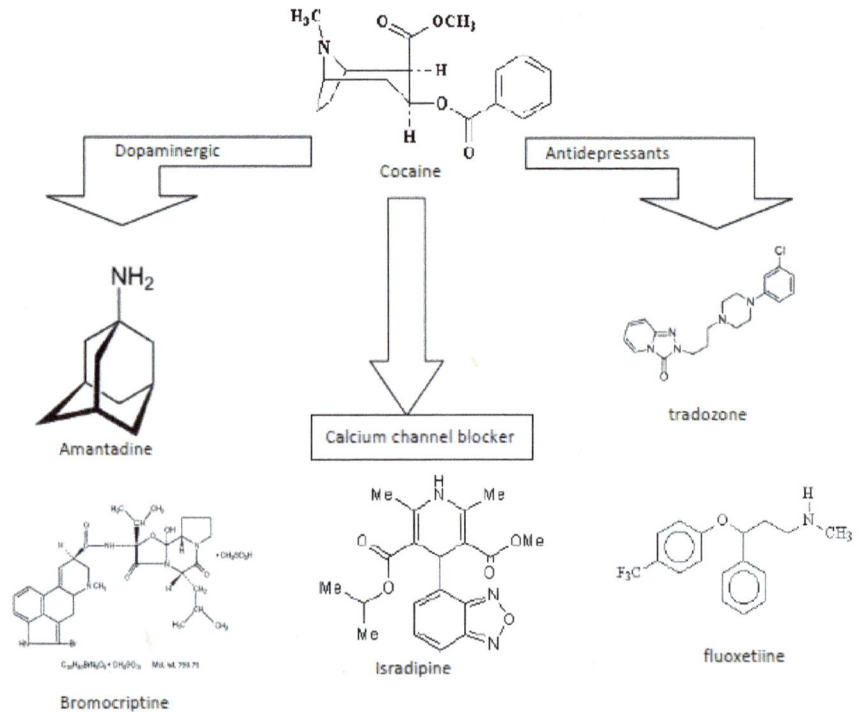

Fig. 7. Classification of medications used for cocaine addiction, based on target and mechanism of action (based on Carrera et al., 2004).

Large array of cocaine analogues and other dopamine uptake inhibitors (see Table 2) including analogues of WIN-35,065, GBR-12909, nomifensine, and benztropine have been developed in the last years. The largest class of compound studies is the class of 3-phenyltropane analogues, of which many hundreds have been made and tested. The analogues RTI-112 and PTT are in preclinical evaluation. Like cocaine, RTI-112 and PTT both have good affinity for all three monoamine transporters, but in contrast to cocaine they enter the brain slowly and are long-lasting. A number of other 3-phenyltropanes are potent and selective for the dopamine transporter relative to inhibition of serotonin and norepinephrine transporters, are long-lasting, and also enter the brain more slowly than cocaine, for example, RTI-113 and RTI-177 (Carrera et al., 2004).

The effect of inhibiting neurotransmitter uptake is to stimulate neurotransmitter receptors; thus the use of direct receptor agonists as substitute agonist medications also has been suggested. Data on dopamine receptor agonists have been extensively reviewed. Animal studies indicate that dopamine receptor agonists such as apomorphine and bromocriptine maintain self-administration in rodents.

Compound	CNS target
RTI-113, RTI-177, GBR-12909	DA uptake inhibitors (selective for DAT)
Mazindol, methyl phenidate, nomifensine, benztropine	DA uptake inhibitors (not selective)
Apomorphine, bromocriptine, SKF38393, quinpirole	DA receptor agonists and partial agonist
Desipramine	Antagonist of cocaine binding that spare DA uptake
Fluoxetine, alaproclate	5HT uptake inhibitors
Quipazine	5HT receptor agonist
Ketanserin, ritanserin, ondansetron	Calcium channel blockers

Table 2. List of some compounds that have been used as pharmacotherapy in cocaine addiction and target identified in Central Nervous System (adapted from Carrera et al., 2004)

The second class of medications used to treat cocaine dependence, antidepressants, are thought to down regulate synaptic catecholamine receptors, and this action is opposite to the presynaptic up-regulation caused by chronic stimulant use. Although antidepressants have a relatively benign side-effect profile, good patient compliance rates, and lack of abuse liability, they have a delayed onset of action ranging from 10 to 20 days. Therefore, the physician may consider beginning antidepressant treatment during early withdrawal and continuing for weeks or longer as clinically indicated. The tricyclic antidepressant desipramine has been studied most extensively as a treatment of cocaine dependence. Early studies of desipramine to treat cocaine dependence showed positive results but placebo-controlled trials have not produced impressive findings. A meta-analysis of placebo-controlled studies by Levin and Lehman showed that although desipramine did not improve retention in treatment, it did produce greater cocaine abstinence relative to placebo. However, treatment with desipramine has induced "early tricyclic jitteriness syndrome" and cocaine craving, as well as relapse to cocaine use in some patients. Therefore, desipramine as pharmacotherapy would hold serious clinical caveats. Additional studies have focused on the involvement of the 5HT3 receptor subtype in the neuropharmacology of cocaine, but the results obtained are somewhat inconsistent. Several 5HT3-selective antagonists, including MDL-72222 and ondansetron were reported to attenuate cocaine-induced locomotor activity in rodents. However, ondansetron failed to block the reinforcing or discriminative-stimulus effects of cocaine in rodents. Several other antidepressants, including fluoxetine, sertraline, and trazodone, that work predominantly through serotonergic mechanisms also have been used as pharmacotherapy for cocaine dependence. Although some reports indicated that treatment with fluoxetine reduced cocaine craving and use in cocaine-abusing heroin addicts, other investigators have not found fluoxetine to be effective in attenuating cocaine use and withdrawal symptoms. Bupropion, a "second-generation" antidepressant, has been studied as pharmacotherapy for cocaine dependence (Heilis and Egli., 2006; Carrera et al., 2004)

Various studies suggest that L-type calcium channel blockers potentially reduce the rewarding effects of cocaine. One such compound, the L-type calcium channel blocker isradipine (Fig. 7), attenuated the cocaine induced dopamine release in the striatum of rats. Another report described isradipine-induced attenuation of condition place preference and the discriminative stimulus properties of cocaine. Also, pretreatment with isradipine resulted in a dose-dependent decrease in intravenous cocaine self-administration. Because of the antihypertensive quality of calcium channel blockers, the potential increase in cardiac output in patients with normal ventricular function could complicate their use as pharmacotherapies for cocaine abuse (Carrera et al., 2004)

Notwithstanding the impressive amount of research effort in this area, a large number of studies using dopaminergic drugs have failed to yield encouraging results. To date, no pharmacotherapeutic agent of this type used on an experimental basis has been shown effectiveness that would merit medical implementation.

7. Perspectives

The fact that GABA and glutamate are so widely present makes it likely that they will be altered during drug addiction. This fact also makes it difficult to treat addiction with drug therapy. Say that a drug affects GABA and glutamate in way that relieves craving. Because GABA and glutamate are so widely present, these drugs could produce a mess of side effects as well. If we had drugs that could selectively stimulate or block certain receptors, then we could treat addiction and avoid doing people more harm than good.

Treatment studies should continue the present emphases on (1) identifying and systematically testing pharmacological agents that may be useful in achieving abstinence from cocaine and reducing the likelihood of relapse; (2) characterizing and understanding the processes and outcomes of existing treatments by using field studies with outcomes studied over a 1-year post treatment period and longer; and (3) testing the efficacy of specific psychosocial interventions such as psychotherapies, behavioral treatments, and relapse prevention strategies. The need for theory-based treatment approaches should be recognized. Promising pharmacotherapies also should be field tested in clinical programs to understand issues related to compliance with medication regimens.

Recent efforts to discover new pharmacs have been oriented to get a vaccine for cocaine addiction. However, to improve existing treatment, there should be a systematic effort to integrate research and treatment. Research should develop and test criteria for client-treatment matching so that the most cost-effective treatments can be provided for cocaine dependent users. Additional research should focus on better understanding motivation as a factor for increasing the retention of cocaine users in treatment. This focus would include use of motivational incentives to enter and remaining treatment. There is a need to better understand the role of self-help in treating cocaine users.

Additional studies for the current cocaine vaccine are planned to confirm and extend the discussed outpatient studies, and there are ongoing developmental studies of alternative adjuvants and vaccine constructs which will likely improve the quantity and quality of antibodies produced, as well as the proportion of high response subjects. Such results would lead to clinical application of these vaccines for in the treatment of cocaine abusers. Better vaccines or newer methods will not be the end of the game for treating substance abuse, however. The motivated cocaine addict will need other interventions such as therapy and rehabilitation programs in order to overcome this seductive addiction. Anti-drug programs in schools should be strengthened, as cocaine addiction often starts before age 20. The criminal justice system should reconsider the wholesale incarceration of cocaine users, and offer help rather than punishment. Let us hope that in the years ahead anti-cocaine vaccination will be one of numerous arrows in our therapeutic quiver to combat drug addiction (Kinsey et al., 2010).

Incorporation of technology into treatment methods is also being explored. Computer-assisted therapies may offer more consistent and convenient delivery of instruction and reinforcement in conjunction with CBT. An additional and innovative approach, to be used with a structured treatment program, is the administration of a therapeutic cocaine vaccine. The vaccine is shown to inhibit the cocaine 'high' through antibodies binding to cocaine in the circulation and inhibiting entry to the brain. However, it does not stop drug cravings. In addition, recent findings suggest that only those subjects who attain high (> 43 ug/L) IgG anticocaine antibody levels benefited from significantly reduced cocaine use. Unfortunately, only 38% of the vaccinated subjects achieved such high IgG levels. Psychosocial therapy is still essential in medication and vaccine studies because the underlying issues of the dependence and use behavior must be addressed or individuals may relapse or resort to misusing another drug. The intent of the vaccine is to immunize motivated patients as part of a comprehensive recovery program and to inhibit the reinforcing activity of cocaine and decrease the likelihood of relapse (Penberthy et al., 2010).

8. Acknowledgements

Authors want to express a special thanks to people who have worked so hard in developing science in our country, Colombia, and specially to three people who now are making amazing science in the kingdom of God, Leonardo Lareo, Gerardo Pérez and Luis Osses. In memoriam of Leonardo, Gerardo and Luis, Professors and friends.

9. References

Anderson, SM, Famous, KR, Sadri-Vakili, G, Kumaresan, V, Schmidt HD, Bass CE, Terwilliger EF, Cha JH, Pierce RC. (2008). CaMKII: A biochemical bridge linking accumbens dopamine and glutamate systems in cocaine seeking. *Nat Neurosci* 11,3 (March 2008), pp. 344-53, ISSN 1097-6256

Ary, A.W.; Szumlinski, K.K. (2007). Regional differences in the effects of withdrawal from repeated cocaine upon Homer and glutamate receptor expression: a two-species comparison. *Brain Res*, 12,1184 (December 2007), pp. 295-305, ISSN 0006-8993

Bachtell, RK, Choi, KH, Simmons, DL, Falcon, E, Monteggia, LM, Neve, RL, Self, DW.(2008). Role of GluR1 expression in nucleus accumbens neurons in cocaine sensitization and cocaine-seeking behavior.*Eur J Neurosci*, 27, 9 (May 2008), pp. 2229-40 ISSN 1460-9568

Ballon J, Feifel D. (2006). A systematic review of modafinil: potential clinical uses and mechanisms of action. J Clin Psychiatry, 67, 4 (april 2006), pp. 554-66. ISSN 0160-6689

Barrett, A. C., Negus, S. S, Mello, N. K., and Caine, S. B. (2005). Effect of GABA Agonists and GABA-A Receptor Modulators on Cocaine- and Food-Maintained Responding and Cocaine Discrimination in Rats. *JPET*, 315, 2 (November 2005), pp. 858-871, ISSN 0022-3565

Barrós-Loscertales, A; Garavan, H; Bustamante, J; Ventura-Campos, N; Llopis, J; Belloch, V; Parcet, M; Ávila, C. (2011).   Reduced striatal volume in cocaine-dependent patients.*Neuroimage* 56, 3 (june 2011), pp. 1021-1026. ISSN 1053-8119.

Berridge, K, Robinson T. (1998). What is the role of dopamine in reward: hedonic impact, reward learning, or incentive salience? *Brain Res Rev*, 28 (December 1998), pp. 309-369, ISSN 0165-0173

Boehm, J. and Malinow, R. (2005).AMPA receptor phosphorylation during synaptic plasticity.*Biochem. Soc. Trans.* 33, pt 6 (December 2005), pp. 1354–1356, ISSN 0300-5127

Boudreau, A.C, and Wolf, M.E. (2005). Behavioral sensitization to cocaine is associated with increased AMPA receptor surface expression in the nucleus accumbens. *J Neurosci* , 25, 40 (October 2005), pp. 9144-9151, ISSN 0270-6474

Boudreau, AC, Reimers, JM, Milovanovic, M, Wolf ME. (2007). Surface AMPA receptors in the rat nucleus accumbens increase during cocaine withdrawal but internalize after cocaine challenge in association with altered activity of mitogen-activated protein kinases. *J Neurosci*, 27,39 (September 2007), pp. 10621–10635, ISSN 0270-6474

Bowers, M.; Chen, B.; Chou, J.; Osborne, M.; Gass, J.; See, R.; Bonci, A.; Janak, P.; Olive, M. (2007). Acamprosate attenuates cocaine- and cue-induced reinstatement of cocaine-seeking behavior in rats. *Psychopharmacology*, 195, 3 (December 2007), pp. 397-406. ISSN 0033-3158Carrera, M; Meijler, M; Janda, K. (2004).Cocaine pharmacology and current pharmacotherapies for its abuse.*Bioorganic & Medicinal Chemistry*,12 (October 2004)pp. 5019-5030. ISSN 0968-0896

Carroll, K. M., Fenton, L. R., Ball, S. A., Nich, C., Frankforter, T. L., Shi, J., Rounsaville, B. (2004). Efficacy of disulfiram and cognitive behavior therapy in cocaine dependent outpatients: a randomized placebo-controlled trial. *Arch Gen Psychiatry*, 61, 3, (march 2004) pp. 264−272. ISSN 0003-990x

Chiamulera, C.; Epping-Jordan, M.P.; Zocchi, A.; Marcon, C.; Cottiny, C.; Tacconi, S.; Corsi, M.; Orzi, F.; Conquet, F. (2001).Reinforcing and locomotor stimulant effects of cocaine are absent in mGluR5 null mutant mice. *Nat. Neurosci*, 4,9 (September 2001), pp. 873-4, ISSN 1097-6256

Conn, P. J., and Pin, J. P. (1997).Pharmacology and functions of metabotropic glutamate receptors.*Annu. Rev. Pharmacol. Toxicol.*37 (1997), pp. 205–237. ISSN 0362-1642

Conrad, KL, Tseng, KY, Uejima JL, Reimers JM, Heng LJ, Shaham Y, Marinelli M, Wolf ME. (2008). Formation of accumbens GluR2-lacking AMPA receptors mediates incubation of cocaine craving. *Nature* 454, (July 2008), pp. 118-121. ISSN0028-0836

Cornish, JL, Kalivas, PW. (2000). Glutamate transmission in the nucleus accumbens mediates relapse in cocaine addiction. *J Neurosci* 20 (May 2000), pp. RC89, ISSN 0270-6474

Cull-Candy, S., Brickley, S., and Farrant, M. (2001). NMDA receptor subunits: diversity, development and disease. *Curr.Opin.Neurobiol,* 11(2001), pp. 327–335,ISSN 0959-4388

Di Chiara, G. (2002). Nucleus accumbens shell and core dopamine: differential role in behavior and addiction. *Behav Brain Res,* 137 (December 2002), pp. 75-114. ISSN 0166-4328

Di Ciano, P, Everitt, BJ. (2001). Dissociable effects of antagonism of NMDA and AMPA/KA receptors in the nucleus accumbens core and shell on cocaine-seeking behavior.*Neuropsychopharmacology,* 25, 3 (September 2001), pp. 341-360, ISSN 1461-1457

Dingledine, R., Borges, K., Bowie, D., and Traynelis, S. F. (1999).The glutamate receptor ion channels.*Pharmacol. Rev.* 51,1 (March 1999), pp. 7–61, ISSN 0031-6997

Edwards, S., Graham, D. L., Bachtell, R. K., and Self, D. W. (2007).Region-specific tolerance to cocaine-regulated cAMP-dependent protein phosphorylation following chronic self-administration.*Eur. J. Neurosci,* 25 (April 2007), pp. 2201–2213,ISSN 1460-9568

Ersche, K; Barnes, A; Jones, S; Morein-Zamir, S; Robbins, T; Bullmore, E. (2011). Abnormal structure of frontostriatal brain systems is associated with aspects of impulsivity and compulsivity in cocaine dependence. *Brain.*134, 7, (july 2011) pp. 2013-2024. ISSN 0006-8950.

Everitt, B.J. and Wolf, M.E. (2002) Psychomotor stimulant addiction: a neural systems perspective. *J. Neurosci,* 22 (May 2002), pp. 3312–3320, ISSN 0270-6474

Fadda P, Scherma M, Fresu A, Collu M, Fratta W. (2003). Baclofen antagonizes nicotine-, cocaine-, and morphine-induced dopamine release in the nucleus accumbens of rat. *Synapse.* 50, 1 (October 2003), pp. 1-6. ISSN 0887-4776

Ferrario, CR, Li X, Wang, X, Reimers, JM, Uejima, JL, Wolf ME. (2010). The role of glutamate receptor redistribution in locomotor sensitization to cocaine. *Neuropsychopharmacology*35 (February 2010), pp. 818–833,ISSN 1461-1457

Floresco, SB, Yang, CR, Phillips, AG, Blaha, CD. (1998). Basolateral amygdala stimulation evokes glutamate receptor-dependent dopamine efflux in the nucleus accumbens of the anesthetised rat. *Eur J Neurosci* 10,4 (April 1998), pp. 1241–1251, ISSN 1460-9568

Fourgeaud, L. Mato Susana, Bouchet, Delphine, Hémar, Agnès, Worley, Paul F, and Manzoni, Olivier J. (2004). A single in vivo exposure to cocaine abolishes endocannabinoid-mediated longterm depression in the nucleus accumbens. *J. Neurosci.* 24, 31 (August 2004), pp. 6939–6945,ISSN 0270-6474

Franklin, T.R., Acton, P.D., Maldjian, J.A., Gray, J.D., Croft, J.R., Dackis, C.A., O'Brien, C.P., and Childress, A.R. (2002). Decreased gray matter concentration in the insular, orbitofrontal, cingulate, and temporal cortices of cocaine patients.*Biol. Psychiatry,*51, 2 (january 2002), pp. 134–142, ISSN 0006-3223

Gass, J.T. and M.F. Olive.(2008). Glutamatergic substrates of drug addiction and alcoholism.*Biochem.Pharmacol.* 75,1 (January 2008), pp. 218–265, ISSN 0006-2952

Ghasemzadeh, M.B., C. Mueller and P. Vasudevan. (2009). Behavioral sensitization to cocaine is associated with increased glutamate receptor trafficking to the postsynaptic density after extended withdrawal period. *Neuroscience* 159 (March 2009), pp. 414–426, ISSN 0306-4522

Goldstein, RA, Volkow, ND. (2002). Drug addiction and its underlying neurobiological basis: neuroimaging evidence for the involvement of the frontal cortex. *Am J Psychiatry,* 159,10 (2002), pp. 1642-1652. ISSN 0002-953X

Gonzalez, G.; Sevarino, K.; Sofuoglu, M.; Poling, J.; Oliveto, A.; Gonsai, K.; George, T.; Kosten, T. (2003). Tiagabine increases cocaine-free urines in cocaine-dependent methadone-treated patients: results of a randomized pilot study. *Addiction,* 98, 11 (November 2003), pp. 1625-32. ISSN 0965-2140.

Gryder, D. S., &Rogawski, M. A. (2003).Selective antagonism of GluR5 kainate-receptor-mediated synaptic currents by topiramate in rat basolateral amygdala neurons.*J Neurosci,* 23, 18 (August 2003) pp. 7069-7074. ISSN 0270-6474

Haile CN, Kosten TR, Kosten TA. (2009). Pharmacogenetic treatments for drug addiction: cocaine, amphetamine and methamphetamine. *Am J Drug Alcohol Abuse.* 35, 3 (June 2009), pp. 161-77. ISSN 0095-2790.

Harris, B. R., Prendergast, M. A., Gibson, D. A., Rogers, D. T., Blanchard, J. A., Holley, R. C.,Fu, M., Hart, S., Pedigo, N., Littleton, J. (2002). Acamprosate inhibits the binding and neurotoxic effects of trans-ACPD, suggesting a novel site of action at metabotropic glutamate receptors. *Alcohol: ClinExp Res* 26, 12, (December 2002), pp. 1779-1793. ISSN 1530-0277

Heilig, M., Egli, M. (2006) Pharmacological treatment of alcohol dependence: Target symptoms and target mechanisms.*Pharmacology & Therapeutics* 111, 3, (September 2006), pp. 855-876. ISSN 0163-7258

Higgins, G. A., Tomkins, D. M., Fletcher, P. J., & Sellers, E. M. (1992). Effect of drugs influencing 5-HT function on ethanol drinking and feeding behavior in rats: studies using a drinkometer system. *NeurosciBiobehav Rev,* 16, 4 (winter 1992) pp. 535-552. ISSN 0147-7634

Hotsenpiller,G., M. Giorgetti and M.E.Wolf. (2001). Alterations in behaviour and glutamate transmission following presentation of stimuli previously associated with cocaine exposure. *Eur. J. Neurosci.* 14, 11 (December 2001), pp. 1843-1855, ISSN 1460-9568

Kalivas, P.W and McFarland, K. (2003).Brain circuitry and the reinstatement of cocaine-seeking behavior.*Psychopharmacology* (Berl), 168 (July 2003), pp. 168:44-56, ISSN 0033-3158

Kalivas, P. W. (2004). Glutamate systems in cocaine addiction.*Current Opinion in Pharmacology,* 4 (February 2004), pp. 23-29, ISSN1471-4892

Kalivas, P.W and O'Brien C. (2008). Drug addiction as a pathology of staged neuroplasticity. *Neuropsychopharmacology,* 33,1 (January 2008), pp. 166-180, ISSN 1461-1457

Kaminski, R. M., Banerjee, M., &Rogawski, M. A. (2004).Topiramate selectively protects against seizures induced by ATPA, a GluR5 kainate receptor agonist. *Neuropharmacology,* 46, 8 (june 2004) pp. 1097-1104. ISSN 0028-3908

Kantak, KM, Black Y, Valencia, E, Green-Jordan, K, Eichembaum, HB. (2002). Dissociable effects of lidocaine inactivation of the rostral and caudal basolateral amygdala on the maintenance and reinstatement of cocaine-seeking behavior in rats.*J Neurosci,* 22, 3 (February 2002), pp. 1126-1136, ISSN 0270-6474

Kinsey, B; Kosten, T; Orson, F. (2010).Anti-cocaine vaccine development.*Expert Rev Vaccines.* 9, 9 (September 2010), pp. 1109-1114. ISSN 1476-0584.

Kirchmayer, U., Davoli, M., &Verster, A. (2003).Naltrexone maintenance treatment for opioid dependence. (Cochrane Review) *In the cochraneLybrary.* 1 (January 2003). ISSN 1464-780X

Klitenick, M. A., DeWitte, P. and Kalivas, P. W. (1992). Regulation of somatodendritic dopamine release in the ventral tegmental area by opioids and GABA: an in vivo microdialysis study. *J. Neurosci,* 12,7 (July 1992), pp. 2623–2632, ISSN 0270-6474

Kourrich, S, Rothwell, PE, Klug, JR, Thomas, MJ. (2007). Cocaine experience controls bidirectional synaptic plasticity in the nucleus accumbens. *J Neurosci,* 27, 30 (July 2007), pp. 7921–7928,ISSN 0270-6474

Kozell, L.B. & C.K. Meshul.(2004). Nerve terminal glutamate immunoreactivity in the rat nucleus accumbens and ventral tegmental area after a short withdrawal from cocaine.*Synapse* 51, 4 (March 2004), pp. 224–232, ISSN 0887-4476

Kozell,B. and K.Meshul. (2003). Alterations in nerve terminal glutamate immunoreactivity in the nucleus accumbens and ventral tegmental area following single and repeated doses of cocaine.*Psychopharmacology* (Berl) 165, 4 (February 2003), pp. 337–345, ISSN 0033-3158

Kreek, M. J., LaForge, K. S., &Butelman, E. (2002).Pharmacotherapy of addictions.*Nat Rev Drug Discov,* 1, 9, (September 2002), pp. 710–726.ISSN 1474-1776.

Johnson B. (2004). An overview of the development of medications including novel anticonvulsants for the treatment of alcohol dependence.*Expert OpinPharmacother,* 5, 9 (September 2004), pp. 1943-55. ISSN 1465-6566

Lau, C.G. and Zukin, R.S. (2007).NMDA receptor trafficking in synaptic plasticity and neuropsychiatric disorders.*Nat. Rev. Neurosci.* 8 (June 2007), pp. 413-426 ISSN 1471-0048

Levin, F.; Lehman, A. F.(1991).Meta-Analysis of Desipramine as an Adjunct in the: Treatment of Cocaine Addiction. J. Clin. Psychopharmacol.11,6 (December 1991), pp. 374-378. ISSN 0271-0479.

Levin FR, Evans SM, Brooks DJ, Garawi F. (2007). Treatment of cocaine dependent treatment seekers with adult ADHD: double-blind comparison of methylphenidate and placebo. Drug *Alcohol Dependence,* 87, 1 (February 2007), pp. 20-29. ISSN 0376-8716

Liu, XY, Chu, XP, Mao, LM, Wang, M, Lan, HX, Li, MH, *et al.* (2006). Modulation of D2R-NR2B interactions in response to cocaine.*Neuron,* 52, 5 (December 2006), pp. 897-909, ISSN 0896-6273

Loftis, J. M., and Janowsky, A. (2002). Cocaine treatment- and withdrawal- induced alterations in the expression and serine phosphorylation of the NR1 NMDA receptor subunit. *Psychopharmacology,* 164 (2002), pp. 349–359, ISSN 0033-3158

Lu, L, Grimm, JW, Shaham, Y, Hope, BT. (2003). Molecular neuroadaptations in the accumbens and ventral tegmental area during the first 90 days of forced abstinence from cocaine self-administration in rats. *J Neurochem* 85, 6 (June 2003), pp. 1604-1613, ISSN 0022-3042

Makris N., Gasic GP, Seidman LJ, Goldstein JM, Gastfriend DR, Elman I, Albaugh DM, Hodge SM, Ziegler DA, Sheahan F, Caviness VS Jr., Tsuang MT, Kennedy DN, Hyman SE, Rosen BR, Breiter HC. (2004). Decreased Absolute Amygdala Volume in Cocaine Addicts. *Neuron,* 44 (November 2004), pp. 729–740, ISSN 0896-6273

Mao, Li-Min, Guo, Ming-Lei, Jin, Dao-Zhong, Fibuch, Eugene E., Choe, Eun Sang, and Wang John Q. (2011). Post-translational modification biology of glutamate receptors and drug addiction.*Frontiers in neuroanatomy*, 5, 19 (March 2011), pp. 1-11, ISSN 1662-5129

Marinelli M, White FJ (2000) Enhanced vulnerability to cocaine self-administration is associated with elevated impulse activity of midbrain dopamine neurons. J Neurosci 20:8876–8885

Matochik, J.A., London, E.D., Eldreth, D.A., Cadet, J.L., and Bolla, K.I. (2003). Frontal cortical tissue composition in abstinent cocaine abusers: a magnetic resonance imaging study. *Neuroimage19*, 3 (july 2003), pp. 1095–1102. ISSN 1053-8119

McCance-Katz E, Kosten T, Jatlow P. (1998).Disulfiram effects on acute cocaine administration. *Drug Alcohol Depend.* 52. 1 (september 1998), pp. 27-39. ISSN 0376-8716

McFarland, K., C.C. Lapish and P.W. Kalivas.(2003). Prefrontal glutamate release into the core of the nucleus accumbensmediates cocaine-induced reinstatement of drug-seeking behavior.*J. Neurosci.* 23 (April 2003), pp. 3531–3537, ISSN 0270-6474

Mitrano, D.A, Arnold, C, Smith, Y. (2008). Subcellular and subsynaptic localization of group I metabotropic glutamate receptors in the nucleus accumbens of cocaine-treated rats.*Neuroscience*, 154, 2 (June 2008), pp. 653-66 ISSN 0306-4522

Meert, T. F. (1993). Effects of various serotonergic agents on alcohol intake and alcohol preference in Wistar rats selected at two different levels of alcohol preference. *Alcohol Alcohol,* 28, 2 (march 1993) pp. 157–170. ISSN 0735-0414

Moran, M.M, McFarland, K, Melendez, R.I, Kalivas, P.W, Seamans, J.K. J. (2005).Cystine/Glutamate Exchange Regulates Metabotropic Glutamate Receptor Presynaptic Inhibition of Excitatory Transmission and Vulnerability to Cocaine Seeking. *J. Neurosci*, 25,27 (July 2005), pp. 6389-6393 ISSN 0270-6474

Neisewander, JL, Baker, DA, Fuchs, RA, Tran-Nguyen, LTL, Palme,r A, Marshall, JF. (2000). Fos protein expression and cocaine seeking behavior in rats after exposure to a cocaine self-administration environment. *J Neurosci*, 20 (January 2000), pp. 798-805 ISSN 0270-6474

Nestler, E. J. (2001).Molecular basis of long-term plasticity underlying addiction. Nature Rev Neurosci, 2, 2 (February 2001), pp. 119-128, ISSN 1471-003X

Nestler, EJ, Barrot, M, Self, DW. (2001). DeltaFosB: a sustained molecular switch for addiction. ProcNatlAcadSci USA 98, 20 (September 2001), pp. 11042-11046 ISSN 0027-8424

Nestler, E. J. (2004).Molecular and cellular mechanisms of opiate and cocaine addiction.*Trends in Pharmacological Sciences*, 25, 4 (April 2004), pp. 210-218, ISSN 0165-6147

Nestler, E. (2005).Neurobiology of drug addiction.*Science & practice perspectives*, 3, 4 (December 2005), pp. 6-10, ISSN 1930-4307

Nestler, E.J. 2005. The Neurobiology of Cocaine Addiction. Sci Pract Perspect. December; 3(1): 4–10.

O'Brien, C. 2001. Drug addiction and drug abuse. In The Pharmacological Basis of Therapeutics. Edited by Hardman J, n Limbird L, Gilman AG. New York: McGraw-Hill; 2001:621-642.

Park, W.K, Bari, A.A, Jey, A. R, Anderson, S. M, Spealman, R. D, Rowlett, J. K, Pierce, R. C. (2002). Cocaine administered into the medial prefrontal cortex reinstates cocaine-seeking behavior by increasing AMPA receptor-mediated glutamate transmission in the nucleus accumbens. *J. Neurosci.* 22,7 (April 2002), pp. 2916–2925, ISSN 0270-6474

Penberthy, J; Ait-Daoud, N; Vaughan, M; Fanning, T. (2010) Review of Treatment for Cocaine Dependence.*Current Drug Abuse Reviews, 3,(march 2010), pp.* 49-62. ISSN 1874-4737.

Pierce, R.C, Bell, R.C, Duffy, K, Kalivas, P.W. (1996). Repeated cocaine augments excitatory amino acid transmission in the nucleus accumbens only in rats having developed behavioral sensitization. *J. Neurosci.* 16 (February 1996), pp. 1550-1560, ISSN 0270-6474

Rist, F., Randall, C. L., Heather, N., & Mann, K. (2005). New developments in alcoholism treatment research in europe. *Alcohol: ClinExp Res.* 29,6 (june 2005) pp. 1127–1132. ISSN 1530-0277

Schmidt, H. D. and Pierce, R. C. (2010).Cocaine-induced neuroadaptations in glutamate transmission Potential therapeutic targets for craving and addiction.*Ann. N.Y. Acad. Sci.* 1187 (January 2010), pp. 35–75, ISNN 0077-8923

Schultz, W. (2002).Getting formal with dopamine and reward.*Neuron,* 36, 2 (October 2002), pp. 241-63, ISSN 0896-6273

Spanagel, R., &Zieglgansberger, W. (1997). Anti-craving compounds for ethanol: new pharmacological tools to study addictive processes. *Trends PharmacolSci,* 18, 2 (February 2007), pp. 54–59. ISSN 0165-6147

Spanagel, R., Pendyala, G., Abarca, C., Zghoul, T., Sanchis-Segura, C., Magnone, M. C., Lascorz, J., Depner, M., Holzberg, D., Soyka, M., Schreiber, S., Matsuda, F., Lathrop, M., Schumann, G., Albrecht, U. (2005). The clock gene Per2 influences the glutamatergic system and modulates alcohol consumption. *Nat Med* 11, 1 (January 2005). Pp. 35–42. ISSN 1078-8956

Stromberg, M. F. (2004). The effect of baclofen alone and in combination with naltrexone on ethanol consumption in the rat.*PharmacolBiochemBehav,* 78, 4 (august 2004) pp. 743–750. ISSN 0091-3057

Sun, X, Zhao, Y, Wolf, M.E. (2005). Dopamine receptor stimulation modulates AMPA receptor synaptic insertion in prefrontal cortex neurons. *J Neurosci,* 25, 32 (August 2005), pp. 7342-7351, ISSN 0270-6474

Suto, N, Tanabe, LM, Austin, JD, Creekmore, E, Pham, CT, Vezina, P. (2004). Previous exposure to psychostimulants enhances the reinstatement of cocaine seeking by nucleus accumbens AMPA. *Neuropsychopharmacology*29 (December 2004), pp. 2149–2159, ISSN 1461-1457

Sutton, M.A., Schmidt, E.F., Choi, K.-H., Schad, C.A., Whisler, K., Simmons, D., *et al.* (2003). Extinction-induced up-regulation in AMPA receptors reduces cocaine-seeking behaviour. Nature, 421 (January 2003), pp, 70–75, ISSN 0028-0836

Szumlinski, K.K, Ary, A.W, Lominac, K.D. (2008). Homers regulate drug-induced neuroplasticity: implications for addiction. Biochem.Pharmacol, 75(January 2008), pp. 112-33, ISSN 0006-2952

Thomas, M.J., P.W. Kalivas and Y. Shaham.(2008). Neuroplasticity in the mesolimbic dopamine system and cocaine addiction.*Br. J. Pharmacol,* 154 (May 2008), pp. 327–342, ISSN 0007-1188

Thomas, MJ, Beurrier, C, Bonci, A, Malenka, RC. (2001). Long-term depression in the nucleus accumbens: A neural correlate of behavioral sensitization to cocaine. *Nat Neurosci,* 4 (December 2001), pp. 1217–1223, ISSN ISSN 1097-6256

Tomkins, D. M., Le, A. D., & Sellers, E. M. (1995).Effect of the 5-HT3 antagonist ondansetron on voluntary ethanol intake in rats and mice maintained on a limited access procedure.*Psychopharmacology*, 117, 4 (February 1995) pp. 479−485. ISSN 0033-3158

Tzschentke, TM and Schmidt, WJ. (2003). Glutamatergic mechanisms in addiction.*Molecular Psychiatry*, 8 (September 2003), pp. 373–382, ISSN 1476-5578

Tzschentke, TM. (2001). Pharmacology and behavioural pharmacology of the mesocortical dopamine system.*ProgNeurobiol*, 63, 3 (February 2001), pp. 241–320, ISSN 0555-4047

Uys, J. D. and LaLumiere, R. T. (2008). Glutamate: The New Frontier in Pharmacotherapy for Cocaine Addiction. *CNS & Neurological Disorders - Drug Targets*, 7, 5 (November 2008), pp. 482-491, ISSN 1871-5273

Volkow, N.D, Wang, G-J, Ma, Y, Fowler, J.S, Wong, C, Ding, Y-S, Hitzemann, R, Swanson, J, and Kalivas, P. (2005). Activation of orbital and medial prefrontal cortex by methylphenidate in cocaineaddicted subjects but not in controls: relevance to addiction. *J. Neurosci*, 25, 15 (April 2005), pp. 3932–3939, ISSN 0270-6474

Winder, D.G, Egli, R.E, Schramm, N.L, Matthews, R.T. (2002).Synaptic plasticity in drug reward circuitry.*CurrMol Med*, 2, 7 (November 2002), pp. 667-676, ISSN 1566-5240

White, H. S., Brown, S. D., Woodhead, J. H., Skeen, G. A., & Wolf, H. H. (1997). Topiramate enhances GABA-mediated chloride flux and GABAevoked chloride currents in murine brain neurons and increases seizure threshold. *Epilepsy Res*, 28, 3 (October 2008) pp. 167−179. ISSN 0920-1211

Wolf, M.E, Ferrario, C.R. (2010). AMPA receptor plasticity in the nucleus accumbens after repeated exposure to cocaine.*NeurosciBiobehav Rev*, 35 (January 2010), pp. 185–211, ISSN 0149-7634

Wolf, M.E, Sun, X, Mangiavacchi, S, Chao, SZ. (2004). Psychomotor stimulants and neuronal plasticity.*Neuropharmacology*, 47, suppl 1 (September 2004), pp. 61–79, ISSN 0028-3908

Xi, Z.X, Ramamoorthy, S, Baker, D.A, Shen, H, Samuvel, D.J, Kalivas, P. (2002), Modulation of group II metabotropic glutamate receptor signaling by chronic cocaine. *J. Pharmacol. Exp. Ther*, 303, 2 (November 2002), pp., 608-15, ISSN 0022-3565

Xi, Z.X. and Stein, E.A. (1998). Nucleus accumbens dopamine release modulation by mesolimbic GABAA receptors-an in vivo electrochemical study. *Brain Res*, 798 (1998), pp. 156-165 ISSN 0006-8993

Ye, J.H and Ren, J. (2006). Cocaine inhibition of GABA(A) current: role of dephosphorylation. *Crit Rev Neurobiol*, 18, 1-2 (2006), pp. 85-94, ISSN 0892-0915

Yücel, M; Solowij, N; Respondek, C; Whittle, S; Fornito, A; Pantelis, C; Lubman, D. (2008). Regional Brain Abnormalities Associated With Long-term Heavy Cannabis Use. *Arch Gen Psychiatry*, 65, 6 (June 2008) pp. 694-701.ISSN 0003-990x.

Zahm DS, Brog JS. 1992. On the significance of subterritories in the "accumbens" part of the rat ventral striatum. Neuroscience 50:751–767

Zhang, X, Lee, T.H, Davidson, C, Lazarus, C, Wetsel, W.C, Ellinwood, E.H. (2007).Reversal of cocaine-induced behavioral sensitization and associated phosphorylation of the NR2B and GluR1 subunits of the NMDA and AMPA receptors. *Neuropsychopharmacology*, 32, 2 (February 2007), pp. 377-387, ISSN 0893-133X

Zona, C., Ciotti, M. T., &Avoli, M. (1997).Topiramate attenuates voltage-gated sodium currents in rat cerebellar granule cells. *NeurosciLett*, 231, 3 (august 1997) pp 123−126. ISSN 0304-3940

7

A Molecular Mechanism of Ethanol Dependence: The Influence of the Ionotropic Glutamate Receptor Activated by N-Methyl-D-Aspartate

Sonia Luz Albarracín Cordero[1,*], Bernd Robert Stab II[1,*],
Felipe Guillen[1,**] and Edgar Antonio Reyes Montano[2,**]
Pontificia Universidad Javeriana, Colombia
Universidad Nacional de Colombia
Colombia

1. Introduction

The World Health Organization (WHO) estimates that there are about 2 billion people world-wide who consume alcoholic beverages (WHO, 2004). Alcohol use is related to a wide range of physical, mental, and social detriments. Additionally, alcohol affects almost every organ in the human body as well as the central nervous system (CNS) (Spanagel, 2009). There are several theories as to how alcohol affects the CNS. They are classified into two main groups depending on the primary target of ethanol. These two groups are lipid and protein theories (Goldstein, 1986). Before the 1990s, different lipid theories postulated that alcohol acted via some perturbation of the membrane lipids in CNS neurons. In particular, the effects on membrane fluidity and the disordering of the bulk lipid phase of membranes were originally attractive hypotheses for alcohol action. However, recently the protein hypothesis has become the predominant theory (Lovinger, 1997). This hypothesis predicts that alcohol acts specifically on membrane proteins such as receptors and ion channels. The main reason for a shift towards the protein theory originates from evidence that alcohol, at concentrations in the 10–20 mM range, directly interferes with the function of several ion channels (K^+, Ca^{2+}) and receptors (Lovinger et al., 1989). These ethanol effects are mediated through a number of neural transmitter systems including γ-aminobutyric acid (GABA) and glutamate (Takadera et al., 2008; Murail et al., 2011).

The GABA receptor is involved in GABA signalling and the ionotropic glutamate receptor complex activated by N-methyl-D-aspartate (iGluR-NMDA) is involved in glutamate signalling. The GABA and NMDA receptors have competing roles in neural excitability and transmission. Activation of GABA receptors results in a decrease in neural activity. In contrast, activation of iGluR-NMDA results in an increase in neural activity. Alcohol has been shown to have opposite effects on these two types of receptors. Alcohol administration leads to increases in GABA receptor activity and decreases in iGluR-NMDA activity (Suzdak et al., 1986; Tsai et

---

* Primary Authors
** Contributing Authors

al., 1995). The GABA receptor is a key inhibitory neurotransmitter receptor in the CNS (Figure 1). There are two types of GABA receptors. The $GABA_A$ receptor is a ligand-gated ion channel receptor and the $GABA_B$ receptor is a G coupled-protein receptor. Both are associated with the influx of chloride ions into the cell upon activation by GABA. Under normal conditions GABA binds to the GABA receptor and the chloride channel opens (Figure 1). This allows negatively charged chloride ions to enter the cell and inhibit neuronal cell activity. The GABA receptor is affected by low concentrations of alcohol (Suzdak et al., 1986). Also, ethanol has been shown to reduce the number of $GABA_A$-receptor sub-units, and GABA receptor polymorphisms have been associated with several alcoholic phenotypes (Mihic et al., 1997; Sander et al., 1999). The effects of alcohol are not limited to the modulation of GABA receptor activity; they also modulate iGluR-NMDA activity.

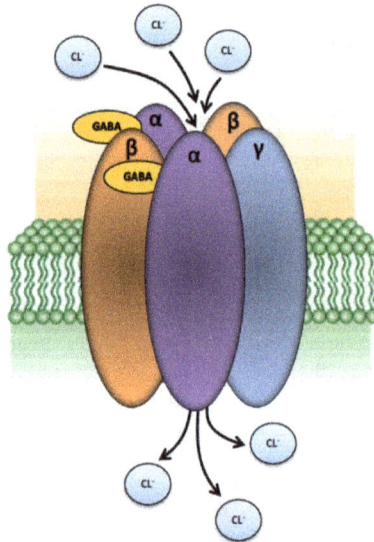

Fig. 1. The GABA receptor composition and potential GABA binding sites. Adapted from Belelli, 2005.

Most GABA receptors are believed to assemble as pentamers with two α subunits, two β subunits, and one γ subunit. The figure shows the influx of Cl- ions into the cell during GABA activation of the GABA receptor. The GABA molecules bind to interfaces between the α and β subunits.

The iGluR-NMDA is one of the most active molecules in the central nervous system that is involved in learning and memory. It has been extensively studied during the last 30 years. iGluR-NMDA function is inhibited by ethanol in a concentration-dependent manner over the range of 5–50 mM. This is also the concentration range that produces intoxication and that is linearly related to the intoxication potency (Ron, 2004). This suggests that ethanol-induced inhibition of responses to the iGluR-NMDA activation may contribute to the neural and the cognitive impairments associated with alcohol intoxication. However, the mechanism(s) of ethanol interference on NMDA receptor function remains in question.

The iGluR-NMDA is a ligand-gated ion channel with a heteromeric assembly of GluN1, GluN2 (A-D), and GluN3 subunits. The GluN1 and GluN2 subunits contain the co-agonist and agonist binding sites for glycine and glutamate respectively. The GluN3 subunit has some modulatory functions on channel activity especially under pathological conditions (Paoletti, 2011; Traynelis et al., 2010). Electrophysiological studies demonstrated ethanol interactions with domains that influence channel activity. This suggested that residues within the transmembrane (TMD) domains were involved. In the search for these possible binding sites of alcohol in the iGluR-NMDA, several putative binding sites were discovered. Utilizing site-directed mutagenesis, several studies reported putative binding sites in the TM3 and TM4 domains of the GluN1 and GluN2 subunits, respectively. Furthermore, the substitution of an alanine for a phenylalanine residue in the TM3 domain of the GluN1 subunit strongly reduced ethanol sensitivity in recombinant iGluR-NMDAs (Ren et al., 2003, Ren et al., 2008).

The iGluR-NMDA functions as a modulator of synaptic response and a molecular coincidence detector. At resting membrane potentials, iGluR-NMDAs are inactive. This is due to a voltage-dependent block of the channel pore by magnesium ions. This prevents ion flow. For example, the depolarization of the post-synaptic cell occurs through a train of impulses arriving at the pre-synaptic terminal. These impulses sustain the activation of α-amino-3-hydroxy-5-methyl-4-isoxazolepropionic acid (AMPA) receptors. AMPA receptors are a non-NMDA-type ionotropic transmembrane receptor for glutamate. This depolarization caused by the influx of sodium ions into the post-synaptic cell leads to the repulsion of magnesium ions in the iGluR-NMDAs. This repulsion of magnesium ions releases the channel inhibition and allows for iGluR-NMDA activation. However, this is not the only factor necessary for iGluR-NMDA channel function. Other factors include the agonist (glutamate) and the co-agonist (glycine) that allows the channel to open. Unlike GluA2-containing AMPA receptors, NMDA receptors are permeable to calcium ions as well as being permeable to other ions such as sodium and potassium. Therefore, iGluR-NMDA activation leads to a calcium influx into the post-synaptic cell. This event is important in the activation of a number of signaling cascades. Depending on the specific impulse received, the iGluR-NMDA is responsible for a wide range of post-synaptic functions that are involved in physiological processes such as long-term potentiation (LTP) and synaptic plasticity (Van Dongen, 2009). These processes have essential functions in learning and memory (Traynelis et al., 2010). In addition, the iGluR-NMDA is involved in different neurodegenerative diseases such as Alzheimer's, Huntington's, and Parkinson's (Ułas et al., 1994; Hallett et al., 2005; Levine et al., 2010; Saft et al., 2010). It is also involved in psychiatric disorders and pathophysiological conditions such as neuropathic pain (Javitt & Zukin, 1991; Collins et al., 2010). Recently, the iGluR-NMDA has been proposed as an important factor that can be altered in several addictions such as drug and alcohol addiction.

Ethanol inhibits iGluR-NMDA activity at very low concentrations that are typically found during alcohol dependence and abuse (Vengeliene et al., 2005). Several studies have investigated the direct involvement of the N-methyl D-aspartate receptor subtype 2B (NR2B)-containing iGluR-NMDA in ethanol dependence. Narita et al. demonstrated that the protein levels of NR2B subunits in the limbic forebrain but not the cerebral cortex were significantly increased during chronic ethanol dependence in mice. These findings suggest that the up-regulation of NR2B subunits during chronic ethanol exposure may be implicated in the initial development of physical dependence on ethanol (Narita et al., 2007). Sheela et al. reported that NR2B mRNA was significantly elevated in cultured mouse cortical neurons during chronic ethanol exposure (intermittent and non-intermittent) and remained elevated 5 days after withdrawal (Sheela et al., 2006). Studies such as these and others demonstrate that ethanol is a potent inhibitor of the iGluR-NMDA in a number of brain regions (Lovinger, et al., 1989; Lovinger, 1995; Weitlauf & Woodward, 2008). The ability of ethanol to inhibit responses to the iGluR-NMDA is dependent on the subunit combination of the iGluR-NMDA. The N-methyl D-aspartate receptor subtypes 1/2A (NR1/NR2A) and 1/2B (NR1/NR2B) combinations are preferentially sensitive to ethanol inhibition (Otton et al., 2009).

Structural information about the putative alcohol-binding sites on proteins such as the iGluR-NMDA continues to be discovered (Peoples & Weight, 1992; Mirshahi & Woodward, 1995). The functional impact of these binding sites also remains to be elucidated. Substitution studies have shown that a complete substitution for ethanol is exerted by iGluR-NMDA antagonists and certain GABA-mimetic drugs acting through different sites within the GABA$_A$ receptor complex. It has been consistently shown in mice, rats, and monkeys that noncompetitive antagonists of the iGluR-NMDA such as dizocilpine (MK-801), phencyclidine (PCP), ketamine, or memantine (which all act as an ion channel blockers) result in a generalized ethanol response. However, competitive iGluR-NMDA antagonists have often shown only partial substitution for ethanol. Moreover, it has been demonstrated that ketamine produced dose-related ethanol-like subjective effects in detoxified alcoholics. This suggests that NMDA receptors mediate the subjective effects, at least in part, of ethanol in humans (Ren et al., 2003).

In recent years the iGluR-NMDA has emerged as one of the most important and relevant molecules in all neural processes and a key structure in all excitable tissues. The iGluR-NMDA participates in almost all physiological, pathological, and pharmacological processes of the postsynaptic neural membrane. In addition, the iGluR-NMDA is a major target of alcohol (ethanol) in the brain and has been implicated in acute tolerance, long-term facilitation (LTF), sensitization, dependence, withdrawal, and craving (Nagy & László, 2002; Trujillo & Akil, 1995; De Witte, 2004). This chapter's focus is to present in a coherent and comprehensive approach as to why the iGluR-NMDA is one of the most important therapeutic targets in alcohol addiction. It will provide important information for understanding the effects produced by ethanol on the iGluR-NMDA such as the signaling pathways involved and the physiological consequences. It will also summarize information regarding the potential use of different iGluR-NMDA modulators as therapeutic treatments for the adverse effects of alcoholism. In addition, the review will summarize key results obtained from preclinical research such as *in vivo* animal models, *in vitro* cellular models, and *ex vivo* organotypic/acute brain slice models that are currently used to investigate CNS addictions.

2. Structural and functional aspects of the iGluR-NMDA

The iGluR-NMDA is a post-synaptic receptor involved in most neural functions that include fundamental processes such as learning, memory, and possibly consciousness (Lebel et al., 2006; Lareo & Corredor, 2007). The NMDARs are heteromeric complexes composed of three major types of subunits: NR1, with eight isoforms generated by the alternative splicing of the Grin1 gene (Perez-Otano et al., 2001); four NR2 subunits (A–D) generated by the genes

Grin2A–D (Sun et al., 2000); and two NR3 subunits generated by the genes Grin3A and Grin3B (Andersson et al., 2001). The stoichiometry of the NMDAR remains unknown. It is also not clear whether the NMDAR is a trimeric, tetrameric, or pentameric subunit complex (Ferrer-Montiel & Montal, 1996; Laube et al., 1998; Rosenmund et al., 1998; Hawkins et al., 1999; Nusser, 2000). However, it is known that the various cellular, biophysical, and pharmacological properties of NMDARs are dependent on the splice variants and the composition of these subunits within the receptor complex (Cull-Candy & Leszkiewicz, 2004; Paoletti & Neyton, 2007). The NMDAR is differentially distributed throughout the CNS and has been shown to mediate the fast synaptic action of the major excitatory neurotransmitter L-glutamate (Cochilla & Alfors, 1999; Nusser, 2000). These receptors are multimodulated. Glycine, polyamines (spermine and spermidine), histamine, and cations can act as positive modulators (McBain & Mayer, 1994; Hirai et al., 1996; Kashiwagi et al., 1997; Paoletti et al., 1997). The NMDA receptors are coupled to high conductance cationic channels that are permeable to Ca^{+2}, K^+, and Na^+ ions (Cushing et al., 1999).

NMDAR subunits contain a long extracellular N-terminal domain, three true transmembrane segments, a re-entrant pore loop, and an intracellular C-terminal domain of variable length (Mayer, 2005). The C-terminus of both NR1 and NR2 subunits interact with several intracellular scaffolding proteins and are subject to phosphorylation. As such, they are involved in the regulation of receptor trafficking and function (Salter & Kalia, 2004; Lau & Zukin, 2007). Glutamate, an agonist, binds to the NR2 subunits while the co-agonist glycine binds to the NR1 subunit. The N-terminal domain of the NR2 subunit is subject to allosteric inhibition by compounds such as ifenprodil and zinc (Figure 2) (Perin-Dureau et al., 2002; Hatton & Paoletti, 2005). Synaptic NMDA receptors are localized in the post-synaptic density where they are structurally organized into large macromolecular complexes that interact with signaling molecules such as kinases and phosphatases. They also interact with other transmembrane proteins such as adhesion proteins and metabotropic glutamate receptors (mGluRs) (Husi et al., 2000). Membrane export and synaptic insertion of NMDA receptors involves intrinsic trafficking signals specific for each subunit, splice variant, and complex interaction between NMDA receptors and a variety of interacting proteins. These interacting proteins include the post-synaptic density protein (PSD95), Drosophila disc large tumor suppressor (Dlg1), and zonula occludens-1 protein (zo-1) also known collectively as PDZ-domain proteins. Membrane insertion and regulated endocytosis of NMDA receptors are also tightly controlled by phosphorylation events (Chen & Roche, 2007; Lau & Zukin, 2007). The synaptic activity of NMDARs influence the number and the subunit composition of other synaptic membrane receptors (Zhou & Baudry, 2006; Lau & Zukin, 2007).

The NMDAR requires simultaneous activation by glutamate and glycine for channel opening (Dingledine et al., 1999). Ion passage also requires depolarization because magnesium directly blocks the ion channel in a voltage-dependent manner. Although the physiological significance remains unknown, the receptor is also modulated by polyamines such as spermine and spermidine in a biphasic manner (Figure 2) (Lynch & Guttmann, 2002). At low micromolar concentrations, polyamines promote channel opening by increasing the affinity of the receptor for glycine as well as by removing tonic proton inhibition (Dingledine et al., 1999). In contrast, polyamines at high concentrations that are probably not achievable in vivo block the channel in a voltage dependent manner. Three other types of endogenous compounds (zinc, redox modulators, and nitric oxide) also inhibit the NMDA receptor allosterically through different sites (Lynch & Guttmann, 2002). Several compounds such as haloperidol, amitriptyline, and amantidine have been characterized for their ability to inhibit NMDA receptors. These diverse pharmacological antagonists produce different effects when given to animals which suggest that the NMDA receptor population within the brain is heterogeneous.

2.1 NMDA receptor complexes: Structure and function

The NMDA type of glutamate receptor is thought to play a role in long-term potentiation, memory formation, and controlling brain development (MacDonald et al., 2006; Ewald & Cline, 2009; Vastagh et al., 2012). NMDA receptor-mediated neurotoxicity is implicated in neurodegeneration associated with epilepsy, ischemia, Huntington's chorea, Alzheimer's disease, and AIDS encephalopathy (Durand et al., 1993; Reyes et al., 2006).

Three gene families encoding NMDA receptor subunits have been identified in rat brain. One family is composed of the NR1 gene. The NR1 gene encodes RNA that undergoes alternate splicing to yield at least eight receptor variants. These variants arise from the splicing of three alternative exons which have been designated as N1, C1, and C2. Exon N1 encodes 21 amino acids that can be inserted into the N-terminal domain. Exons C1 and C2 are adjacent and encode the last portion of the C-terminal domain. Exon C1 encodes 37 amino acids and exon C2 encodes 38 amino acids before reaching a stop codon followed by an additional 239 nucleotides from the 3' non-coding region. The splicing out of exon C2 removes the first stop codon. This yields an open reading frame that encodes an unrelated sequence C2' which consists of 22 amino acids before a second stop codon is reached. The NR1 subunit is essential for channel activity and has glycosylated and de-glycosylated functionally active forms (Reyes et al., 2006).

There are four subtypes (A–D) of the NR2 subunit which bind glutamate (Figure 2). These subunits confer the majority of pharmacological and biophysical properties associated with NMDA receptor (NMDAR) subtypes (Chen & Wyllie, 2006). Since the cloning of NMDAR subunits, the identification of many native NMDARs has been elucidated by comparing the properties of native receptors with those of known recombinant subunit compositions. These studies determined that NR2A and NR2B-containing NMDARs are widely expressed throughout the CNS while NR2C-containing NMDARs are mainly expressed in the cerebellum. Expression levels of NR2D subunits peak around the first week of postnatal development and are thought to be retained in certain neurons that express receptors with properties indistinguishable from recombinant receptors containing only NR1 and NR2D subunits (Monyer et al., 1992; Momiyama et al., 1996; Misra et al., 2000). Activation of NR1/NR2D NMDARs at synaptic sites are thought to produce long lasting synaptic events since recombinant forms deactivate with a time constant of several seconds following rapid synaptic-like glutamate application (Vicini et al., 1998; Wyllie et al., 1998; Wyllie, 2008). The NR2 subunits contain divergent sequences that regulate unique protein-protein interactions and distinct receptor trafficking properties. For example, the NR2A and NR2B intracellular C-terminal domains contain trafficking motifs that regulate NMDAR endocytosis and intracellular trafficking (Tang et al., 2010).

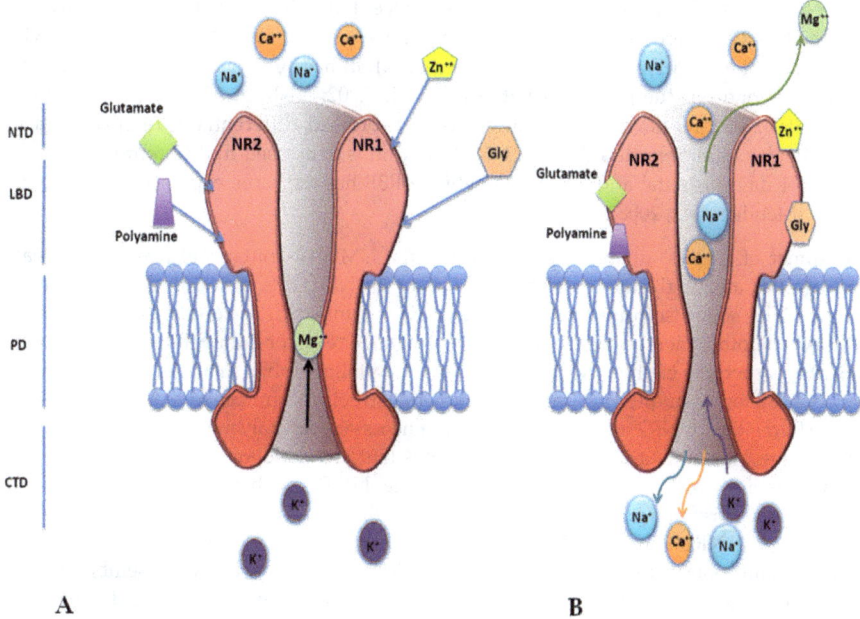

Fig. 2. NMDA receptor composition and potential ligand binding sites.

Most NMDARs are believed to assemble as tetramers that associate two NR1 and two NR2 subunits in a "dimer of dimers" quaternary structure. The diagram shows an assembly with the heterodimer NR1/NR2. For clarity, only one of the two NR1/NR2 heterodimers is shown. The extracellular region is composed of the N-terminal domain (NTD) and ligand binding domain (LBD). Allosteric modulators such as zinc interact with the NTD. Competitive agonists such as glycine, glutamate, and polyamines interact with the LBD. The intermembrane region is composed of the Pore Domain (PD). The Mg^{2+} ion is the endogenous pore blocker of the PD. The intracellular region is composed of the C-terminal domain (CTD). The CTD is involved in receptor trafficking and cell signaling processes.

The successful cloning of NR3, the third subunit of the NMDA receptor, has taken the complexity of NMDA receptors to a new level. NR3 subunits have been identified in rat brains in two variants known as NR3A and NR3B (Méndez et al., 2008; Ciabarra et al., 1995; Sucher et al., 1995). The NR3 subunits have been reported in GenBank as L34938 and U29873, respectively. NR3A has 27% similarity to the other NMDA receptor subunits and 23% similarity to other non-NMDA receptor proteins. Despite this low homology, NR3A was grouped under the NMDA receptor because the CTD and the region upstream of M1 are structurally related to other NMDA receptor subunits (Ciabarra et al., 1995; Moreno et al., 2010; Vargas et al., 2010). The NR3B subunit was initially discovered in 1995. Its complete characterization was published later by other groups (Forcina et al., 1995;

Sevarino et al., 1996; Matsuda et al., 2003; Méndez, 2008). NR3B is also the most similar to NR3A with 47% similarity in amino acid sequence, but it has only 17-21% similarity to NR1 and NR2. There is greater similarity between NR3 and NR1 than with NR2 (Andersson et al., 2001). The mouse homolog of NR3B has 1003 residues whereas the rat homolog is one residue shorter (Chatterton et al., 2002; Nishi et al., 2001; Low & Wee, 2010). NR3 subunits have been reported to be expressed differentially in space and in time. Méndez et al. reported that the NR3A subunit is expressed in different proportions between 1 day postnatal and adult rats, while NR3B has the same expression at both age groups (Méndez et al., 2008).

The "dimer of dimers" quaternary structure of the NMDAR contains at least 2 glutamate binding sites and 2 glycine-binding sites (Figure 2). NMDARs can also assemble with 2 different NR1 splice isoforms and 2 different NR2 subunits. Studies on the AMPA receptor (AMPAR), another member of the ionotropic glutamate receptor family, have given insights into the structure of the NMDA receptor. Crystallographic analyses coupled with electrophysiologic studies indicate a tetrameric structure similar to AMPARs. In the NMDAR, regions of NR2 and NR1 subunits are necessary for transmitting allosteric signals between the glutamate and glycine-binding sites that are analogous to the areas of dimer interactions in AMPARs. This suggests that the NMDARs have similar dimer-dimer interactions. Therefore, collected research suggests that functional NMDAR complexes are tetramers of 2 NR1 and 2 NR2 subunits with an evolutionary link between glutamate receptors and potassium channels (Figure 2). The actual process of assembly of the individual subunits into the functional channel has not been well characterized. However, critical residues in this process are known to be located in the N-terminal domain of the NMDAR (Prybylowski & Wenthold, 2004).

2.2 Stoichiometry

The stoichiometry of NMDA receptors has not been completely established, but the consensus is that they are mostly tetramers composed of two NR1 subunits and two NR2 subunits (Paoletti & Neyton, 2007; Ulbrich & Isacoff, 2008) (Figure 3). NMDARs assemble from two glycine-binding NR1 subunits with two glutamate-binding NR2 subunits to form glutamate-gated excitatory receptors that mediate synaptic transmission and plasticity (Figure 2, 3). The role of glycine-binding NR3 subunits is less clear. In *Xenopus laevis* oocytes, two NR3 subunits co-assemble with two NR1 subunits to form a glycine-gated receptor; such a receptor has yet to be found in mammalian cells. The NR1, NR2, and NR3 appear to co-assemble into tri-heteromeric receptors in neurons, but it is not clear whether this occurs in oocytes (Figure 3). To test the rules that govern subunit assembly in NMDA receptors, Ulbrich and Isacoff developed a single-molecule fluorescence co-localization method. They found that NR1, NR2, and NR3 follow an exclusion rule that yields separate populations of NR1/NR2 and NR1/NR3 receptors on the surface of oocytes. In contrast, co-expression of NR1, NR3A, and NR3B yields tri-heteromeric receptors with a fixed stoichiometry of two NR1 subunits with one NR3A subunit and one NR3B subunit (Figure 3). Therefore, at least part of the regulation of subunit stoichiometry appears to be caused by internal retention. Cell-to-cell differences in these rules may help sculpt distinct physiological properties (Ulbrich & Isacoff, 2008).

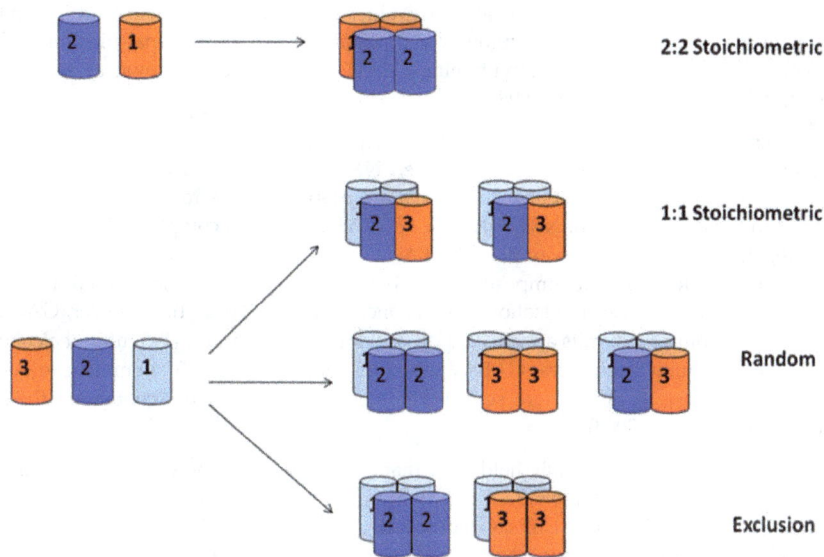

Fig. 3. The different assembly scenarios for NMDA receptors:

Scenario (i) is a 2:2 stoichiometric assembly where two NR1 (orange) and two NR2 (blue) subunits co-assemble. Scenario (ii) is a 1:1 stoichiometric assembly where two NR1 (light blue) subunits assemble with one NR2 (blue) and one NR3 (orange) subunit. Scenario (iii) is a random assembly where two NR1 (light blue) subunits assemble randomly with two NR2 (blue) or two NR3 (orange) subunits, or one NR2 (blue) and one NR3 (orange) subunit. Scenario (iv) is an exclusion rule where two NR1 (light blue) subunits assemble with either two NR2 (blue) or two NR3 (orange) subunits but never form a tri-heteromeric receptor (adapted from Ulbrich & Isacoff, 2008).

3. The impact of alcohol on the NMDA receptor

Alcohol has a complex pharmacology that acts by disrupting distinct receptor or effector proteins via direct or indirect interactions (protein theory). At very high concentrations, it might even change the composition of lipids in the surrounding membrane (lipid theory). At concentrations in the 5–20 mM range, (which constitutes the legal intoxication range for driving in many countries) alcohol directly interferes with and/or influences the function of several membrane receptors. Lovinger et al. showed that NMDA function was inhibited by alcohol in a concentration dependent manner in the range of 5-50 mM. The amplitude of the NMDA-activated current was reduced 61% by 50 mM alcohol (Lovinger et al., 1989). Also, the potency of several alcohols to inhibit the NMDA-activated current is linearly related to their intoxicating potency. This suggests that alcohol-induced inhibition of NMDA receptor activation may contribute to the neural and cognitive impairments associated with intoxication. Several other ionotropic receptors have also been characterized as primary targets of alcohol. These other ionotropic receptors include $GABA_A$ and glycine receptors that have their functions enhanced by alcohol (Mihic, 1999). Alcohol has also been shown to potentiate the function of other non-ionotropic receptors such as neuronal nicotinic ACh receptor (nAChR) and 5-hydroxytryptamine 3 (5-HT3) that is also known as serotonin (Lovinger, 1999; Narahashi et al., 1999).

The influence of alcohol on ionotropic receptors depends on the alcohol concentration and receptor subunit composition. For example, NMDA receptors composed of either NR1/NR2A or NR1/NR2B subunit complexes are more sensitive to alcohol's inhibitory effects than those composed of NR1/NR2C or NR1/NR2D subunit complexes (Kalluri et al., 1998; Allgaier, 2002). Another example is GABA$_A$. GABA$_A$ receptors are composed of α, β, γ, and δ subunits. Most subunit compositions of GABA$_A$ receptors are deficient in δ subunits and only display responses to alcohol at high concentrations (460 mM). However, GABA$_A$ receptors containing δ subunits are affected by very low concentrations (1–3 mM) of alcohol. Also in $\alpha4\beta\delta$ subunit complexes, GABA$_A$ receptors containing the $\beta3$ subunit have been found to be almost 10 times more sensitive to alcohol than receptors containing the $\beta2$ subunit (Wallner et al., 2003).

In summary, despite the generally held view that alcohol is a non-specific pharmacological compound recent studies demonstrate that it specifically targets certain receptors such as NMDA, GABA, 5-HT3, and nAChRs. Concentrations as low as 1 mM produce alterations in the function of these ionotropic receptors. The complex interaction of alcohol on these receptors is generally characterized by the inhibition of NMDA receptors and by the inhibition of GABA receptors. This complex interaction of alcohol with different receptors is responsible for the psychotropic effects seen with alcohol consumption. These pathways involved in the effects of alcohol on the brain continue to be elucidated.

3.1 The stages of alcohol effects and NMDAR function

The effects of alcohol can be categorized into several stages. These stages are referred to as initiation of alcohol consumption (acute alcohol effects), maintenance of alcohol consumption (chronic alcohol effects and loss of control), craving and alcohol seeking (withdrawal), and relapse to alcohol use (compulsive alcohol consumption) (Wolffgramm et al., 2000; Heyne et al., 1998; Heyne et al., 2000; Ferko, 1994). The glutamatergic system which is a fast-signaling system important for information processing has been shown to play a pivotal role in these stages. The glutamatergic system is composed of at least three major types of glutamate receptors: the AMPA receptor, the NMDA receptor, and the kainate receptor. The NMDA receptor has been demonstrated to have major influence in the first and last stages of alcohol effects and minor or no influence in the middle stages. The AMPA receptor has been shown to have a major influence in the craving and reinstating of alcohol seeking stage (middle stage).

In the initiation of alcohol consumption stage, glutamate has been shown to enhance the central depressant action of alcohol because glutamate can alter the alcohol induced loss of righting reflex (LORR) (Petrakis et al., 2004). NMDARs are associated with decreases in LORR response time and are primary targets of alcohol. This suggests that altered NMDAR function contributes to the initial pathophysiological response during acute alcohol exposure (Ge et al., 2007). Accordingly, NMDAR antagonists are capable of preventing initial alcohol responses. This was shown by the elimination of alcohol-induced conditioned place preference in rats during administration of dizocilpine (a non-competitive NMDAR antagonist). It was also shown by the attenuation of alcohol self-administration in a free-choice operant task with administration of 2-amino-5-phosphopentanoic acid (a competitive NMDAR antagonist) microinjections (Biala & Kotlinska, 1999; Rassnick et al., 1992).

Nitric oxide (NO) production has also been correlated to the initiation of alcohol consumption stage. The glutamatergic/NMDA receptor system is closely linked to NO production. NO is an intracellular and extracellular messenger which is produced by nitric oxide synthase (NOS) (Bredt et al., 1990). The stimulation of NMDARs leads to a calcium influx within the cell and the binding of calcium to calmodulin activates neuronal NOS (nNOS) activity (Spanagel et al., 2002). Other studies have also implicated NOS activity in the modulation of alcohol mediated effects on the CNS (Spanagel et al., 2002; Deng & Deitrich, 2007). Alcohol has been shown to increase inducible NOS (iNOS) activity in glial cells and inhibit nNOS activity in neurons. The link between the NMDA receptor system and NO production implies that both iNOS and nNOS activity within the brain may also be involved in the modulation of acute alcohol effects. NOS activity has also been implicated in the maintenance of alcohol consumption stage (Deng & Deitrich, 2007).

In the maintenance of alcohol consumption stage, adaptive responses occur such as changes in the number and/or affinity of synaptic glutamate receptors or their subunits (Henniger et al., 2003; Vengeliene et al., 2008). These adaptive responses act to counterbalance the acute inhibitory effect of alcohol on iGluR-NMDA function (Nagy et al., 2003; Wu et al., 2010). However, studies suggest that iGluR-NMDA has no influence during this stage. For example, NR2A subunit deletion in mice does not affect voluntary alcohol intake (Boyce-Rustay & Holmes, 2006). Also studies utilizing knockout mice (GluR1 and GluR3 deletions) did not have any effect on either home cage alcohol drinking or operant self-administration (Cowen et al., 2003; Sanchis-Segura & Spanagel, 2006). In contrast, two studies did report that antagonists against the non-ionotropic receptor mGluR5 were capable of reducing alcohol-reinforced responding in mice and alcohol-preferring P/Fawn-Hooded rats (Cowen et al., 2005; Schroeder et al., 2005). This suggests a role for non-ionotropic receptors during this stage of alcohol effects.

In the craving and alcohol seeking stage, adaptive responses in the glutamatergic system cause hyper-excitability in the Central Nervous System (CNS) during withdrawal or conditioned withdrawal. Animal studies have shown that the overactivation of glutamate receptors contributes to the generation of hyper-excitability (Grant et al., 1990; Gulya et al., 1991; Davidson et al., 1995; Grant, 1999). Human studies have supported this hyper-excitability by demonstrating that excitatory neurotransmitters were elevated in the cerebrospinal fluid of alcohol-dependent patients (Tsai & Coyle, 1998). These adaptive responses may represent one mechanism that causes alcohol cravings (Gass & Olive, 2008). Both NMDA receptors and non-NMDA ionotropic glutamate receptors such as AMPA receptors have major roles during this stage (Bachteler et al., 2005; Sanchis-Segura et al., 2006). More specifically, as in the previous stage, mGluRs have also been implicated in this alcohol-craving/seeking behavior. For example, mGluR5 receptor antagonists have been effective in attenuating alcohol cravings (Bäckström et al., 2004). In regards to the NMDA receptor, ethanol withdrawal has been shown to potentiate NMDA-induced damage to the hippocampus by increases in mRNA expression of the NR2 subunit which is correlated with withdrawal seizures (Davidson et al., 1993; Follesa & Ticku, 1996). Also, the competitive

NMDA receptor antagonist, CGP-39551, is a potent inhibitor of withdrawal seizures and hyperexcitability (Liljequist, 1991; Ripley & Little, 1995).

In the last stage, relapse to alcohol use, one major hypothesis proposes that the glutamatergic system is critically involved (Gass & Olive, 2008). Several studies have demonstrated a major role for the NMDA receptors during this stage. For example, the clinical drug acamprosate, known to attenuate hyper-glutamatergic activity, was capable of reducing the alcohol deprivation effect (ADE) in Wistar rats under home cage and operant conditions (Spanagel et al., 1996; Spanagel et al., 2005; Heyser et al., 1998). Furthermore, Hölter et al. demonstrated that chronic treatment with a non-competitive NMDA receptor antagonist selectively abolished the increased alcohol intake during the ADE (Hölter et al., 2000). Similarly, reduction of relapse-like alcohol drinking after a deprivation phase was reported during the administration of competitive and non-competitive antagonists of the NMDA receptor (Vengeliene et al., 2005).

3.2 Acute and chronic alcohol exposure

Acute and chronic effects of alcohol exposure on NMDARs have been observed in hippocampal brain slices in which resistance develops 5-15 min after exposure to ethanol (100 mM) (Miyakawa et al., 1997; Yaka et al., 2003; Nelson et al., 2005). However, the mechanisms of this resistance are not fully understood. Wu et al. proposes that time and dose dependent effects of ethanol produce adaptive changes in the NMDAR which may also occur during exposure to ethanol in *ex vivo* conditions. These changes may be the basis for the functional adaptation of these receptors to alcohol exposure (Wu et al., 2011). It has been shown that changes in the process of adaptation can also occur as a result of NMDAR overexpression, or by other signaling mechanisms that are mediated by selective dephosphorylation of the NMDAR after acute or chronic alcohol exposure (Roberto et al., 2004; Lack et al., 2007; Clapp et al., 2010; Wu et al., 2011).

The NMDAR is considered one of the primary molecular targets of ethanol in the brain. Ethanol inhibits NMDAR function via a non-competitive mechanism and induces the dephosphorylation of NR2 subunits (Wirkner et al., 2000; Suvarna et al., 2005; Wang et al., 2007). For example, NR2A and NR2B in hippocampal and cortical brain slices were characterized after acute ethanol exposure. They exhibited a decrease in tyrosine phosphorylation levels. Both the inhibition of NMDAR function and the decrease in tyrosine phosphorylation of NR2 subunits produced by acute ethanol exposure were blocked by protein tyrosine phosphatases (PTP) inhibitors (Alvestad et al., 2003; Ferrani-Kile et al., 2003). This suggests that ethanol's inhibition of NMDAR function is a result of a decrease in tyrosine phosphorylation of NMDARs by ethanol enhancement of PTP activity (Mahadev & Vemuri, 1999).

NMDARs have also been strongly implicated in synaptic development and cellular models of learning and memory such as long-term potentiation (LTP) and long-term depression (LTD) (Medina et al., 2001; Malenka & Bear, 2004). It has been shown that ethanol inhibits the induction of several forms of neural plasticity such as LTP in the hippocampus, dorsal striatum, and bed nucleus of the stria terminalis while enhancing LTD in the hippocampus (Blitzer et al., 1990; Morrisett et al., 1993; Pyapali et al., 1999; Hendricson et al., 2002; Weitlauf et al., 2004; Hendricson et al., 2007; Yin et al., 2007). Such mechanisms of synaptic plasticity could subsequently lead to the reorganization of neural circuitry by altering gene and protein expression of neuronal receptors such as NMDAR. LTP and LTD have thus become important candidate mechanisms for alcohol induced alterations of neural circuit function in alcohol addiction (Hyman & Malenka, 2001). These studies have proposed the intriguing possibility that disruptions and subsequent adaptive changes in glutamate signaling through NMDARs may contribute to adaptations in brain function. These adaptions in return may produce ethanol tolerance and/or dependence similar to processes involved in experience-dependent plasticity.

The ability of ethanol to inhibit NMDAR function is dependent on various factors including the NR1 splice variant that is co-assembled with NR2 subunits (Jin & Woodward, 2006). While homomeric NR1 subunits form an active ion channel that conducts Na^+ and Ca^{2+} currents, the incorporation of NR2 subunits allows this channel to be modulated by the Src family of kinases (SFKs), phosphatases, and other small molecules such as ethanol. Therefore, NMDAR complexes containing subunits NR1/NR2A or NR1/NR2B are more sensitive to the inhibitory effects of alcohol than complexes that contain the subunits NR1/NR2D or NR1/NR2C. Additionally, given the differential distribution of NMDAR subunits in the brain, alcohol affects certain brain regions more than others. For example, the NR1/NR2B subtype that is mainly expressed in forebrain regions is more sensitive to the inhibitory effects of ethanol (Allgaier, 2002; Smothers et al., 2001; Popp, 1998).

Recently, it has been found that acute ethanol exposure inhibits NMDAR function by modifying STriatal enriched protein tyrosine phosphatase (STEP) activity. STEP is a brain-specific protein that is thought to play a critical role in synaptic plasticity (Fitzpatrick & Lombroso, 2011). The genetic deletion of STEP61, the active form of STEP within the brain, leads to marked attenuation of acute ethanol inhibition of NMDAR currents. Also, STEP61 negatively regulates Fyn and p38 mitogen-activated protein kinase (p38 MAPK). Both of these proteins are members of the NMDAR super molecular complex. The adaptation of NMDAR responses to acute alcohol is associated with 1) a partial inactivation of STEP61, 2) an activation of p38 MAPK, and 3) a requirement for NR2B activity. Together this data indicates that altered STEP61 and p38 MAPK signaling contributes to the modulation of ethanol inhibition of NMDAR activity in brain neurons (Wu et al., 2011).

The functional activity of the NMDAR is increased by SFKs, but its activity is also regulated by protein tyrosine phosphatases (Pelkey et al., 2002; Salter & Kalia, 2004; Snyder et al., 2005; Paul et al., 2007). STEP61 co-immunoprecipitates with NMDARs suggesting a strong physical association between these two molecules as a signaling unit (Pelkey et al., 2002; Braithwaite et al., 2006; Xu et al., 2009). Inhibition of STEP61, the only actively expressed isoform of STEP in the hippocampus, has been shown to enhance NMDAR function and to attenuate ethanol inhibition of the NMDA receptor (Pelkey et al., 2002; Hicklin et al., 2011). Acute ethanol exposure has been shown to decrease phosphorylation at the tyrosine (Y) 1472 phosphorylation site of the NR2B subunit without altering its protein levels (Alvestad et al., 2003; Wu et al., 2010). Y-1472 is a site in the C-terminal tail of the NR2B subunit where STEP61 has been shown to interact. This suggests that acute ethanol treatment activates STEP61 which is involved in the dephosphorylation of the Y-1472 site (Paul et al., 2007; Braithwaite et al., 2006). In accordance, several studies have also shown that the inhibition of NMDAR currents by the action of ethanol requires the participation of STEP61. When STEP61 activity is repressed, ethanol's ability to inhibit NMDAR current is attenuated

(Alvestad et al., 2003; Wu et al., 2010; Hicklin et al., 2011). During the adaptive response increased levels of STEP33 and phospho-p38 mitogen-activate protein kinase (pp38 MAPK) along with decreased levels of STEP61 were correlated with the failure of acute alcohol exposure to inhibit NMDAR currents (Wu et al., 2010; Wu et al., 2011). STEP33 is produced by the cleavage of STEP61. This cleavage process may be one of the mechanisms involved in the partial inhibition of STEP61 during the adaptive phase of alcohol exposure. Studies such as these have suggested that the adaptive resistance of NMDAR currents to acute ethanol inhibition likely involves NR2B subunit activity.

The mechanism of resistance to acute and chronic alcohol exposure during the adaptive response is not well understood. Several studies have reported increases in the expression level of several subunits of the NMDAR such as NR1, NR2A, and NR2B during the adaptive phase under chronic alcohol exposure conditions (Snell et al., 1996; Roberto et al., 2004; Roberto et al., 2006; Lack et al., 2007). Other studies have reported increases in the accumulation of synaptic NMDARs during this phase as well (Carpenter-Hyland et al., 2004; Clapp et al., 2010). For example, hippocampal neurons exposed to ethanol chronically for 7 days demonstrated an increase and accumulation of synaptic NMDARs that was quickly reversed once ethanol exposure ceased (Clapp et al., 2010). This suggests that alcohol inhibition of NMDAR activity regulates the expression and accumulation of NMDARs. In contrast, other studies reported no changes in the expression levels of the NMDAR or its subunits. Instead these studies showed an increased inhibition of NMDAR activity using NR2B antagonists and concluded that resistance may be attributed to increases in NR2B activity (Ferreira et al., 2001; Wu et al., 2010). Even though increases in NR2B activity have not been directly verified, increases in STEP33 and pp38 as mentioned previously are characteristic of excessive NMDAR activation (Floyd et al., 2003; Hardingham, 2009; Xu et al., 2009).

Other mechanisms involved in the adaptive response have been proposed but proven to be untrue. For example, several studies proposed that tolerance could occur in presynaptic neurons, postsynaptic neurons, or both (Wu et al., 2001). Thus, the inhibitory actions of ethanol on postsynaptic glutamate receptors could be counteracted by an increase in presynaptic glutamate release. This hypothesis was tested via a paired pulse facilitation (PPF) experiment. The PPF ratio proves to be inversely proportional to the amount of neurotransmitter release in neurons (Dobrunz & Stevens, 1997; Dittman et al., 2000; Wu et al., 2001). No significant effects of chronic ethanol in the PPF ratio were seen. This suggested that chronic ethanol did not significantly alter the pre-synaptic mechanisms of NMDA neurotransmission. Another group of studies proposed that alterations in the Mg^{2+} blockade were responsible for the alcohol resistance seen during the adaptive phase. However, acute ethanol inhibition of NMDAR currents did not significantly differ in low Mg^{2+} and control Mg^{2+} conditions. This demonstrated that alterations in the Mg^{2+} blockade were unlikely to be responsible for this adaptive response as well (Alvestad et al., 2003; Hicklin et al., 2011; Wu et al., 2011).

Studies in humans have shown that individuals with low initial sensitivity (high resistance) to acute ethanol effects on cognition are at greater risk for becoming alcohol dependent (Schuckit & Smith, 2001). However, other studies have shown that those individuals that develop greater acute ethanol tolerance (low initial resistance) also have a greater risk for alcohol dependence (Newlin & Renton, 2010). Even though the underlying mechanisms for alcohol dependence are not clear, the general consensus is that STEP61 and p38 MAPK activities have critical roles in the modulation of acute and chronic alcohol exposure. These studies also suggest that NR2B subunit antagonists are likely to be effective in regulating the acquisition of functional tolerance to the acute and chronic inhibitory effects of ethanol.

3.3 Mechanisms of alcohol-induced brain damage

The mechanisms of alcohol-induced brain damage and abstinence-induced regeneration are complex (Crews et al., 1998; Farber et al., 2004). The extent of neurodegeneration and potential regeneration varies by brain region and is dependent on many factors including pattern of intake (Crews & Nixon, 2009). Alcoholics display cycles of excessive ethanol intake, abstinence, and relapse behavior. For example, Bell et al showed that high alcohol drinking rats consumed significantly more alcohol upon re-exposure than control rats after a period of alcohol abstinence (Bell et al., 2008). Another studied showed that repeated alcohol deprivation cycles increased the severity of relapse within rats (Rodd et al., 2008). These studies suggest a strong correlation between abstinence and relapse that perpetuate the detrimental cycle of alcohol consumption.

Chronic exposure to ethanol causes an adaptive increase in NMDA receptor sensitivity both *in vivo* and *in vitro*. This leads to an increased vulnerability to the glutamate-induced cytotoxic response (excitotoxicity) (Dodd et al., 2000). This sensitization of neuronal cells is one of the most important factors in the mechanism underlying ethanol-induced brain damage. Increased calcium influx through NMDA receptors, as a result of hyper-sensitivity, is tightly coupled to the increase in calcium influx within the mitochondria. This results in the increased production of reactive oxygen species and oxidative damage that eventually attenuates mitochondrial function. Primary inhibition of the mitochondrial respiratory chain can also indirectly induce further NMDA receptor stimulation and damage (Matsumoto et al., 2001).

Various studies show the effect of alcohol on the induction of brain damage. Cell culture models *in vitro* suggest that chronic ethanol intake inhibits the NMDARs which over time results in a hyper-sensitivity that is alleviated by alcohol withdrawal (Chandler et al., 1993; Chandler et al., 2006, Chandler et al., 1999). These studies suggest that neurotoxicity occurs through NMDARs during withdrawal (Butler et al., 2008; Smith et al., 2008). However, other studies *in vivo* using different NMDAR antagonists such as MK801 (dizocilpine), memantine, and DNQX failed to reduce binge ethanol neurotoxicity. Surprisingly, some doses even increased neurodegeneration (Collins et al., 2010; Corso et al., 1998; Crews et al., 2004; Hamelink et al., 2005). These studies suggest that the mechanism of ethanol-induced brain damage is not glutamate excitotoxicity. Therefore, ethanol-induced brain damage in the binge model occurs during intoxication. Other studies also support the hypothesis that alcohol-induced neurodegeneration occurs primarily during intoxication and is related to increased oxidative stress and pro-inflammatory signaling (Qin et al., 2008). Abstinence after binge ethanol intoxication results in brain cell genesis that could contribute to the return to normal brain function and structure found in abstinent humans (Crews & Nixon, 2009).

Additionally, transcription factors such as the cAMP responsive element-binding protein (CREB) and the nuclear factor κB (NF-κB) regulate the gene expression that increases plasticity and survival of damaged neurons (Walton & Dragunow, 2000; Mabuchi et al.,

2001; Hara et al., 2003). In the presence of ethanol changes can be seen in DNA binding protein activities such as increased DNA binding by NF-κB and reduced DNA binding by CREB. NMDAR activation by synaptic glutamate release is associated with decreased DNA binding by CREB as a result of a decrease in CREB phosphorylation (pCREB) (Papadia & Hardingham, 2007). This decrease in pCREB has also been observed in an *in vivo* model of alcohol consumption where rats were treated with ethanol. Therefore, pCREB is reduced during intoxication (Bison & Crews, 2003). NMDAR inhibition is caused by saturation with ethanol and is expected to enhance neurodegeneration and inhibit neurogenesis. During ethanol withdrawal there is a notable increase in pCREB, 3 days post-withdrawal, which is consistent with the neurogenesis observed (Bison & Crews, 2003). Therefore, it is possible that during abstinence NMDAR activity recovers leading to an increase in the pCREB activated transcription of genes involved in plasticity, cell growth, cell proliferation, and neurogenesis. However, oxidative stress and pro-inflammatory cytokines could attenuate the regeneration process due to imbalances generated by brain cell damage (Collins & Neafsey, 2011; Qin et al., 2008).

3.3.1 Alcoholic neurodegeneration and glial cells

Studies in nonhuman primate adolescents show alcohol-induced changes during neurogenesis in the hippocampus. Alcohol significantly reduced the number of different neural progenitor cell types 1, 2a, and 2b as well as glial progenitor cells (Taffe et al., 2010). This suggests that alcohol interferes with the division and migration of progenitor cells in the hippocampus preneuronal region. Thus, the effect of alcohol decreases neurogenesis and increases degeneration. These results demonstrate that the neurogenic niche of the hippocampus during adolescence is very vulnerable to alcohol. It also demonstrates that alcohol decreases the turnover of neurons in the hippocampus by altering the process of neural development. This effect diminishes slowly and can be seen two months after alcohol abstinence. These findings could explain the deficit in the hippocampus associated with cognitive tasks that may be associated with increased DNA binding of NF-kB and reduced DNA binding of CREB (Fulton et al., 2009, Taffe et al., 2010).

Alcohol-related neuronal loss has been documented in specific regions of the cerebral cortex (superior frontal association cortex), hypothalamus, and cerebellum (Harper et al., 2003; Baker et al., 1999). Glial cells, also contribute to neurodegeneration because astroglial degeneration has been reported during ethanol exposure (Miguel-Hidalgo et al., 2006, Miguel-Hidalgo & Rajkowska, 2003). Glial cells are non-neuronal cells that provide physical and functional support for neurons and are essential for normal neuronal cell function. The loss of glial cells results in a deficiency of metabolic and trophic support for neuronal cells. For example, loss of glial cells leads to the inactivation of neurotransmitters such as glutamate and loss of ionic homeostasis, particularly K+ (Bezzi & Volterra, 2001; Volterra & Meldolesi, 2005; Obara et al., 2008). This loss directly enhances the deleterious effects of ethanol on neurons. An increase in the glial fibrillary acidic protein (GFAP), a glial-specific cell marker, has been reported after brain injury which suggests activation of glial proliferation in response to damage (Eng et al., 1992; Norton et al., 1992). Studies have demonstrated reduced glial cell proliferation and reduced expression of GFAP by ethanol exposure in astrocyte cultures (Crews et al., 2004; Guerri & Renau-Piqueras, 1997). In addition, acute alcohol exposure or acute alcohol-induced brain damage results in gliosis (enlargement and increased proliferation of astrocytes) and increases in GFAP levels (Crews et al., 2004; Evrard et al., 2006). In contrast, chronic ethanol exposure results in decreased levels of GFAP (Duvernoy et al., 1981; Franke et al., 1997; Miguel-Hidalgo, 2005; Udomuksorn et al., 2011).

Postmortem studies in patients with alcohol dependence showed low glial densities in the Pre-Frontal Cortex (PFC). However, in these patients glutamine sythetase (GS) levels as well as GFAP levels were significantly higher (Miguel-Hidalgo et al., 2010). One hypothesis for this activation of astrocytes in alcoholism involving increased GS/GFAP expression may be due to the repeated acute exposure to alcohol or to periods of withdrawal that defines alcoholism. This augmentation of GS expression in astrocytes of alcoholics is supported by augmented GS immunoreactivity detected in the PFC of alcohol-consuming rats three days after withdrawal from alcohol (Miguel-Hidalgo, 2005). In this animal model, the GS immunoreactivity was significantly correlated with the amount of ethanol ingested in the days before withdrawal. It has been suggested that astrocytes play a critical role in controlling glutamatergic activity and take up most of the synaptically released glutamate that terminates neurotransmitter activity. Glutamate can then be delivered to neurons via the glutamate–glutamine cycle (Danbolt, 2001). Therefore, changes in the glial expression of GS/GFAP suggest an impairment of certain aspects of glutamatergic processing during alcohol exposure and withdrawal. Further research should determine whether the morphological plasticity and GS/GFAP expression are induced more readily in chronic alcoholics despite a paradoxical association of chronic alcohol intake with low glial or astrocyte density (Korbo, 1999; Miguel-Hidalgo et al., 2002; Miguel-Hidalgo et al., 2006).

3.4 Clinical studies: The role of NMDA receptor antagonists ketamine and memantine

Several studies have suggested that NMDA receptor antagonists are an effective method of treatment for alcohol disorders. Ketamine, a NMDA receptor antagonist, has been evaluated in subjects with a strong family history of ethanol dependence versus subjects with no such family history (Petrakis, 2004). This study demonstrated that during ketamine infusion individuals with a family history of ethanol dependence showed an attenuated response in terms of perceptual alterations and dysphoric mood relative to those without such a family history. This study reaffirms NMDAR dysfunction as an important contributing factor of alcohol dependence. Another study by Phelps et al. investigated whether a family history of alcohol dependence influences ketamine's initial antidepressant effect. The study reported that subjects with a family history of alcohol dependence showed significantly greater improvement in MADRS (Montgomery-Asberg Depression Rating Scale) scores compared with subjects who had no family history of alcohol dependence. The study concluded that a family history of alcohol dependence appears to predict a rapid initial anti-depressant response to NMDA receptor antagonists (Phelps, 2009). The precise reasons underlying the better response of the family history of alcohol dependence (FHP) group to ketamine remains unknown but reaffirms NMDARs association with LTD. Another study compared the ethanol-related effects of ketamine and thiopental on both NMDA and GABA$_A$ receptor activity. This study reported that the ethanol-like effects of ketamine were greater than that of thiopental (Dickerson, 2008). The results obtained are important because ketamine (a NMDAR antagonist) produced alcohol alterations in perception that were not produced by thiopental (a GABA$_A$ receptor agonist). This also reaffirms the role of the NMDAR in alcohol dependence.

Memantine, another NMDAR antagonist, also has been evaluated in clinical trials for the treatment of alcoholism. The first study was conducted by Bisagra et al. by evaluating the acute effects of memantine on the subjective, physiological, and performance effects of alcohol in moderate (10–30 drinks per week) alcohol drinkers. This study reported that pre-treatment with memantine attenuated the craving for alcohol before alcohol administration but not after alcohol was given. It demonstrated that memantine increased the dissociative effects of alcohol without altering its sedative, stimulant, and overall intoxicating effects. It reported that memantine had no effect on alcohol-induced impairment in performance, physiological changes, or pharmacokinetics. This study also showed that memantine increased subjective reports of dissociation, confusion, stimulation, and impaired motor coordination on the balance task (Bisaga & Evans, 2004). Due to the high comorbidity shared between alcoholism and depression Muhonen et al. also evaluated memantine as well as escitalopram, a selective serotonin reuptake inhibitor (SSRI), for the treatment of comorbid with alcohol dependence. This study reported that both treatments significantly reduced the baseline level of depression and anxiety according to Montgomery-Asberg Depression Rating Scale (MADRS) and Hamilton Rating Scale for Anxiety (HAM-A). This evidence provides safety and potential efficacy of memantine and escitalopram for major depressive disorder in patients with comorbid alcohol dependence (Muhonen, 2008).

4. Conclusion

Approximately 2 billion people world-wide consume alcoholic beverages. Alcohol use is related to a wide range of physical, mental, and social detriments. Additionally, alcohol affects almost every organ in the human body as well as the central nervous system. The protein theory is the generally accepted theory on how alcohol affects the CNS. This theory proposes that alcohol acts specifically on membrane protein receptors such as the iGluR-NMDA. The iGluR-NMDA is one of the most active molecules in the central nervous system and has been shown to be directly inhibited in a non-competitive manner by alcohol. It is a post-synaptic receptor critical in most neural activities such as learning and memory.

NMDARs are hetermeric complexes composed of three major types of subunits NR1, NR2, and NR3. Alcohol effects on the NMDAR are dependent on the NMDAR subunit composition as well as alcohol concentration. The major effects of alcohol on the NMDAR activity are thought to be conferred by alcohol's direct interaction with the NR2 subunits of the NMDA receptor. The effects of alcohol can be categorized into several stages. These stages are referred to as initiation of alcohol consumption, maintenance of alcohol consumption, craving and reinstating of alcohol seeking, and relapse to alcohol use. A combination of ionotropic receptors such as NMDAR, non-ionotropic receptors, and other receptors of the glutamatergic system are intimately involved in the acquisition of alcohol dependence. The NMDAR has a critical role in the stages of initiation of alcohol consumption and relapse to alcohol use. In response to the NMDA receptors role in alcohol addiction several NMDAR antagonists have been used in clinical trials to alleviate alcohol dependence. These antagonists include ketamine and memantine. Both have been shown to be successful in alleviating some of the symptoms of alcohol dependence. Future research should focus on the continued characterization of the NMDAR structure as well as its structural variation in different tissue compartments within the brain. Also, further studies are needed to elucidate the interactions of alcohol on specific NMDAR subunits and characterize their effects on NMDAR activity. This will be crucial in developing novel therapeutic targets against alcohol addiction.

5. References

Allgaier, C. (2002). Ethanol sensitivity of NMDA receptors. *Neurochem Int*, 41, 6 (December 2002), pp. 377–382, ISSN 0197-0186

Alvestad, R.M., Grosshans, D.R., Coultrap, S.J., Nakazawa, T., Yamamoto, T., and Rowning, M.D., (2003). Tyrosine dephosphorylation and ethanol inhibition of N-Methyl-aspartate receptor function. *J Biol Chem*, 278, 13, (March 2003), pp. 11020-11025, ISSN 0021-9258

Andersson, O., Stenqvist, A., Attersand, A. and von Euler, G. (2001). Nucleotide sequence, genomic organization, and chromosomal localization of genes encoding the human NMDA receptor subunits NR3A and NR3B. *Genomics*, 78, 3, (December 2001), pp. 178–184, ISSN 0888-7543

Bachteler, D., Economidou, D., Danysz, W., Ciccocioppo, R., Spanagel, R. (2005). The effects of acamprosate and neramexane on cue-induced reinstatement of ethanol-seeking behavior in rat. *Neuropsychopharmacology*, 30, 6 (June 2005), pp. 1104–1110, ISSN 0893-133X

Bäckström, P., Bachteler, D., Koch, S., Hyytiä, P., Spanagel, R. (2004). mGluR5 antagonist MPEP reduces ethanol-seeking and relapse behavior. *Neuropsychopharmacology*, 29, 5 (May 2004), pp. 921–928, ISSN 0893-133X

Baker, K., Harding, A., Halliday, G., Kril, J., and Harper C. (1999). Neuronal loss in functional zones of the cerebellum of chronic alcoholics with and without Wernicke's encephalopathy. *Neuroscience*, 91, 2, 429-438, ISSN 0306-4522

Belelli, D., Lambert, J.J. (2005). Neurosteroids: endogenous regulators of the GABA(A) receptor. *Nat Rev Neurosci*, 6, 7, (July 2005), pp. 565-75 ISSN 1471-0048

Bell RL, Rodd ZA, Schultz JA, Peper CL, Lumeng L, Murphy JM, McBride WJ. Effects of short deprivation and re-exposure intervals on the ethanol drinking behavior of selectively bred high alcohol-consuming rats. *Alcohol*, 42, 5, (August 2008), pp. 407-416, ISSN 0741-8329

Bezzi, P., and Volterra, A. (2001). A neuron-glia signalling network in the active brain. *Curr Opin Neurobiol*, 11, 3, (Jun 2001), pp. 387-394, ISSN 0959-4388

Biala, G., and Kotlinska, J. (1999). Blockade of the acquisition of ethanolinduced conditioned place preference by N-methyl-D-aspartate receptor antagonists. *Alcohol*, 34, 2 (March-april 1999), pp 175–182, ISSN 0735-0414

Bisaga, A., and Evans, S.M. (2004). Acute effects of memantine in combination with alcohol in moderate drinkers. *Psychopharmacology (Berl)*, 172, 1, (February 2004), pp. 16-24, ISSN 0033-3158

Bison, S., and Crews, F. (2003). Alcohol withdrawal increases neuropeptide Y immunoreactivity in rat brain. *Alcohol Clin Exp Res*, 27, 7, (July 2003), pp. 1173-1183, ISSN 1530-0277

Blitzer, R.D., Gil, O., and Landau, E.M. (1990). Long-term potentiation in rat hippocampus is inhibited by low concentrations of ethanol. *Brain Res*, 24, 537, (December 1990), pp. 203-208, ISSN: 0006-8993

Boyce-Rustay, and J., Holmes, A. (2006). Ethanol-related behaviors in mice lacking the
    NMDA receptor NR2A subunit. *Psychopharmacology* (Berl), 187, 4 (September 2006),
    pp. 455–466, ISSN 0033-3158

Braithwaite, S.P., Paul, S., Nairn, A.C., and Lombroso, P.J. (2006). Synaptic plasticity: one
    STEP at a time. *Trends Neurosci*, 29, 8 (August 2006), pp. 452-458, ISSN 0166-2236

Butler, T.R., Smith, K.J., Self, R.L., Braden, B.B., Prendergast, M.A. (2008). Sex differences in
    the neurotoxic effects of adenosine A1 receptor antagonism during ethanol
    withdrawal: reversal with an A1 receptor agonist or an NMDA receptor antagonist.
    Alcohol Clin Exp Res, 32, 7 (July 2008), pp. 1260-1270, ISSN 1530-0277

Carpenter-Hyland, E.P., Woodward, J.J., and Chandler, L.J. (2004). Chronic ethanol induces
    synaptic but not extrasynaptic targeting of NMDA receptors. *J Neurosci*, 8, 24,
    (September 2004), pp. 7859-7868, ISSN 0270-6474.

Chandler, L.J., Dean, N., and Greg, S. (1999). Chronic Ethanol Upregulates NMDA and
    AMPA, but Not Kainate Receptor Subunit Proteins in Rat Primary Cortical
    Cultures. *Alcohol Clin Exp Res*, 23, 2, (February 1999), pp. 363-370, ISSN 1530-0277

Chandler, L.J., Carpenter-Hyland, E., Hendricson, A.W., Maldve, R.E., Morrisett, R.A.,
    Zhou, F.C., Sari, Y., Bell, R., and Szumlinski, K.K.(2006). Structural and functional
    modifications in glutameric synapses following prolonged ethanol exposure.
    Alcohol Clin Exp Res, 30, 2, (February 2006), pp. 368-376, ISSN 1530-0277

Chandler, L.J., Newsom, H., Sumners, C., and Crews, F. (1993). Chronic ethanol exposure
    potentiates NMDA excitotoxicity in cerebral cortical neurons. *J Neurochem*, 60, 4,
    (April 1993), pp. 1578-1581, ISSN 0022-3042

Chatterton, J.E., Awobuluyi, M., Premkumar, L.S., Takahashi, H., Talantova, M., Shin, Y.,
    Cui, J., Tu, S., Sevarino, K.A., Nakanishi, N., et al. (2002). Excitatory glycine
    receptors containing the NR3 family of NMDA receptor subunits. *Nature*, 415
    (February 2002), pp. 793–798, ISSN 0028-0836

Chen, B.-S., and Roche, K. W. (2007). Regulation of NMDA receptors by phosphorylation.
    Neuropharmacology, 53 (September 2007), pp. 362-368, ISSN 0028-3908

Chen, P.E., and Wyllie, D.J.A. (2006). Pharmacological insights obtained from structure-
    function studies of ionotropic glutamate receptors. *Br. J. Pharmacol*, 547 (April
    2006), pp. 839–853, ISSN 0007-1188

Ciabarra, A., Sullivan, J., Gahn, L., Pecht, G., Heinemann, S., Sevarino, K. (1995). Cloning
    and characterization of chi-1: A developmentally regulated member of a novel class
    of the ionotropic glutamate receptor family. *J Neurosci*, 15, 10 (October 1995), pp.
    6498–6508, ISSN 0270-6474.

Clapp, P., Gibson, E.S., Dell'acqua, M.L., and Hoffman, P.L. (2010). Phosphorylation
    regulates removal of synaptic N-methyl-D-aspartate receptors after withdrawal
    from chronic ethanol exposure. *J Pharmacol Exp Ther*, 332, 3, (Mar 2010), pp. 720-729,
    ISSN 0022-3565

Cochilla, A.J., and Alford, S. (1999). NMDA receptor-mediated control of presynaptic
    calcium and neurotransmitter release. *J Neurosci*, (January 1999), 19, 1, pp. 193-205,
    ISSN 0270-6474

Collins, M.A., Neafsey, E.J., Wang, K., Achille, N.J., Mitchell, R.M., Sivaswamy, S. (2010).
    Moderate ethanol preconditioning of rat brain cultures engenders neuroprotection
    against dementia-inducing neuroinflammatory proteins: possible signaling
    mechanisms. *Mol Neurobiol*, 41, (June 2010), pp. 420-425, ISSN: 0893-7648

Collins S., Sigtermans M.J., Dahan A., Zuurmond W.W., Perez R.S. (2010). NMDA receptor antagonists for the treatment of neuropathic pain. *Pain Med*, 11, 11, (November 2010), pp. 1726-1742, ISSN 1526-4637

Collins, M.A., and Neafsey, E.J. (2011). Neuroinflammatory Pathways in Binge Alcohol-Induced Neuronal Degeneration: Oxidative Stress Cascade Involving Aquaporin, Brain Edema, and Phospholipase A2 Activation. *Neurotox Res*, (September 2011), [Epub ahead of print], ISSN 1476-3524

Collins, M.A., Zou, J.Y., Neafsey, E.J. (1998). Brain damage due to episodic alcohol exposure in vivo and in vitro: furosemide neuroprotection implicates edema-based mechanism. *FASEB J.*, 12 (February 1998), pp. 221-230, ISSN: 1530-6860

Corso, T.D., Mostafa, H.M., Collins, M.A., and Neafsey, E.J. (1998). Brain neuronal degeneration caused by episodic alcohol intoxication in rats: effects of nimodipine, 6,7-dinitro-quinoxaline-2,3-dione, and MK-801. *Alcohol Clin Exp Res*, 22, 1, (February 1998), pp. 217-224, ISSN 1530-0277

Cowen, M.S., Djouma, E., Lawrence, A.J. (2005). The metabotropic glutamate 5 receptor antagonist 3-[(2-methyl-1,3-thiazol-4-yl)ethynyl]-pyridine reduces ethanol self-administration in multiple strains of alcohol-preferring rats and regulates olfactory glutamatergic systems. *J Pharmacol Exp Ther*, 315, 2 (November 2005), pp. 590–600, ISSN 0022-3565

Cowen, M.S., Schroff, K.C., Gass, P., Sprengel, R., Spanagel, R. (2003). Neurobehavioral effects of alcohol in AMPA receptor subunit (GluR1) deficient mice. *Neuropharmacology*, 45, 3, (September 2003), pp. 325–333, ISSN 0028-3908

Crews F.T., Steck JC, Chandler LJ, Yu CJ, Day A. (1998). Ethanol, stroke, brain damage, and excitotoxicity. *Pharmacol Biochem Behav*, 59, 4, (April 1998), pp. 981-991, ISSN 0091-3057

Crews, F.T., Collins, M.A., Dlugos, C., Littleton, J., Wilkins, L., Neafsey, E.J., Pentney, R., Snell, L.D., Tabakoff, B., Zou, J., and Noronha, A. (2004). Alcohol-induced neurodegeneration: when, where and why? *Alcohol Clin Exp Res*, 28, 2, (February 2004), pp. 350-364, ISSN 1530-0277

Crews, F.T., and Nixon, K. (2009). Mechanisms of neurodegeneration and regeneration in alcoholism. *Alcohol and Alcoholism*, 44, 2,(March 2009), pp. 115-127, ISSN 0735-0414

Cull-Candy S, Brickley S, Farrant M. (2001). NMDA receptor subunits: diversity, development and disease. *Curr Opin Neurobiol*, 11, 3, (Jun 2001), pp. 327-335, ISSN 0959-4388

Cull-Candy, S.G., and Leszkiewicz, D.N. (2004). Role of distinct NMDA receptor subtypes at central synapses. *Sci STKE*, 255, (October 2004) pp. re16, ISSN 1525-8882

Cushing, A., Price-Jones, M.J., Graves, R., Harris, A.J., Hughes, K.T., Bleakman, D., and Lodge, D. (1999). Measurement of calcium flux through ionotropic glutamate receptors using Cytostar-T scintillating microplates. *J Neurosci Methods*, 1, 90, (August 1999), pp. 33-36, ISSN 0165-0270

Danbolt, N.C. (2001). Glutamate uptake. *Prog Neurobiol*, 65, 1, (September 2001), pp. 1-105, ISSN 0301-0082

De Witte P. (2004). Imbalance between neuroexcitatory and neuroinhibitory amino acids causes craving for ethanol. *Addict Behav*, 29, 7, (September 2004), pp. 1325-1339, ISSN 0306-4603

Davidson, M.D., Wilce ,P., Shanley, B.C. (1993). Increased sensitivity of the hippocampus in ethanol-dependent rats to toxic effect of N-methyl-D-aspartic acid in vivo. *Brain Research*, 606, 1, (March 1993), pp. 5-9, ISSN 0006-8993

Deng, X. S., Deitrich R. A. (2007). Ethanol metabolism and effects: nitric oxide and its interaction. *Curr Clin Pharmacol,* 2, 2, (May 2007), pp. 145-53, ISSN 1574-8847

Dickerson, D., Pittman, B., Ralevski, E., Perrino, A., Limoncelli, D., Edgecombe, J., Acampora, G., Krystal, J.H., and Petrakis, I. (2010). Ethanol-likeeffects of thiopental and ketamine in healthyhumans. *J Psychopharmacol,* 24, 2, (February 2010), pp.203-211, ISSN 0269-8811

Dingledine, R., Borges, K., Bowie, D., and Traynelis, S.F. (1999). The glutamate receptor ion channels. *Pharmacol Rev,* 51 (March 1999), pp. 7–61, ISSN 0031-6997

Dittman, J. S., Kreitzer, A. C., and Regehr, W. G. (2000). Interplay between facilitation, depression, and residual calcium at three presynaptic terminals. *J Neurosci,* 20, 4, (February 2000), pp. 1374-85, ISSN 0270-6474

Dobrunz, L. E., and Stevens, C. F. (1997). Heterogeneity of release probability, facilitation, and depletion at central synapses. *Neuron,* 18, 6 (June 1997), pp. 995–1008, ISSN 0896-6273

Dodd, P.R. Beckmann, A.M. Davidson, M.S. Wilce, P.A. (2000). Glutamate-mediated transmission, alcohol, and alcoholism. *Neurochem Int,* 37, (2000), pp. 509-533, ISSN 0197-0186

Durand, G.M., Bennett, M.V.L., Zukin, R.S. (1993). Splice variants of the N-methyl-d-aspartate receptor NR1 identify domains involved in regulation by polyamines and protein kinase C. *Proc Natl Acad Sci USA* 90 (July 2003), pp. 6731–6735, ISSN 0027-8424

Eng, L.F., Yu, A.C., and Lee, Y.L. (1992). Astrocytic response to injury. *Prog Brain Res,* 94, pp. 353-365, ISSN 0006-8993

Evrard, S.G., Duhalde-Vega, M., Tagliaferro, P., Mirochnic, S., Caltana, L.R., and Brusco, A. (2006). A low chronic ethanol exposure induces morphological changes in the adolescent rat brain that are not fully recovered even after a long abstinence: an immunohistochemical study. *Exp Neurol,* 200, 2, (August 2006), pp. 438-459, ISSN 0014-4886

Ewald R.C., Cline H.T. (2009). NMDA Receptors and Brain Development. In: Biology of the NMDA Receptor. *Frontiers in Neuroscience,* Boca Raton (FL): CRC Press, ISBN 13: 978142004414

Farber N.B., Heinkel C., Dribben W.H., Nemmers B., Jiang X. (2004). In the adult CNS, ethanol prevents rather than produces NMDA antagonist-induced neurotoxicity. *Brain Res,* 1028, 1, (November 2004),pp. 66-74, ISSN 0006-8993

Ferko, A. (1994). Interaction between L-glutamate and ethanol on the central depressant properties of ethanol in mice. *Pharmacol Biochem Behav,* 47, 2 (February 1994), pp. 351–354, ISSN 0091-3057

Ferrani-Kile, K., Randall, P., Leslie, S. (2003). Acute ethanol affects phosphorylation state of the NMDA receptor complex: implication of tyrosine phosphatases and protein kinaseA. Brain research. *Molecular brain research,* 115, 1 (July 2003), pp. 78-86, ISSN 0169-328X

Ferreira, V.M., Frausto, S., Browning, M.D., Savage, D.D., Morato, G.S., and Valenzuela, C.F. (2001). Ionotropic glutamate receptor subunit expression in the rat hippocampus: lack of an effect of a long-term ethanol exposure paradigm. *Alcohol Clin Exp Res,* 25, 10, (October 2001), pp. 1536-1541, ISSN 0145-6008

Ferrer-Montiel, A. V. & Montal, M. (1996). Pentameric subunit stoichiometry of a neuronal glutamate receptor. *Proc. Natl. Acad. Sci. USA,* 93, 7 (April 1996), pp. 2741–2744, ISSN 0027-8424

Fitzpatrick, C.J., and Lombroso, P.J. (2011). The Role of Striatal-Enriched Protein Tyrosine
    Phosphatase (STEP) in Cognition. *Front Neuroanat*, 5, 47, (July 2011), Epub, ISSN
    1662-5129

Floyd, D.W., Jung, K.Y., and McCool, B.A. (2003). Chronic Ethanol Ingestion Facilitates N-
    Methyl-D-aspartate Receptor Function and Expression in Rat Lateral/Basolateral
    Amygdala Neurons. *J Pharmacol Exp Ther*, 307, pp. 1020-1029, ISSN 0022-3565

Follesa, P., Ticku, M.K. (1996). Chronic ethanol-mediated up-regulation of the N-methyl-D-
    aspartate receptor polypeptide subunits in mouse cortical neurons in culture.
    Journal of Biological Chemistry, 271, 23, (June 1996), pp. 13297-13299.

Forcina, M., Ciabarra, A., Seravino, K. (1995). Cloning of chi-2: a putative member of the
    ionotropic glutamate receptor superfamily. *Soc Neurosci Abstr*, 21 (June 1995), pp.
    438-3, ISSN 0190-5295

Franke, H., Kittner, H., Berger, P., Wirkner, K., and Schramek, J. (1997). The reaction of
    astrocytes and neurons in the hippocampus of adult rats during chronic ethanol
    treatment and correlations to behavioral impairments. *Alcohol*, 14, 5, (September
    1997), pp. 445-454, ISSN 0741-8329

Fulton, T., Crews, F.T., and Nixon, K. (2009). Mechanisms of Neurodegeneration and
    Regeneration in Alcoholism. *Alcohol and Alcoholism*, 44, 2, (March-april 2009), pp.
    115-127, ISSN 0735-0414

Gass, J.T., Olive, M.F. (2008). Glutamatergic substrates of drug addiction and alcoholism.
    Biochem Pharmacol, 75, 1 (January 2008), pp. 218–265, ISSN 0006-2952

Ge, Z.J., Zhang, L.C., Zeng, Y.M., Da, T.J., Wang, J.K., Cui, G.X., Tan, Y.F., Zhao, Y.P., and
    Liu, G.J. (2007). Involvement of NMDA receptors in thiopental-induced loss of
    righting reflex, antinociception and anticonvulsion effects in mice. *Pharmacology*, 80,
    2-3, (May 2007), pp. 127-133, ISSN 1432-2072

Goldstein, D.B. (1986). Effect of alcohol on cellular membranes. *Ann Emer Med* 15, 9
    (September 1986), pp. 1013-1018, ISSN 0196-0644

Grant, K. (1999). Strategies for understanding the pharmacological effects of ethanol with
    drug discrimination procedures. *Pharmacol Biochem Behav*, 64, 2 (October 1999), pp.
    261–267, ISSN 0091-3057

Grant, K.A., Valverius, P., Hudspith, M., Tabakoff, B. (1990). Ethanol withdrawal seizures
    and the NMDA receptor complex. *European Journal of Pharmacology*, 176, 3,
    (November 1990), pp. 289-296, ISSN 0014-2999

Guerri, C., and Renau-Piqueras, J. (1997). Alcohol, astroglia, and brain development. *Mol
    Neurobiol*, 15, 1, (August 1997), pp. 65-81, ISSN 0893-7648

Gulya, K., Grant, K.A., Valverius, P., Hoffmann, P.L., Tabakoff, B. (1991). Brain regional
    specificity and time-course of changes in the NMDA receptor-ionophore complex
    during ethanol withdrawal. *Brain Research*, 547, 1, (April 1991), pp. 129-134, ISSN
    0006-8993

Hallett, P.J., Dunah A.W., Ravenscroft, P., Zhou, S., Bezard, E., Crossman, A.R., Brotchie,
    J.M., Standaert, D.G. (2005). Alterations of striatal NMDA receptor subunits
    associated with the development of dyskinesia in the MPTP-lesioned primate
    model of Parkinson's disease. *Neuropharmacology*, 48,4, (March 2005), pp.503-516,
    ISSN 0028-3908

Hamelink, C., Hampson, A., Wink, D.A., Eiden, L.E., and Eskay, R.L. (2005). Comparison of
    cannabidiol, antioxidants, and diuretics in reversing binge ethanol-induced
    neurotoxicity. *J Pharmacol Exp Ther*, 314, 2, (Aug 2005), pp. 780-788, ISSN 0022-3565

Harper, C., Dixon, G., Sheedy, D., and Garrick, T. (2003). Neuropathological alterations in alcoholic brains. Studies arising from the New South Wales Tissue Resource Centre. *Prog Neuropsychopharmacol Biol Psychiatry,* 27, 6, (September 2003), pp. 951-961, ISSN 0006-3223

Hatton, C.J, and Paoletti, P. (2005). Modulation of triheteromeric NMDA receptors by N-terminal domain ligands. *Neuron,* 46 (April 2005), pp. 261–274, ISSN 0896-6273

Hendricson, A.W., Maldve, R.E., Salinas, A.G., Theile, J.W., Zhang, T.A., Diaz, L.M., and Morrisett, R.A. (2007). Aberrant synaptic activation of N-methyl-D-aspartate receptors underlies ethanol withdrawal hyperexcitability. *J Pharmacol Exp Ther,* 321, 1, (April 2007), pp. 60-72, ISSN 0022-3565

Hendricson, A.W., Miao, C.L., Lippmann, M.J., and Morrisett, R.A. (2002). Ifenprodil and ethanol enhance NMDA receptor-dependent long-term depression. *J Pharmacol Exp Ther,* 301, 3, (June 2002), pp. 938-944, ISSN 0022-3565

Henniger, M.S., Wotjak, C.T., and Hölter, S.M. (2003). Long-term voluntary ethanol drinking increases expression of NMDA receptor 2B subunits in rat frontal cortex. *European Journal of Pharmacology,* 470, 1-2, (May 2003), pp. 470-433, ISSN 0014-2999

Heyne A., Wolffgramm J. (1998). The development of addiction to d-amphetamine in an animal model: same principles as for alcohol and opiate. *Psychopharmacology (Berl),* 140, 4, (December 1998), pp. 510-8, ISSN 1432-2072

Heyne A., May T., Goll P., Wolffgramm J. (2000). Persisting consequences of drug intake: towards a memory of addiction. *J Neural Transm,* 107, 6, (2000), pp. 613-38, ISSN 1435-1463

Heyser, C.J., Schulteis, G., Durbin, P., Koob, G.F. (1998). Chronic acamprosate treatment eliminates the alcohol deprivation effect while having limited effects on baseline responding for ethanol in rats. *Neuropsychopharmacology,* 18, 2 (February 1998), pp. 125–133, ISSN 0893-133X

Hicklin, T.R., Wu, P.H., Radcliffe, R.A., Freund, R.K., Goebel-Goody, S.M., Correa, P.R., Proctor, W.R., Lombroso, P.J., and Browning, M.D. (2011). Alcohol inhibition of the NMDA receptor function, long-term potentiation, and fear learning requires STEP. *Proc Natl Acad Sci (USA),* 108, 16, (April 2011), pp. 6650-6655, ISSN 0027-8424

Hirai, H., Kirsch, J., Laube, B., Betz, H., and Kuhse, J. (1996). The glycine binding site of the N-methyl-D-aspartate receptor subunit NR1: identification of novel determinants of co-agonist potentiation in the extracellular M3-M4 loop region. *Proc Natl Acad Sci U S A,* 93, 12, (June 1996), pp. 6031-6036, ISSN 0027-8424

Hölter, S.M., Danysz, W., Spanagel, R. (2000). Novel uncompetitive N-methyl-D-aspartate (NMDA)-receptor antagonist MRZ 2/579 suppresses ethanol intake in long-term ethanol-experienced rats and generalizes to ethanol cue in drug discrimination procedure. *J Pharmacol Exp Ther,* 292, 2 (February 2000), pp. 545–552, ISSN 0022-3565

Husi, H,. Ward, M.A., Choudhary, J.S., Blackstock, W.P., Grant, S.G. (2000). Proteomic analysis of NMDA receptor-adhesion protein signaling complexes. *Nature Neuroscience,* 3 (July 2000), pp. 661 – 669, ISSN 1097-6256

Hyman, S.E., and Malenka, R.C. (2001). Addiction and the brain: the neurobiology of compulsion and its persistence. *Nat Rev Neurosci,* 2, 10, (Oct 2001), pp. 695-703, ISSN 1471-003X

Javitt, D.C., Zukin S.R. (1991). Recent advances in the phencyclidine model of schizophrenia. *Am J Psychiatry,* 148, 10, (October 1991), pp. 1301-1308, ISSN 1535-7228

Kalluri, H.S., Mehta, A.K., and Ticku, M.K. (1998). Up-regulation of NMDA receptor
    subunits in rat brain following chronic ethanol treatment. *Molecular Brain Research*,
    58, 1-2, (July 1998), pp. 221-224, ISSN 0169-328X

Lack, A.K., Diaz, M.R., Chappell, A., DuBois, D.W. and McCool, B.A. (2007). Chronic
    ethanol and withdrawal differentially modulate pre- and postsynaptic function at
    glutamatergic synapses in rat basolateral amygdala. *J Neurophysiol*, 98, 6 (December
    2007), pp. 3185-3196, ISSN 0022-3077

Lareo, L.R. and Corredor, C. (2006). Molecular correlate of consciousness. In: *Consciousness
    and Learning Research*, S. K. Turrini (Ed) Nova Publishers, New York. pp. 97–117,
    ISSN 0196-6006

Lau, C.G. and Zukin, R.S. (2007). NMDA receptor trafficking in synaptic plasticity and
    neuropsychiatric disorders. *Nat. Rev. Neurosci*, 8 (June 2007), pp. 413-426, ISSN
    1471-003X

Laube, B., Kuhse, J. & Betz, H. (1998). Evidence for a tetrameric structure of recombinant
    NMDA receptor. *J. Neurosci*, 18, 8, (Apr 1998), pp. 2954–2961, ISSN 0270-6474

Lebel, D., Sidhu, N., Barkai, E. and Quinlan, E.M. (2006). Learning in the absence of
    experience-dependent regulation of NMDAR composition. *Learn. Mem*, 13, 5,
    (October 2006), pp. 566–570, ISSN 1072-0502

Levine, MS, Cepeda C, André VM. (2010). Location, location, location: contrasting roles of
    synaptic and extrasynaptic NMDA receptors in Huntington's disease. *Neuron 28*,
    65, (January 2010), pp. 145-147, ISSN: 0896-6273

Liljequist, S. (1991). NMDA receptor antagonists inhibit ethanol-produced locomotor
    stimulation in NMRI mice. *Alcohol*, 8, 4, (July 1991), pp. 309-312, ISSN 0741-8329

Lovinger, D.M., White, G., Weight, F.F. (1989). Ethanol inhibits NMDA-activated ion current
    in hippocampal neurons. *Science*, 243 (March 1989), pp. 1721–1724, ISSN 0036-8075

Lovinger, D.M. (1995). Developmental decrease in ethanol inhibition of N-methyl-
    Daspartate receptors in rat neocortical neurons: Relation to the actions of
    ifenprodil. *J Pharmacol Exp Ther*, 274, 1, (July 1995), pp. 164-172, ISSN 0022-3565

Lovinger, D.M. (1997). Alcohols and neurotransmitter gated ion channels: past, present, and
    future. *Naunyn Schmiedebergs Arch Pharmacol*, 356, 3, (September 1997), pp. 267-82,
    ISSN 1432-1912

Lovinger, D.M. (1999). 5-HT3 receptors and the neural actions of alcohols: an increasingly
    exciting topic. *Neurochem Int*, 35, 2 (August 1999), pp. 125–130, ISSN 0197-0186

Low, C., Wee, K. (2010). New insights into the not-so-new NR3 subunits of N-methyl-D-
    aspartate receptor: localization, structure, and function. *Mol Pharmacol*, 78, 1 (July
    2010), pp. 1-11, ISSN 0026-895X

Lynch, D.R., and Guttmann, R.P. (2002). Excitotoxicity: perspectives based on NMDA receptor
    subtypes. *J Pharmacol Exp Ther*, 300 (March 2002), pp. 717–723, ISSN 0022-3565.

MacDonald, J.F., Jackson, M.F., and Beazely, M.A. (2006). Hippocampal long-term synaptic
    plasticity and signal amplification of NMDA receptors. *Crit Rev Neurobiol*, 18, 1-2,
    pp. 71-84, ISSN 0892-0915

Mahadev, K., Vemuri, M. (1999). Effect of pre- and postnatal ethanol exposure on protein
    tyrosine kinase activity and its endogenous substrates in rat cerebral cortex. *Alcohol*,
    17, 3 (April 1999), pp. 223-9, ISSN 0741-8329

Malenka, R.C., and Bear, M.F. (2004). LTP and LTD: an embarrassment of riches. *Neuron*, 44,
    1, (September 2004), pp. 5-21. ISSN 0896-6273

Matsuda, K., Fletcher, M,. Kamiya, Y., and Yuzaki, M. (2003). Specific assembly with the NMDA receptor 3B subunit controls surface expression and calcium permeability of NMDA receptors. *J Neurosci*, 23, 31 (November 2003), pp. 10064-10073, ISSN 0270-6474

Matsumoto, I. Burke, L. Inoue, Y. Wilce, P.A. (2001). Two models of ethanol withdrawal kindling. *Nihon Arukoru Yakubutsu Igakkai Zasshi*, 36 (2001), pp. 53–64, ISSN 1341-8963

Mayer, M.L. (2005b). Glutamate receptor ion channels. *Curr Opin Neurobiol*, 15 (October 2005b), pp. 282–288, ISSN 0959-4388

Medina, A.E., Liao, D.S., Mower, A.F., and Ramoa, A.S. (2001). Do NMDA receptor kinetics regulate the end of critical periods of plasticity? *Neuron*, 32, 4, (November 2001), pp. 553-555 ISSN 0896-6273

Méndez, G., Reyes, E., Poutou, R., Quevedo, B., Lareo, L. (2008). Purification of IgY against the NR3 subunit of the rat brain NMDA receptor. *Rev.MVZ Córdoba*, 13, 1 (February 2008), pp. 1146-1156, ISSN 0122-0268

Miguel-Hidalgo, J.J. (2005). Lower packing density of glial fibrillary acidic protein-immunoreactive astrocytes in the prelimbic cortex of alcohol-naive and alcohol-drinking alcohol-preferring rats as compared with alcohol-nonpreferring and Wistar rats. *Alcohol Clin Exp Res*, 29, 5, (May 2005), pp. 766-772, ISSN 1530-0277

Miguel-Hidalgo, J.J., Alvarez, X.A., Cacabelos, R., and Quack, G. (2002). Neuroprotection by memantine against neurodegeneration induced by beta-amyloid(1-40). *Brain Res*, 958, 1, (Dec 2002), pp. 210-221, ISSN 0006-8993

Miguel-Hidalgo, J.J., and Rajkowska G. (2003). Comparison of prefrontal cell pathology between depression and alcohol dependence. *J Psychiatr Res*, 37, 5, (September 2003), pp. 411-420, ISSN 0022-3956

Miguel-Hidalgo, J.J., Overholser, J.C., Meltzer, H.Y., Stockmeier, C.A., and Rajkowska, G. (2006). Reduced glial and neuronal packing density in the orbitofrontal cortex in alcohol dependence and its relationship with suicide and duration of alcohol dependence. *Alcohol Clin Exp Res*, 30, 11, (November 2006), pp. 1845-1855, ISSN 1530-0277

Miguel-Hidalgo, J.J., Waltzer, R., Whittom, A.A., Austin, M.C., Rajkowska, G., and Stockmeier, C.A. (2010). Glial and glutamatergic markers in depression, alcoholism, and their comorbidity. *J Affect Disord*, 127, 1-3, (December 2010), pp. 230-240, ISSN 0165-0327

Mihic S.J., Harris R.A. (1997). GABA and the GABAA receptor. *Alcohol Health Res World* 21, 2 (1997), pp. 127-31, ISSN 0090-838X

Mihic, S. (1999). Acute effects of ethanol on GABAA and glycine receptor function. *Neurochem Int*, 35, 2 (August 1999), pp. 115–123, ISSN 0197-0186

Mirshahi T., and Woodward J.J. (1995) Ethanol sensitivity of heteromeric NMDA receptors: Effects of subunit assembly, glycine and NMDAR1 Mg2+-insensitive mutants. *Neuropharmacology* 34, 3 (March 1995), pp. 347-355, ISSN 0028-3908

Misra, C.h., Brickley, S., Farrant, M., and Cull-Candy, S. (2000). Identification of subunits contributing to synaptic and extrasynaptic NMDA receptors in Golgi cells of the rat cerebellum. *The Journal of Physiology*, 524 (April 2000), pp. 147-162, ISSN 0022-3751

Miyakawa, T., Yagi, T., Kitazawa, H., Yasuda, M., Kawai, N., Tsuboi, K., and Niki, H. (1997) Fyn kinase as a determinant of ethanol sensitivity: Relation to NMDA-receptor function. *Science*, 278 (October 1997), pp. 698-701, ISSN 0036-8075

Momiyama, A., Feldmeyer, D., Cull-Candy, S.G. (1996). Identification of a native low-conductance NMDA channel with reduced sensitivity to Mg2+ in rat central neurones. *J Physiol (Lond)*, 494 (July 1996), pp. 479–492, ISSN 0022-3751

Monyer, H., Sprengel, R., Schoepfer, R., Herb, A., Higuchi, M., Lomeli, H., Burnashev, N., Sakmann, B., Seeburg, P.H. (1992). Heteromeric NMDA receptors: Molecular and functional distinctions of subtypes. *Science (Wash DC)*, 256 (May 1992), pp. 1217–1221, ISSN 0036-8075

Moreno, F., Reyes, E., Lareo, L. (2010). Computational study of the evolutionary relationships of the ionotropic receptors NMDA, AMPA and kainate in four species of primates. *Universitas Scientiarum*. 15, 3 (October 2010), pp. 183-193, ISSN 0122-7483

Morrisett, R.A., and Swartzwelder, H.S. (1993). Attenuation of hippocampal long-term potentiation by ethanol: a patch-clamp analysis of glutamatergic and GABAergic mechanisms. *J Neurosci*, 13, 5, (May 1993), pp. 2264-2272. ISSN 0270-6474

Muhonen, L.H., Lönnqvist, J., Juva, K., and Alho, H. (2008). Double-blind, randomized comparison of memantine and escitalopram for the treatment of major depressive disorder comorbid with alcohol dependence. *J Clin Psychiatry*, 69, 3, (Mar 2008), pp. 392-399, ISSN 0160-6689

Murail, S., Wallner, B., Trudell, J.R., Bertaccini, E., Lindahl, E. (2011). Microsecond Simulations Indicate that Ethanol Binds between Subunits and Could Stabilize an Open-State Model of a Glycine Receptor. *Biophys J*, 100 (April 2011), pp. 1642-1650, ISSN 0006-3495

Nagy J, László L. (2002). Increased sensitivity to NMDA is involved in alcohol-withdrawal induced cytotoxicity observed in primary cultures of cortical neurones chronically pre-treated with ethanol. *Neurochem Int*, 40,7, (June 2002), pp. 585-591, ISSN 0364-3190

Nagy J, Kolok S, Dezso P, Boros A, Szombathelyi Z. (2003). Differential alterations in the expression of NMDA receptor subunits following chronic ethanol treatment in primary cultures of rat cortical and hippocampal neurones. *Neurochem Int*, 42, 1, (January 2003), pp. 35-43, ISSN 0364-3190

Narahashi, T., Aistrup, G.L., Marszalec, W., Nagata, K. (1999). Neuronal nicotinic acetylcholine receptors: a new target site of ethanol. *Neurochem Int*, 35, 2 (August 1999), pp. 131-141, ISSN 0197-0186

Nelson, T.E., Ur, C.L., and Gruol, D.L. (2005). Chronic intermittent ethanol exposure enhances NMDA-receptor-mediated synaptic responses and NMDA receptor expression in hippocampal CA1 region. *Brain Research*, 1048, 1-2, (Jun 2005), pp. 69-79, ISSN 00068993

Newlin, D.B., and Renton, R.M. (2010). High risk groups often have higher levels of alcohol response than low risk: the other side of the coin. *Alcohol Clin Exp Res*, 34, 2, (February 2010), pp. 199-202, ISSN 0145-6008

Nishi, M., Hinds, H., Lu, H.P., Kawata, M., and Hayashi, Y. (2001). Motoneuron-specific expression of NR3B, a novel NMDA-type glutamate receptor subunit that works in a dominant-negative manner. *J Neurosci*, 21, (December 2001), pp. 23:RC185, ISSN 0270-6474

Norton, W.T., Aquino, D.A., Hozumi, I., Chiu, F.C., and Brosnan, C.F. (1992). Quantitative aspects of reactive gliosis: a review. *Neurochem Res,* 17, 9, (September 1992), pp. 877-885, ISSN 1573-6903

Nusser, Z. (2000). AMPA and NMDA receptors: similarities and differences in their synaptic distribution. *Curr. Opin. Neurobiol.* 10, 3, (June 200), pp. 337–341, ISSN 0959-4388

Obara, M., Szeliga, M., and Albrecht, J. (2007). Regulation of pH in the mammalian central nervous system under normal and pathological conditions: facts and hypotheses. *Neurochem Int,* 52, 6, (May 2008), pp. 905-19, ISSN 0197-0186

Paoletti, P., Ascher, P., and Neyton, J. (1997). High-affinity zinc inhibition of NMDA NR1-NR2A receptors. *J Neurosci,* 17, 15, (August 1997), pp. 5711-5725, ISSN 0270-6474

Paoletti, P., and Neyton, J. (2007). NMDA receptor subunits: function and pharmacology. *Curr Opin Pharmacol,* 7 (February 2007), pp. 39–47, ISSN 1471-4892

Paoletti P. (2011). Molecular basis of NMDA receptor functional diversity. *Eur J Neurosci,* 33, 8, (April 2011), pp. 1351-1365, ISSN 1359-5962

Paul, S., Olausson, P., Venkitaramani, D.V., Ruchkina, I., Moran, T.D., Tronson, N., Mills, E., Hakim, S., Salter, M.W., Taylor, J.R., and Lombroso, P.J. (2007). The striatal-enriched Protein tyrosine phosphatase gates long-term potentiation and fear memory in the lateral amygdala. *Biol Psychiatry,* 61, 9 (May 2007), pp. 1049-1061, ISSN 0006-3223

Pelkey, K.A., Askalan, R., Paul, S., Kalia, L.V., Nguyen, T.H., Pitcher, G.M., Salter, M.W., and Lombroso P.J. (2002). Tyrosine phosphatase STEP is a tonic brake on induction of long-term potentiation. *Neuron,* 34, 1 (March 2002), pp. 127-138, ISSN 0896-6273

Peoples R.W., Weight FF. (1992). Ethanol inhibition of N-methyl-D-aspartate-activated ion current in rat hippocampal neurons is not competitive with glycine. *Brain Res,* 7,571, (February 1992), pp. 342-344, ISSN 0006-8993

Perez-Otano, I., Schulteis, C. T., Contractor, A., Lipton, S. A., Trimmer, J. S., Sucher, N. J. and Heinemann, S.F. (2001). Assembly with the NR1 subunit is required for surface expression of NR3A-containing NMDA receptors. *J. Neurosci,* 21, 4, (February 2001), pp. 1228–1237, ISSN 0270-6474

Perin-Dureau, F., Rachline, J., Neyton, J., Paoletti, P. (2002). Mapping the binding site of the neuroprotectant ifenprodil on NMDA receptors. *J Neurosci,* 22, 14 (July 2002), pp. 5955-65, ISSN 0270-6474

Petrakis, I.L., Limoncelli, D., Gueorguieva, R., Jatlow, P., Boutros, N.N., Trevisan, L., et al. (2004). Altered NMDA glutamate receptor antagonist response in individuals with a family vulnerability to alcoholism. *Am J Psychiatry,* 161, 10 (October 2004) 1776–1782, ISSN 0002-953X

Phelps, L.E., Brutsche, N., Moral, J.R., Luckenbaugh, D.A., Manji, H.K., and Zarate, C.A. Jr. (2009). Family history of alcohol dependence and initial antidepressant response to an N-methyl-D-aspartate antagonist. *Biol Psychiatry,* 65, 2, (January 2009), pp. 181-184, ISSN 0006-3223

Popp, R.L., Lickteig, R., Browning, M.D., and Lovinger, D.M. (1998). Ethanol sensitivity and subunit composition of NMDA receptors in cultured striatal neurons. *Neuropharmacology,* 37, 1, pp. 45-56, ISSN 0028-3908

Prybylowski, K., Wenthold, R. (2004). N-Methyl-D-aspartate receptors: subunit assembly and trafficking to the synapse. *J Biol Chem,* 279, 11 (March 2004), pp. 9673-6, ISSN 0021-9258

Qin, L., He, J., Hanes, R.N., Pluzarev, O., Hong, J.S., and Crews, F.T. (2008). Increased systemic and brain cytokine production and neuroinflammation by endotoxin following ethanol treatment. J *Neuroinflammation*, 18, (March 2008), pp. 5-10, ISSN 1742-2094

Reyes-Montaño, E.A, Lareo, L.R., Chow, D-C., Pérez-Gómez, G. (2006). Immunolocalization and Biochemical Characterization of N-methyl-D-aspartate Receptor Subunit NR1 from Rat Brain. *The Protein Journal*, 25, 2 (February 2006), pp. 95-108, ISSN 1572-3887

Ripley, T.L., Little, H.J. (1995). Effects on ethanol withdrawal hyperexcitability of chronic treatment with a competitive N-methyl-D-aspartate receptor antagonist. J *Pharmacol Exper Therap*, 272, 1, (January 1995), pp. 112-118, ISSN. 0022-3565

Roberto, M., Bajo, M., Crawford, E., Madamba, S.G., and Siggins, G.R. (2006). Chronic Ethanol Exposure and Protracted Abstinence Alter NMDA Receptors in Central Amygdala. *Neuropsychopharmacology*, 31,5, (May 2006), pp. 988-996, ISSN 0893-133X

Roberto, M., Schweitzer, P., Madamba, S.G., Stouffer, D.G., Parsons, L.H., Siggins, G.R. (2004) Acute and chronic ethanol alter glutamatergic transmission in rat central amygdala: An in vitro and in vivo analysis. *J Neurosci*, 24, 7 (February 2004), pp. 1594-1603, ISSN 0270-6474

Rodd ZA, Bell RL, Kuc KA, Murphy JM, Lumeng L, McBride WJ. Effects of concurrent access to multiple ethanol concentrations and repeated deprivations on alcohol intake of high alcohol-drinking (HAD) rats. *Addict Biol*, (2008), Submitted, ISSN 1369-1600

Ron, D. (2004). Signaling Cascades Regulating NMDA Receptor Sensitivity to Ethanol. *Neuroscientist*, 10 (August 2004), pp. 325-336, ISSN 0306-4522

Saft C, Epplen JT, Wieczorek S, Landwehrmeyer GB, Roos RA, de Yebenes JG, Dose M, Tabrizi SJ, et al. (2011). NMDA receptor gene variations as modifiers in Huntington disease: a replication study. *PLoS Curr*, 4, 3, (October 2011), RRN1247, ISSN 2157-3999

Salter, M.W., and Kalia, L.V. (2004). Src kinases: a hub for NMDA receptor regulation. *Nat. Rev. Neurosci.*, 5 (April 2004), pp. 317–328, ISSN 1471-003X

Sanchis-Segura, C., Spanagel, R. (2006). Behavioural assessment of drug reinforcement and addictive features in rodents: an overview. *Addict Biol*, 11, 1 (March 2006), pp. 2–38, ISSN 1355-6215

Sander T., Ball D., Murray R., Patel J., Samochowiec J., Winterer G., Rommelspacher H., Schmidt L.G., Loh E.W. (1999). Association analysis of sequence variants of GABA(A) alpha6, beta2, and gamma2 gene cluster and alcohol dependence. *Alcohol Clin Exp Res* 23 (March 1999), pp. 427-31, ISSN 1720-8319

Schroeder, J.P., Overstreet, D.H., Hodge, C.W. (2005). The mGluR5 antagonist MPEP decreases operant ethanol self-administration during maintenance and after repeated alcohol deprivations in alcohol-preferring (P) rats. *Psychopharmacology (Berl)*, 179, 1 (April 2005), pp. 262–270, ISSN 0033-3158

Schuckit, M.A., and Smith, T.L. (2001). The clinical course of alcohol dependence associated with a low level of response to alcohol. *Addiction*, 96, 6 (June 2001), pp. 903-910, ISSN 0965-2140

Sevarino, K., Ciabarra, A., Forcina, M. (1996). χ-1 and χ-2, members of a novel class of the glutamate receptor superfamily. *Soc Neurosci Abstr*, 22 (October 1995), pp. 59219, ISSN 0190-5295

Smith, K.J., Butler, T.R., Self, R.L., Braden, B.B., Prendergast, M.A. (2008). Potentiation of N-methyl-D-aspartate receptor-mediated neuronal injury during methamphetamine withdrawal in vitro requires co-activation of IP3 receptors. *Brain Res*, 1187, 2, (January 2008), pp. 67-73, ISSN: 0006-8993

Smothers, C.T., Clayton, R., Blevins, T., and Woodward, J.J. (2001). Ethanol sensitivity of recombinant human N-methyl-D-aspartate receptors. *Neurochem Int*, 38, 4, (April 2001), pp. 333-340, ISSN 0197-0186

Snell, L.D., Nunley, K.R., Lickteig, R.L., Browning, M.D., Tabakoff, B., and Hoffman, P.L. (1996). Regional and subunit specific changes in NMDA receptor mRNA and immunoreactivity in mouse brain following chronic ethanol ingestion. *Mol Brain Res*, 40, 1, (August 1996), pp. 71-78, ISSN 0169-328X

Snyder, E.M., Nong, Y., Almeida, C.G., Paul, S., Moran, T., Choi, E.Y., Nairn, A.C., Salter, M.W., Lombroso, P.J., Gouras, G.K., and Greengard, P. (2005). Regulation of NMDA receptor trafficking by amyloid-beta. *Nat Neurosci*, 8 (March 2005), pp. 1051-1058, ISSN 0896-6273

Spanagel, R. (2009). Alcoholism: A Systems Approach From Molecular Physiology to Addictive Behavior. *Physiol Rev*, 89 (April 2009), pp. 649–705, ISSN 0031-9333

Spanagel, R., Hölter, S., Allingham, K., Landgraf, R., Zieglgänsberger, W. (1996). Acamprosate and alcohol: I. Effects on alcohol intake following alcohol deprivation in the rat. *Eur J Pharmacol*, 305, 1-3, (June 1996), pp. 39–44, ISSN 0014-2999

Spanagel, R., Sigmund, S., Cowen, M., Schroff, K.C., Schumann, G., Fiserova, M. et al. (2002). The neuronal nitric oxide synthase (nNOS) gene is critically involved in neurobehavioral effects of alcohol. *J Neurosci*, 22, 19, (October 2002), pp. 8676–8683, ISSN 0270-6474

Sucher, N., Brose, N., Deitcher, D., Awobuluyi, M., Gasic, G., Bading, H., Cepko, C., Greenberg, M., Jahn, R., Heinemann, S. (1993). Expression of endogenous NMDAR1 transcripts without receptor protein suggests post-transcriptional control in PC12 cells. *J Biol Chem*, 268 (October 1993), pp. 22299–22304, ISSN 0021-9258

Suvarna, N., Borgland, S.L., Wang, J., Phamluong, K., Auberson, Y.P., Bonci, A., and Ron, D. (2005). Ethanol alters trafficking and functional N-methyl-D-aspartate receptor NR2 subunit ratio via H-Ras. *J Biol Chem*, 280, 36, (September 2005), pp. 31450-31459, ISSN 0021-9258

Suzdak P.D., Schwartz R.D., Skolnick P., Paul S.N. (1986). Ethanol stimulates gamma-aminobutyric acid receptor-mediated chloride transport in rat brain synaptoneurosomes. *Proc Natl Acad Sci U S A*, 83 (1986), pp. 4071-5 ISSN 0027-8424

Taffe, M.A., Kotzebue, R.W., Crean, R.D., Crawford, E.F., Edwards, S., and Mandyam, C.D. (2010). Long-lasting reduction in hippocampal neurogenesis by alcohol consumption in adolescent nonhuman primates. *Proc Natl Acad Sci U S A*, 107, 24, (June 2010), pp. 11104-11109, ISSN 0027-8424

Takadera, T., Ohyashiki. T. (2008). Benzyl alcohol inhibits N-methyl-D-aspartate receptor-mediated neurotoxicity and calcium accumulation in cultured rat cortical neurons. *J Biomed Sci*, 15 (August 2008), pp. 767-770, ISSN 1937-6871

Tang, T., Badger, J., Roche, P., Roche, K. (2010). Novel Approach to Probe Subunit-specific Contributions to N-Methyl-D-aspartate (NMDA) Receptor Trafficking Reveals a Dominant Role for NR2B in Receptor Recycling. *J Biol Chem*, 285, 27 (July 2010), pp. 20975-81, ISSN 0021-9258

Trujillo KA, Akil H. (1995). Excitatory amino acids and drugs of abuse: a role for N-methyl-D-aspartate receptors in drug tolerance, sensitization and physical dependence. *Drug Alcohol Depend,* 38, 2, (May 1995), pp. 139-154, ISSN 0376-8716

Tsai G., Gastfriend D.R., Coyle J.T. (1995). The glutamatergic basis of human alcoholism. *Am J Psychiatry*, 152 (March 1995), pp. 332-40, ISSN 1535-7228

Tsai, G., Coyle, J.T. (1998) The role of glutamatergic neurotransmission in the pathophysiology of alcoholism. *Annu Rev Med*, 49, (February 1998), pp. 173-184, ISSN 0066-4219

Udomuksorn, W., Mukem, S., Kumarnsit, E., Vongvatcharanon, S., and Vongvatcharanon, U. (2011). Effects of alcohol administration during adulthood on parvalbumin and glial fibrillary acidic protein immunoreactivity in the rat cerebral cortex. *Acta Histochem*, 113, 3, (May 2011), pp. 283-289, ISSN 0044-5991

Ulbrich, M., Isacoff, E. (2008). Rules of engagement for NMDA receptor subunits. *Proc Natl Acad Sci U S A*, 105, 37 (September 2008), pp. 14163-8, ISSN 0027-8424

Ułas J, Weihmuller FB, Brunner LC, Joyce JN, Marshall JF, Cotman CW. (1994). Selective increase of NMDA-sensitive glutamate binding in the striatum of Parkinson's disease, Alzheimer's disease, and mixed Parkinson's disease/Alzheimer's disease patients: an autoradiographic study. J Neurosci. 14, 11, (November 1994), pp. 6317-6324, ISSN-0270-6474

Vargas, N., Reyes, E., Lareo, L. (2010). In silico approach to the evolution of ionotropic glutamate receptor gene family in four primate species. *Universitas Scientiarum*, 15, 3 (October 2010), pp. 194-205, ISSN 0122-7483

Vastagh C, Gardoni F, Bagetta V, Stanic J, Zianni E, Giampa' C, Picconi B, Calabresi P,. (2012). NMDA receptor composition modulates dendritic spine morphology in striatal medium spiny neurons. *J Biol Chem*, (April 2012), [Epub ahead of print], ISSN 0021-9258

Vengeliene, V., Bachteler, D., Danysz, W., Spanagel, R. (2005). The role of the NMDA receptor in alcohol relapse: a pharmacological mapping study using the alcohol deprivation effect. *Neuropharmacology*, 48 (May 2005), pp. 822-829, ISSN 0028-3908

Vengeliene, V., Bilbao, A., Molander, A., and Spanagel, R. (2008). Neuropharmacology of alcohol addiction. Br *J Pharmacol.* 154, 2 (May 2008), pp. 299–315, ISSN 0007-1188

Vicini, S., Wang, J.F., Li, J.H., Zhu, W.J., Wang, Y.H., Luo, J.H., Wolfe, B.B., and Grayson, D.R. (1998). Functional and pharmacological differences between recombinant N-methyl-D-aspartate receptors. *J Neurophysiol*, 79 (February 1998), pp. 555–566, ISSN 0022-3077

Volterra, A., and Meldolesi, J. (2005). Astrocytes, from brain glue to communication elements: the revolution continues. *Nat Rev Neurosci*, 6, 8, (August 2005), pp. 626-640, ISSN 1471-003X

Wallner, M., Hanchar, H.J., Olsen, R.W. (2003). Ethanol enhances alpha 4 beta 3 delta and alpha 6 beta 3 delta gamma-aminobutyric acid type A receptors at low concentrations known to affect humans. *Proc Natl Acad Sci USA*, 100, 25 (December 2003), pp. 15218–15223, ISSN 0027-8424

Wang, J., Carnicella, S., Phamluong, K., Jeanblanc, J., Ronesi, J.A., Chaudhri, N., Janak, P.H., Lovinger, D.M., and Ron, D. (2007). Ethanol induces long-term facilitation of NR2B NMDA receptor activity in the dorsal striatum: implications for alcohol drinking behavior. *J Neurosci*, 27, 13, (March 2007), pp. 3593-3602, ISSN 0270-6474

Weitlauf, C., Egli, R.E., Grueter, B.A., and Winder, D.G. (2004). High-frequency stimulation induces ethanol-sensitive long-term potentiation at glutamatergic synapses in the dorsolateral bed nucleus of the stria terminalis. *J Neurosci*, 24, 25, (June 2004), pp. 5741-5747, ISSN 0270-6474

Weitlauf C., Woodward J.J. (2008). Ethanol selectively attenuates NMDAR-mediated synaptic transmission in the prefrontal cortex. Alcohol Clin Exp Res. (April 2008), 32, 4, pp. 690-698, ISSN 0145-6008

Wirkner, K., Eberts, C., Poelchen, W., Allgaier, C., and Illes, P. (2000). Mechanism of inhibition by ethanol of NMDA and AMPA receptor channel functions in cultured rat cortical neurons. *Naunyn Schmiedebergs Arch Pharmacol*, 362, 6, (December 2000), pp. 568-576, ISSN 0028-1298

Wolffgramm J., Galli G., Thimm F., Heyne A. (2000). Animal models of addiction: models for therapeutic strategies? *J Neural Transm*, 107, 6, (2000), pp. 649-68, ISSN 1435-1463

World Health Organization. (2004). Departamental of Mental Health and Substance abuse. WHO Global Status Report on Alcohol 2004. Geneva. 2004

Wu, P., Coultrap, S., Browning, M., Proctor, W. (2011) Functional Adaptation of the NMDA receptor to acute ethanol inhibition is modulated by striatal-enriched protein tyrosine phosphatase and p38 mitogen activated protein kinase. *Molecular Pharmacology*, 80, 3 (September 2011), pp. 529-37, ISSN 0026-825X

Wu, P.H., Coultrap, S., Browning, M.D., and Proctor, W.R. (2010). Correlated changes in NMDA receptor phosphorylation, functional activity, and sedation by chronic ethanol consumption. *J Neurochem*, 115, 5, (December 2010), pp 1112-1122, ISSN 1471-4159

Wyllie, D. (2008). 2B or 2B and 2D? – That is the question. *J. Physiol*, 586, 3 (February 2008), pp. 693, ISSN 0022-3751

Wyllie, D.J.A., Béhé, P., and Colquhoun, D. (1998). Single-channel activations and concentration jumps: comparison of recombinant NR1a/NR2A and NR1a/NR2D NMDA receptors. *J Physiol*, 510 (July 1998), pp. 1–18, ISSN 0022-3751

Xu, J., Kurup, P., Zhang, Y., Goebel-Goody, S.M., Wu, P.H., Hawasli, A.H., Baum, M.L., Bibb, J.A., and Lombroso, P.J. (2009). Extrasynaptic NMDA receptors couple preferentially to excitotoxicity via calpain-mediated cleavage of STEP. *J Neurosci*, 29, 29, (July 2009), pp. 9330-9343, ISSN 0270-6474

Yaka, R., Phamluong, K., and Ron, D. (2003). Scaffolding of Fyn kinase to the NMDA receptor determines brain region sensitivity to ethanol. *J Neurosci*, 23, 9, (May 2003), pp. 3623-3632, ISSN 0270-6474

Zhou, M., and Baudry, M. (2006), Developmental Changes in NMDA Neurotoxicity Reflect Developmental Changes in Subunit Composition of NMDA Receptors. *J. Neurosci*, 26, 11, (March 2006), pp. 2956-2963, ISSN 0270-6474

8

Role of Multifunctional FADD (Fas-Associated Death Domain) Adaptor in Drug Addiction

Alfredo Ramos-Miguel, María Álvaro-Bartolomé,
M. Julia García-Fuster and Jesús A. García-Sevilla
University of the Balearic Islands
Spain

1. Introduction

Human drug addictions are chronic medical disorders characterized by tolerance and dependence to the abused substance, incentive sensitization, loss of control over drug use that becomes compulsive, relapse (Belin & Everitt, 2010), and in some cases high mortality. A large body of research has established that the majority of drugs leading to addiction stimulate dopamine release through the meso-cortico-limbic circuit in laboratory animals and humans (e.g. see Badiani et al., 2011). Brain neuroadaptations along the reward system are a focus of current research, especially those induced in the prefrontal cortex of human addicts (Goldstein & Volkow, 2011). These persistent neuroplastic events appear to be major causes for compulsive drug-seeking behavior despite the negative effects (e.g., neurotoxicity) induced by drugs of abuse in humans (Nutt et al., 2007).

It is generally accepted that some addictive drugs can induce cell death in the human brain, following observations that neurons and astrocytes die when exposed to drugs of abuse (Cunha-Oliveira et al., 2008; Büttner, 2011). Neurotoxicity and neuroplasticity acting together in the addicted brain might explain the dampened cognition and the reinforced behaviors driving to drug consumption. The best-studied cell-killing machinery is the so-called programmed cell death or apoptosis (Galluzzi et al., 2011). *In vivo* studies have reported controversial data for drugs of abuse regulating the apoptotic machinery in the brain (Tegeder & Geisslinger, 2004). Moreover, other findings have revealed important roles of pro-apoptotic proteins in the molecular mechanisms mediating synaptic and structural plasticity in the brain (Gilman & Mattson, 2002). Indeed, proteins belonging to the extrinsic apoptotic pathway have gained special interest in the study of neuroplastic machinery for their functional duality, promoting either apoptosis or cell survival and differentiation (Park et al., 2005; Tourneur and Chiocchia, 2010). Thus, Fas-associated death domain (FADD) protein is the most proximal adaptor molecule that mediates the signaling of death receptors belonging to the tumor necrosis factor receptor superfamily (TNFRSF), such as Fas or TNFRSF6 receptor (Tourneur and Chiocchia, 2010). Although the main role of FADD adaptor is to engage cell death through the extrinsic apoptotic pathway (Galluzzi et al., 2011), it also mediates non-apoptotic actions in cell systems *in vitro* (Park et al., 2005) and has a critical role in embryogenesis (Imtiyaz et al., 2009). In the CNS, Fas receptor dysregulation is associated with a number of disease states, including neurodegenerative disorders (Sharma et al., 2000). Fas stimulation can also promote neurite outgrowth and neuronal branching, which suggests the induction of neuroplastic responses in neurons (Lambert et al., 2003; Reich et al., 2008). Notably, FADD can translocate to the nucleus, a process favoured by its phosphorylation, and regulate nuclear factors, possibly altering the genetic profile of the cell, and promoting differentiation, neuroplasticity, and/or other anti/non-apoptotic actions.

All these features made of FADD an intriguing molecule for the study of brain neurotoxicity and/or neuroplasticity induced by drugs of abuse. This chapter reviews current evidence on the new roles of brain FADD in the complex neurobiology of drug addiction. After a brief overview on Fas/FADD complex and specific features of FADD protein, the involvement of multifunctional FADD and associated signalling in the acute and chronic effects of opiates, cocaine and cannabinoids are summarized from biochemical and behavioral studies performed in rat, mouse and human brains.

2. Relevant features of FADD protein

2.1 Fas/FADD complex: Pro-apoptotic function

In the standard model of Fas-mediated cell death (binding of FasL resulting in receptor trimerization; Algeciras-Schimnich et al., 2002), Fas and FADD are bound through homotypic death domain (DD) interactions (Fas/FADD complex) (Fig. 1A). Then FADD can recruit death effector domain (DED)-containing initiator pro-caspase 8 (and other molecules such as FLIP and PEA-15) to form a death inducing signalling complex (DISC), which finally promotes the activation of death-effector caspases (mainly caspase-3) with the final cleavage of downstream vital cellular substrates. Recently, two models of Fas/FADD-DISC (Scott et al., 2009; Wang et al., 2010) and a likely 5 Fas:5 FADD stoichiometry (Fig. 1A; Wang et al., 2010) have been proposed based on the crystal structures of the proteins. Therefore, FADD

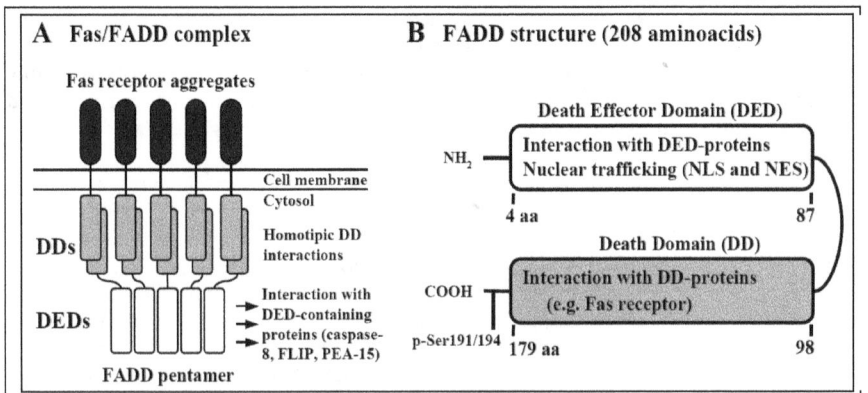

Fig. 1. (A) Fas/FADD-DISC complex. (B) FADD protein structure and domains (DD and DED). NLS: nuclear localization signals; NES: nuclear export signals. FLIP: FADD-like interleukin-1β-converting enzyme-inhibitory protein; PEA-15: phosphoprotein enriched in astrocytes of 15 kDa.

can form functional homo-oligomers of high molecular mass (oligomeric signalling complexes) which have been shown to increase the efficiency of Fas apoptotic signalling in normal and cancer cells (Sandu et al., 2006). Cell death in the CNS shares the same basic mechanisms operating in peripheral cells. Thus, brain apoptosis can be initiated through the extrinsic (Fas receptor) and intrinsic (mitochondrial) pathways, which converge to the activation of executioner caspases (Sastry and Rao, 2000).

2.2 FADD phosphorylation: Nuclear localization and functional implications

The structure of FADD displays, outside its C-terminal DD region (Fig. 1B), a single serine phosphorylation site (p-Ser191 in mouse, p-Ser194 in human; p-Ser194 or p-Ser195 in rat; Zhang et al., 2004; García-Fuster et al., 2008a). This phosphorylation of FADD, mainly mediated by casein kinase 1α (CK1α), is essential for the non-apoptotic actions of this multifunctional protein, such as the regulation of cell growth and differentiation (Alappat et al., 2005).

Although FADD was initially thought to be a cytoplasmic protein, it contains nuclear localization and export signals (NLS/NES; Fig. 1B) that allow its nuclear translocation (Gómez-Angelats and Cidlowski, 2003). Some studies have even reported that FADD is predominantly stored in the nucleus of resting cells, being redistributed to the cytoplasm upon Fas receptor activation (Föger et al., 2009). In any case, p-FADD is the main protein species translocated to the nucleus (Screaton et al., 2003). Nuclear p-FADD is involved in the anti-apoptotic actions of the molecule through the modulation of critical factors (Screaton et al., 2003; Alappat et al., 2005).

2.3 FADD adaptor in the brain: Immunodetection of protein forms and regional distribution

In rat, mouse and human brain tissue, various commercially available antibodies tested against FADD (up to seven) readily immunolabeled a ≈51-kDa band corresponding to its dimeric form (Fig. 2A, left panel). To a lesser extent, these antibodies also reacted against the monomeric (≈20-23 kDa) and other FADD species of higher magnitude (≈92-116 kDa) (García-Fuster et al., 2008a). In contrast, different antibodies against p-FADD recognized 92-116-kDa bands corresponding to oligomeric p-FADD species (Fig. 2A, right panel). Noteworthy, these higher FADD structures fit well with the recently proposed pentameric model of DISC association (see Fig. 1A; Wang et al., 2010). In addition, some of these antibodies immunodetected the monomeric p-FADD species (García-Fuster et al., 2008a; Ramos-Miguel et al., 2009) (Fig. 2A, right panel). The ability of these phospho-directed antibodies to label p-FADD species was challenged with the alkaline phosphatase assay, which demonstrated the specificity of these antibodies to bind to the p-sites of the protein (Fig. 2A, right panel). Therefore, in brain tissue, it is likely that non-p-FADD is more stable as a dimer, and its phosphorylation switches FADD self-associative properties. Thus, these FADD (dimers) and p-FADD (monomers and oligomers) forms were initially selected to assess the role of multifunctional FADD protein in the molecular mechanisms of drug addiction. To note that some p-FADD species (e.g. ≈45 kDa form; Fig. 2A. right) most probably represent degradation products of higher mass p-oligomers. These and other technical issues are largely discussed in previous reports (García-Fuster et al., 2008a).

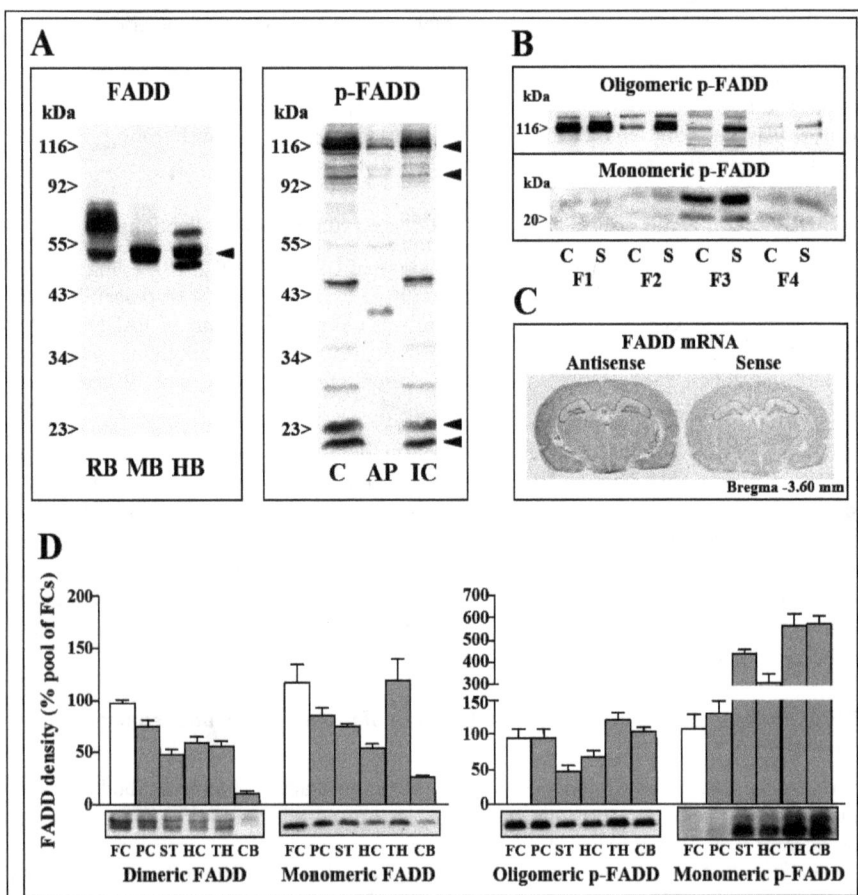

Fig. 2. (A/B) Immunodetection of FADD protein forms (arrow heads: monomeric, dimeric and oligomeric nonphosphorylated and phosphorylated species) in brain total homogenate (RB: rat cortex; MB: mouse cortex; HB: human cortex; C: rat striatum, control sample; AP: alkaline phosphatase; IC: inhibited control, alkaline phosphatase plus sodium pyrophosphate) and subcellular compartments (rat cortex; F1: cytosol; F2: membranes; F3: nucleus; F4: cytoskeleton), in which the acute effect of sufentanil (S: 0.015 mg/kg, s.c., 30 min) on p-FADD is shown (C: control saline). Protein sizes (kDa) as visualized in Western blots. (Modified from García-Fuster et al., 2007a, 2008a). (C) Detection of FADD mRNA in rat brain (anatomical level: Bregma -3.60 mm) by in situ hybridization. Note that FADD mRNA (antisense probe) showed very low expression in the brain, except for hippocampal regions and cortex (see García-Fuster et al., 2009). To verify specificity of binding a sense control probe was hybridized in test tissue. (Modified from García-Fuster et al., 2006). (D) Regional distribution of FADD protein forms in the rat brain (FC: frontal cortex, region of reference; PC: parietal cortex; ST: corpus striatum; HC: hippocampus; TH: thalamus; CB: cerebellum).

FADD is expressed in neurons and glial cells (Hartmann et al., 2002; Bi et al., 2008; Tewari et al., 2008). FADD mRNA expression is homogeneous along the brain tissue, as visualized by *in situ* hybridization (Fig. 2C), with slight increased labeling in cortical areas and hippocampus. However, the distribution of FADD protein (monomeric and dimeric species) in rat brain regions is uneven, with a greater content in the cerebral cortex than in cerebellum (Fig. 2D, left). In contrast, p-FADD (monomeric and oligomeric p-species) is highly expressed in cerebellum (Fig. 2D, right). Thus, the ratio of p-FADD to FADD (monomeric species) was much greater in the cerebellum (CB: 22.4) than in cortical areas (FC: 0.91; PC: 1.58) (Fig. 2D). Subcortical regions also display high p-FADD/FADD ratios (ST: 5.87; HC: 5.61; TH: 4.98) (Fig. 2D). The physiological relevance of the marked variation of p-FADD/FADD ratio across brain regions remains to be determined. To note that FADD and p-FADD are well expressed in brain regions (e.g., the frontal cortex and corpus striatum) more closely associated with the behavioral effects of drug of abuse (Fig. 2D). In the human brain, a dynamic relationship between monomeric and oligomeric p-FADD forms has been observed (Ramos-Miguel et al., 2009). Notably, some opiate and cannabinoid drugs, but not cocaine, have been shown to induce the interconversion between FADD and p-FADD (increasing the ratio p-FADD/FADD), which may favor the induction of non-apoptotic (neuroplastic) actions (see below and Fig. 6).

At the subcelullar level, FADD and p-FADD (rat, mouse and human brains) are expressed in cytosol and nucleus, and to a lesser extent in membranes (García-Fuster et al., 2007a, 2008a; Ramos-Miguel et al., 2009; Álvaro-Bartolomé et al., 2010) (Fig. 2B and 11D). To note that the monomeric form of p-FADD is particularly well expressed in the nucleus (Fig. 2B) (Ramos-Miguel et al., 2009). Nuclear p-FADD has been reported to play important roles in the molecular mechanisms of opiate addiction in humans (Ramos-Miguel et al., 2009), possibly by regulating nuclear factors such as methyl-CpG binding domain protein 4 (Screaton et al., 2003) and nuclear factor kappaB (Schinske et al., 2011).

2.4 FADD adaptor: Apoptotic and non-apoptotic signalling pathways

Besides the role of FADD in the cascades of apoptotic signaling in drug addiction (García-Fuster et al., 2007a, 2008b; Ramos-Miguel et al., 2009; Álvaro-Bartolomé et al., 2011), several pathways have been postulated to link FADD with some forms of behavioral plasticity induced by drugs of abuse, especially heroin/morphine (Ramos-Miguel et al., 2009, 2010, 2011) and cocaine (García-Fuster et al., 2009, 2011; Álvaro-Bartolomé et al., 2011) (Fig. 3).

These signalling pathways involve, *inter alia*, the extracellular signal-regulated kinase (ERK), the kinase Akt1 or protein kinase B (PKB), and phosphoprotein enriched in astrocytes of 15 kDa (PEA-15), which interactions with FADD are discussed below (see section 3.3) in the context of the acute/chronic effects of opiates, cocaine and cannabinoids (Fig. 3).

3. Role of FADD adaptor in opiate addiction

Opiate addiction is associated with various forms of neurotoxicity, which can result in serious brain dysfunction in most subjects (Yücel et al., 2007; Bütnner, 2011). Moreover, heroin addicts often develop severe immunodeficiencies that could be the result of apoptotic cell death in the immune system (Kreek, 1990; Govitrapong et al., 1998). In fact, morphine was reported to increase, through a naloxone-sensitive mechanism, the expression of Fas receptor mRNA in mouse splenocytes and in human blood lymphocytes (Yin et al., 1999). However, the possibility of opiate-induced cell death in the mature brain, including the brains of human addicts, still is a debated issue (Boronat et al., 2001; Tegeder and Geisslinger, 2004; Liao et al., 2005; Cunha-Oliveira et al., 2008; García-Fuster et al., 2008b; Tramullas et al., 2008; Zhang et al., 2008).

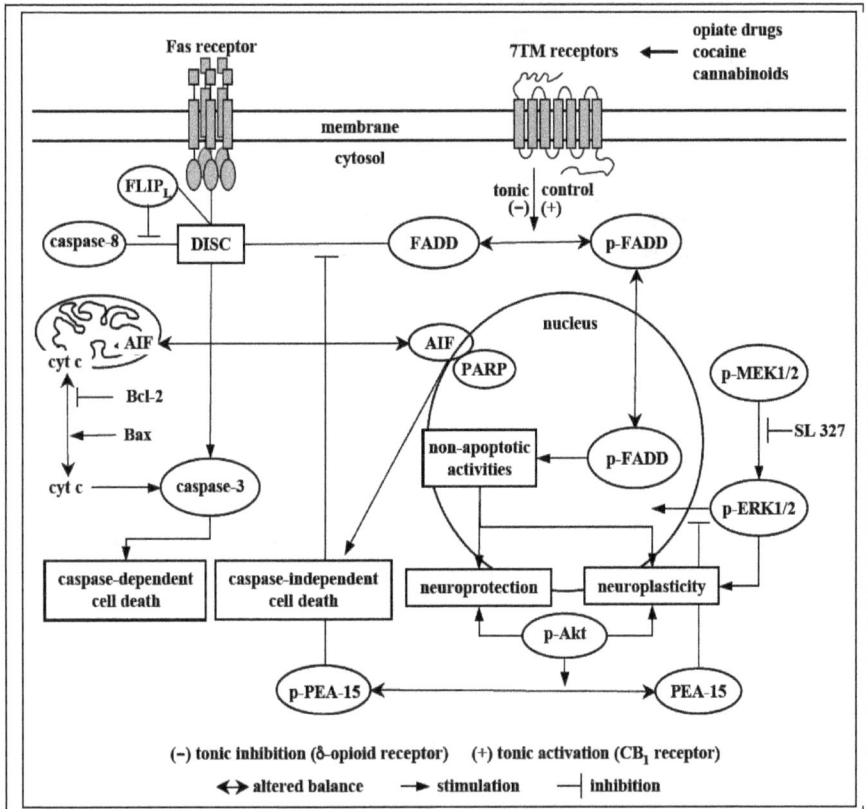

Fig. 3. Schematic diagram illustrating the complex interactions between the multifunctional protein FADD (pro-apoptotic, anti-apoptotic and/or neuroplastic actions) and pro-survival MAP kinases (MEK-ERK) and Akt1/PEA-15 signalling in opiate, cocaine and cannabinoid addiction. See the main text for specific details and comments.

3.1 Regulation of basal Fas/FADD complex by opioid receptors: Anti-apoptotic δ-opioid receptor tone

A relevant interaction between the opioid system and Fas/FADD complex in the brain was disclosed using gene-targeted mice lacking μ-, δ-, or κ-opioid receptors (García-Fuster et al., 2007b). Thus, wild-type (WT) and knock-out (KO) mice were compared to investigate the existence of endogenous opioid tones regulating the basal contents of Fas receptor and FADD adaptor in the brain.

The results indicated that μ- and κ-receptors do not exert a significant tonic control on Fas/FADD complex expression levels in the mouse brain (i.e., no major target changes in μ- and κ-KO mice). In δ-KO mice, however, Fas aggregates (Fas forms triggering receptor signalling) and FADD adaptor were markedly increased in the cortex (Fig. 4) and corpus striatum. Moreover, the basal content of monomeric p-FADD (the FADD species implicated in non-apoptotic signals) was also up-regulated in the cortices of δ-KO mice, which is in line with the observed increase of FADD in these animals (Fig. 4). In this context, it is worth mentioning that inhibitory δ-opioid receptors possess a high level of constitutive (ligand-independent) activity (Costa and Herz, 1989; Neilan et al., 1999), which could control the basal level of some associated signalling molecules such as the Fas/FADD complex.

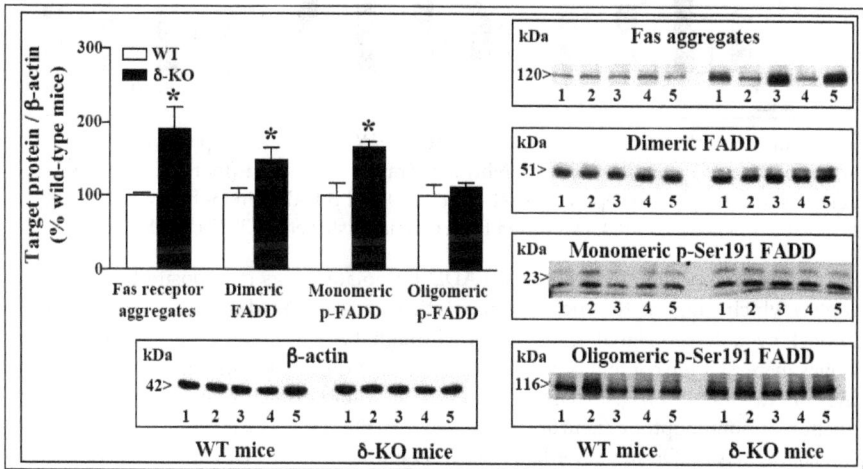

Fig. 4. Fas receptor aggregates, FADD adaptor, and p-FADD (monomeric and oligomeric forms) in the cerebral cortex of WT mice and δ-opioid receptor KO mice. *At least p<0.05 *versus* WT. (Modified from García-Fuster et al., 2007b).

Taken together, the findings in δ-KO mice strongly suggest that the functioning of pro-apoptotic Fas/FADD complex *in vivo* is partly under an inhibitory tonic control of brain δ-opioid receptors (i.e., removal of a negative endogenous opioid tone results in Fas/FADD up-regulation; see Fig. 3) (García-Fuster et al., 2007b). The anti-apoptotic δ-opioid receptor tone on Fas/FADD complex could play an important role in the neuroprotection afforded by δ-opioid receptor agonists (Narita et al., 2006).

3.2 Acute, chronic and withdrawal effects of opiate drugs on FADD and associated signalling in the brain

Acute and chronic treatments of rats with various opiate drugs (heroin, morphine, SNC-80, U-50488-H, pentazocine), as well as the induction of opiate withdrawal states, were initially shown to result in increases or decreases of various Fas receptor forms in the brain (Boronat et al., 2001q; García-Fuster et al., 2003, 2004). Thus, heroin/morphine addiction in rats was associated with up-regulation of both native and aggregated forms, thereby suggesting the induction of pro-apoptotic actions in the brain (García-Fuster et al., 2003, 2004). In contrast, similar treatments with morphine and selective μ-(fentanyl, sufentanil), δ-(SNC-80) and κ-(U-50488-H) opioid receptor agonists were associated with receptor-specific reductions of FADD, except for the chronic treatments that show tachyphylaxis to the acute drug effects in the brain (Fig. 5) (García-Fuster et al., 2007a).

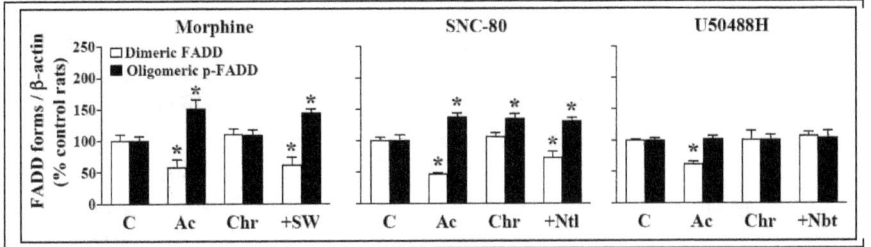

Fig. 5. Acute (Ac), chronic (Chr) and spontaneous (+SW) or antagonist precipitated (naltrindole, Ntl; nor-binaltorphimine, Nbt) withdrawal effects of μ-(morphine), δ-(SNC-80) and κ-(U50488H) opioid receptor agonists on FADD and p-FADD in rat brain cortex. *At least $p<0.05$ versus control (C). (Modified from García-Fuster et al., 2007a, 2008a).

As a matter of fact, the modulation of FADD by opiate drugs is opposite to that of Fas receptor, which suggests that possible apoptotic signals engaged by Fas activation would be offset by a lesser signal transduction through FADD adaptor. Indeed, μ/δ-opiate agonists increased the content of p-FADD in the brain (Fig. 5; see also Fig. 2B for the acute effect of sufentanil on p-FADD in subcellular compartments), which suggests the induction of non-apoptotic (neuroplastic) effects by these drugs (see Fig. 3) (García-Fuster et al., 2007a, 2008a). On the other hand, SNC-80-induced down-regulation of FADD in rat brain (cortex and striatum) was blunted after the inhibition of the MEK-ERK pathway *in vivo*, which demonstrates the direct involvement of this anti-apoptotic signalling in FADD regulation (García-Fuster et al., 2007a). On the other hand, the molecular mechanism by which seven transmembrane (7TM) receptors interact with FADD (i.e., G protein dependent or independent process; see Fig. 3) remains to be fully determined (see García-Fuster et al., 2008a).

Remarkably, morphine, sufentanil and SNC-80 (acute, chronic and/or withdrawal effects) up-regulated the content of p-FADD with a concomitant decrease of total FADD in rat brain cortex (Fig. 6A), indicating that these drugs promote an increase in the ratio of p-FADD to FADD (a proposed index of non-apoptotic activity). The inverse relationship between p-FADD and FADD is likely to be due to changes in the phosphorylation status, possibly mediated by CK1α, of the adaptor molecule induced by opiate drugs (García-Fuster et al., 2008a; Ramos-Miguel et al., 2009). These findings support the concept of an interconversion between non-phosphorylated FADD and phosphorylated FADD after exposure to opiate drugs, which appears to be a relevant molecular mechanism in morphine-induced neuroplasticity (see below). A similar inverse correlation between p-FADD and FADD has been observed for the acute effects of the CB_1 receptor agonist WIN55212-2 (Fig. 6B), but not for the psychostimulant cocaine (Fig. 6C).

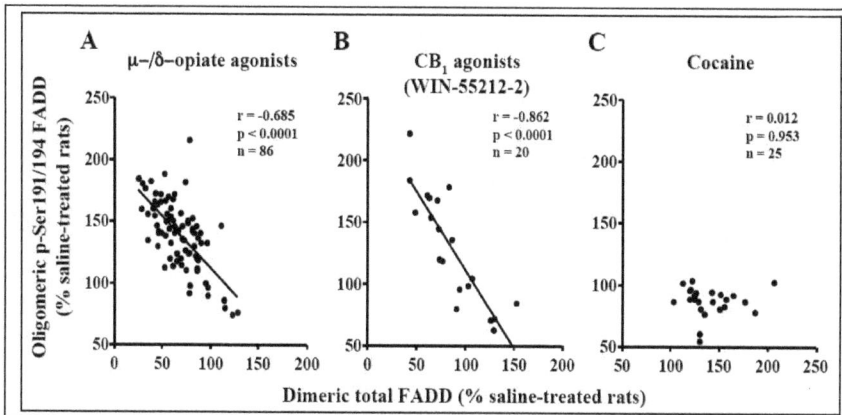

Fig. 6. Inverse correlation between the contents of p-FADD and FADD in rat or mouse brain cortex (each point corresponds to an animal). (A) Opiate agonists: effects of acute (30 and 100 mg/kg) and chronic (10-100 mg/kg; 6 days) morphine, and spontaneous morphine withdrawal (1-3 days); effects of acute sufentanil (15-30 mg/kg); effects of acute SNC-80 (10-30 mg/kg). (B) CB_1 receptor agonist: effects of acute WIN55212-2 (0.5-8 mg/kg). (C) Effects of acute cocaine (3-30 mg/kg). (Modified from García-Fuster et al., 2008a, 2009; Álvaro-Bartolomé et al., 2010).

3.3 FADD phosphorylation correlates with morphine-evoked behaviors

Recent findings have revealed a direct role of p-FADD in the molecular mechanisms leading to the expression of unconditioned morphine-induced psychomotor sensitization (Ramos-Miguel et al., 2010) and to the expression of spontaneous morphine abstinence syndrome (Ramos-Miguel et al., 2011) in rats.

To develop sensitization to morphine (Ramos-Miguel et al., 2010), rats were subjected to a standard treatment protocol (Fig. 7A, left) in which they received saline (controls) or morphine (10 mg/kg/day) for 5 days in absence of environmental cues. After 3 (day 8 of the treatment; Fig. 7A) or 14 days of spontaneous saline/morphine withdrawal (SW3 and SW14, respectively), all rats received a morphine challenge (10 mg/kg) to assess the expression of locomotor sensitization, which was observed at SW3 (Fig. 7A) but not at SW14 (Ramos-Miguel et al., 2010). In parallel to morphine-induced behavioral sensitization, striatal FADD was modulated at SW3, but not at SW14. Thus, p-FADD was up-regulated (Fig. 7A, right) whereas FADD content was decreased (not shown) at SW3. Therefore, the ratio p-FADD/FADD (a postulated marker of neuroplasticity) was increased (2.6-fold) in rat striatum. Similarly, ERK activity was also enhanced in the same striatal samples (Fig. 7A, right). Notably, inhibition of MEK-ERK signalling attenuated the expression of morphine-induced psychomotor sensitization and fully prevented the up-regulation of p-FADD at SW3 (Fig. 7A). The Akt1/PEA-15 pathway, which may link ERK and FADD functions (see Fig. 3), was also activated at SW3, being dependent on the integrity of MEK-ERK signalling (Fig. 7A, right). Taken together, these findings reveal a major role of p-FADD, interacting with MEK/ERK and Akt1/PEA-15, in mediating the short-lasting expression of unconditioned psychomotor sensitization induced by morphine in rats.

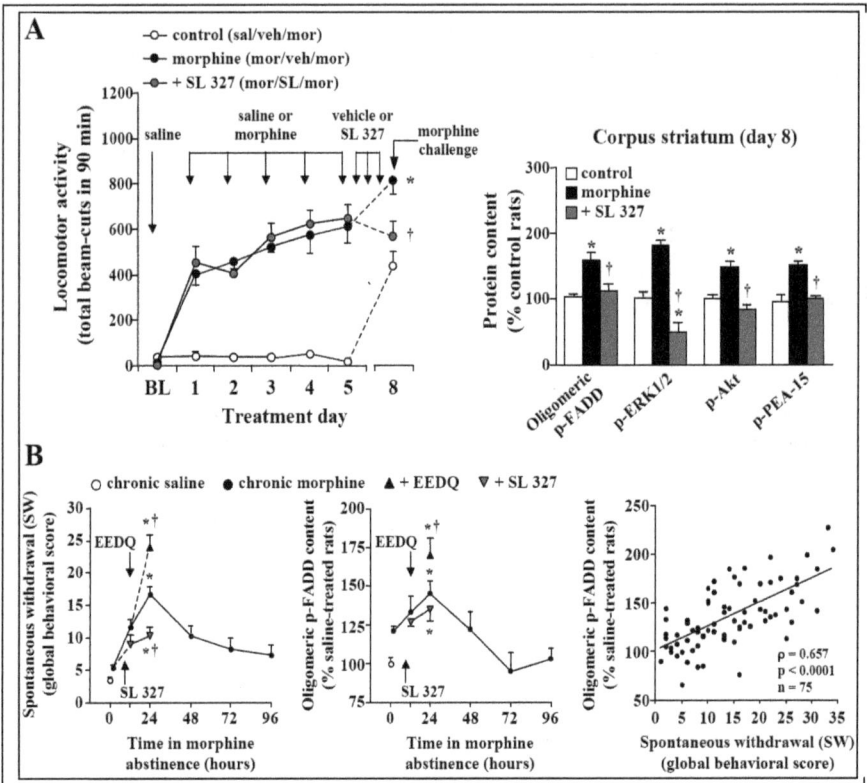

Fig. 7. (A) FADD phosphorylation and expression of unconditioned morphine-induced psychomotor sensitization. Note that day 8 of the treatment corresponds to SW3 (see text). (B) FADD phosphorylation and intensity of spontaneous morphine abstinence syndrome. BL, baseline; SL327, an inhibitor of MEK in vivo; EEDQ, an alkylating of α_2-adrenoceptors. *At least $p<0.05$ *versus* controls, †at least $p<0.05$ *versus* morphine-treated rats. (Modified from Ramos-Miguel et al., 2010, 2011).

To explore the role of FADD in the mechanisms of morphine-induced physical dependence, the regulation of cortical p-FADD was investigated during the development of spontaneous opiate withdrawal (SW) in morphine-dependent rats (10-100 mg/kg for 6 days) (Ramos-Miguel et al., 2011). Notably, cortical p-FADD mirrored the time course of morphine SW (12-96 h; peak at 24 h) (Fig. 7B, left), which resulted in a striking correlation between p-FADD and the intensity of morphine abstinence (Fig. 7B, right). On the other hand, the involvement of α_2-adrenoceptors in opiate addiction is well-known, and the stimulation of these inhibitory receptors induces anti-withdrawal effects in morphine-dependent animals and in human addicts. Interestingly, the inactivation of brain α_2-adrenoceptors (EEDQ at SW12) (Fig. 7B, left) further enhanced morphine abstinence intensity and cortical p-FADD content at SW24 (Fig. 7B, right and middle panels). The disruption of ERK signalling (SL 327 at SW4 and SW8) did not alter morphine abstinence at SW12, but did attenuate the behavioral syndrome at SW24 (Fig. 7B, left). ERK inhibition, however, did not prevent the up-regulation of p-FADD at SW12 and SW24 (Fig. 7B, middle panel). Taken together, these findings reveal that cortical p-FADD, mainly through an interaction with α_2-adrenoceptors, plays a functional role in the behavioral expression of morphine abstinence in rats.

Together, these studies indicate that relevant behavioral adaptations induced by repeated morphine exposure in rats correlate with an increased p-FADD/FADD ratio in the cerebral cortex, which strongly suggests that multifunctional FADD is involved in the complex molecular mechanisms of opiate-induced neuroplasticity.

3.4 Regulation of apoptotic pathways and associated signalling in brains of opiate addicts: p-FADD and neuroplasticity

Recent studies have investigated the role of Fas receptor, FADD adaptor and its phosphorylation, other pro- and anti-apoptotic proteins, and FADD-associated signalling pathways, in postmortem brains of long-term opiate addicts (García-Fuster et al., 2008b; Ramos-Miguel et al., 2009). The prefrontal cortex (Brodmann's area 9, middle frontal gyrus; PFC/BA9) was the region selected for examination because it is directly related with the mesocorticolimbic dopaminergic system and the rewarding and addictive properties of opiates and other drugs of abuse.

First, the hypothesis was tested that human opiate addiction is associated with an increased cell death in the brain (García-Fuster et al., 2008b). In a well-characterized cohort (n=48) of heroin or methadone abusers (including the assessment of opiates and metabolites in blood, urine, and hair samples), the content of Fas receptor in PFC/BA9 did not differ from that in age-, gender-, and postmortem delay-matched controls (Fig. 8A). In contrast, FADD adaptor was down-regulated in the same brain samples of short- and long-term opiate addicts (Fig. 8A). Furthermore, initiator caspase-8 was not altered, but FLIP$_L$ content, a dominant inhibitor of caspase-8, was increased in long-term opiate addicts.

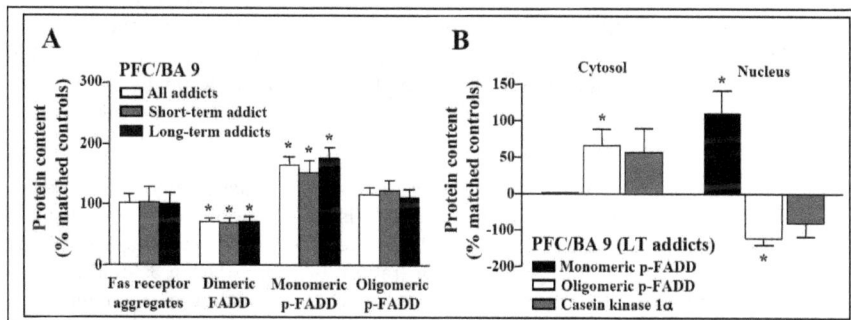

Fig. 8. (A) Contents of Fas receptor aggregates, FADD adaptor, and p-FADD in the prefrontal cortex/Brodmann's area 9 (PFC/BA 9; total homogenate samples) of short- and long-term opiate abusers. (B) Subcellular content (increases or decreases in cytosol and nucleus) of p-FADD and CK1α in the PFC/BA9 of long-term (LT) opiate addicts. *At least $p<0.05$ versus matched controls. (Modified from García-Fuster et al., 2008b; Ramos-Miguel et al., 2009).

In the intrinsic mitochondrial pathway, pro-apoptotic Bax and AIF (apoptosis-inducing factor) were unchanged, cytochrome c (a potent caspase-3 activator) was reduced, and anti-apoptotic Bcl-2 augmented in long-term opiate addicts. Importantly, the content of executioner caspase-3/active fragments and the pattern of cleavage of nuclear PARP-1 (poly-(ADP-ribose)-polymerase-1), a hallmark of apoptosis, were very similar in opiate addicts and control subjects.

Taken together, these findings indicate that the molecular machineries of canonical apoptotic pathways are not abnormally activated enough in the PFC/BA9 of opiate abusers to suggest higher rates of cell death in this brain region. Instead, the long-term adaptations of FADD and cytochrome c (down-regulation) and those of FLIP$_L$ and Bcl-2 (up-regulation) could be related to the induction of non-apoptotic actions including phenomena of neuroplasticity in brains of opiate addicts.

Therefore, the role of p-FADD and FADD-associated signalling pathways involved in neuroplasticity was investigated (Ramos-Miguel et al., 2009) in the same cohort and brain region of opiate abusers (García-Fuster et al., 2008b). In these subjects, the content of monomeric, but not oligomeric, p-FADD was markedly increased in the PFC/BA9 of short- and long-term opiate abusers (Fig. 8A, total homogenate samples). At the subcellular level (PFC/BA9), long-term opiate addiction was associated with up-regulation of monomeric p-FADD and down-regulation of oligomeric p-FADD in the nucleus (Fig. 8B). In the cytosol, in contrast, oligomeric p-FADD was increased (Fig. 8B). Along this line, CK1α, the enzyme that mediates p-FADD, was found co-localized with FADD in cytosol and nucleus (Fig. 8B). These findings appear to indicate that FADD is phosphorylated (and oligomerized) in the cytosol of cortical cells (PFC/BA9), and translocates to the nucleus, where it is disaggregated to monomers to develop its nuclear functions (see Fig. 3).

In long-term opiate addicts, on the other hand, marked down-regulation of ERK1/2, JNK1/2 (c-Jun N-terminal Kinase), PEA-15 and Akt1 signalling were observed in the PFC/BA9 (total homogenate and subcellular compartments) (Ferrer-Alcón et al., 2004; Ramos-Miguel et al., 2009). Remarkably, down-regulation of ERK1/2 and Akt1 in the PFC of chronic opiate addicts could also play a major role in the induction of tolerance to opiate reward (Ramos-Miguel et al., 2009). A complex cross-talk between FADD/p-FADD and Akt1/PEA-15 and ERK1/2 signalling would take place in the brain to finally result in the induction of neuroplasticity without an abnormal rate of cell death in the PFC/BA9 of chronic opiate addicts (see Fig. 3).

Taken together, the results of these studies (García-Fuster et al., 2008b; Ramos-Miguel et al., 2009) clearly indicate that opiate addiction in humans is associated with an altered balance between p-FADD (content increased) and FADD (content decreased) in brain, which may favor the neuroplastic actions of FADD adaptor (ratio p-FADD/FADD: a 3.3-fold increase over matched controls). In fact, relevant roles of p-FADD in modulating morphine-induced behavioral plasticity have been demonstrated in the rat brain (see subheading 3.3.).

4. Role of FADD adaptor in cocaine addiction

Cocaine and/or its oxidative metabolites (e.g. norcocaine) can induce various forms of neurotoxicity (Büttner, 2011), including apoptotic effects in both cultured cells (Xiao et al.,

2000; Cunha-Oliveira et al., 2008) and the developing brain (Novikova et al., 2005). However, the aberrant activation of several cell death mechanisms by cocaine, including those mediated by the Fas/FADD complex, in the adult rat brain remains inconclusive (Dietrich et al, 2005; García-Fuster et al., 2009). Nevertheless, self-exposure to cocaine in humans was recently shown to enhance the degradation of a DNA-repairing enzyme in the PFC/BA9 of long-term addicts, which is compatible with the induction of aberrant cell death by the psychostimulant (Álvaro-Bartolomé et al., 2011).

4.1 Acute, chronic and withdrawal effects of cocaine on FADD and associated signalling in the brain

Acute treatments of rats with cocaine (7.5-30 mg/kg) modulated FADD protein forms in brain cortex, increasing the content of FADD and moderately decreasing that of p-FADD with the lower doses (Fig. 9A) (García-Fuster et al., 2009; Álvaro-Bartolomé et al., 2011). In contrast to opiate and cannabinoid drugs, cortical FADD and p-FADD do not correlate after acute cocaine (Fig. 6C), suggesting that psychostimulants favours the expression of pro-apoptotic FADD form (increased). Acute cocaine increased FADD in all subcellular compartments where it was expressed, with the greater effects in the cytosol and nucleus (García-Fuster et al., 2009). Dopamine D_2 receptors were involved in FADD activation by cocaine as pretreatment with raclopride, a D_2-type receptor antagonist, fully prevented the acute cocaine-induced increase of FADD in rat brain cortex (Fig. 9B). Pretreatment with a D_1-type receptor antagonist (SCH-23390) did not block the acute effect of cocaine on FADD (Fig. 9B). In fact, SCH-23390 by itself increased cortical FADD (Fig. 9B), an effect possibly mediated by its agonistic properties at 5-HT1c/2c receptors (García-Fuster et al., 2009).

A non-contingent experimenter-administered regimen of chronic cocaine in rats (15 or 40 mg/kg, for 6-7 days), known to induce behavioral sensitization, induced tachyphylaxis to the acute modulatory effect of the psychostimulant on cortical FADD (Fig. 9C). Cocaine withdrawal (1-7 days) was associated with a transient reduction in cortical FADD, which was significant 3 days after discontinuation of the chronic treatment (Fig. 9C) (García-Fuster et al., 2009; Álvaro-Bartolomé et al., 2011). It is worth noting that there was a positive correlation between FADD protein and the levels of FADD mRNA in rat brain cortex ($r=0.43$; $n=29$; $p<0.05$, see García-Fuster et al., 2009).

Acute cocaine (20 mg/kg) stimulated p-Thr34 DARPP-32 (dopamine- and cAMP-regulated phosphoprotein of 32 kDa) in rat brain cortex, consistent with the engagement of dopamine signalling. Chronic cocaine (40 mg/kg for 6 days) and cocaine withdrawal (3 days), however, were not associated with activation of cortical p-DARPP-32 (tachyphylaxis after the repeated treatment). Interestingly, chronic cocaine and abstinence, but not acute cocaine, increased the content of t-DARPP (a truncated 30 kDa isoform of DARPP-32 with striking anti-apoptotic actions; El-Rifai et al., 2002) in rat brain cortex. Moreover, acute cocaine, but not the chronic/abstinence treatments, stimulated Akt1 in rat brain cortex. Neither treatment with cocaine (acute, chronic, and abstinence) altered the basal stimulation of anti-apoptotic PEA-15 and pro-apoptotic JNK1/2 signaling (Álvaro-Bartolomé et al., 2011).

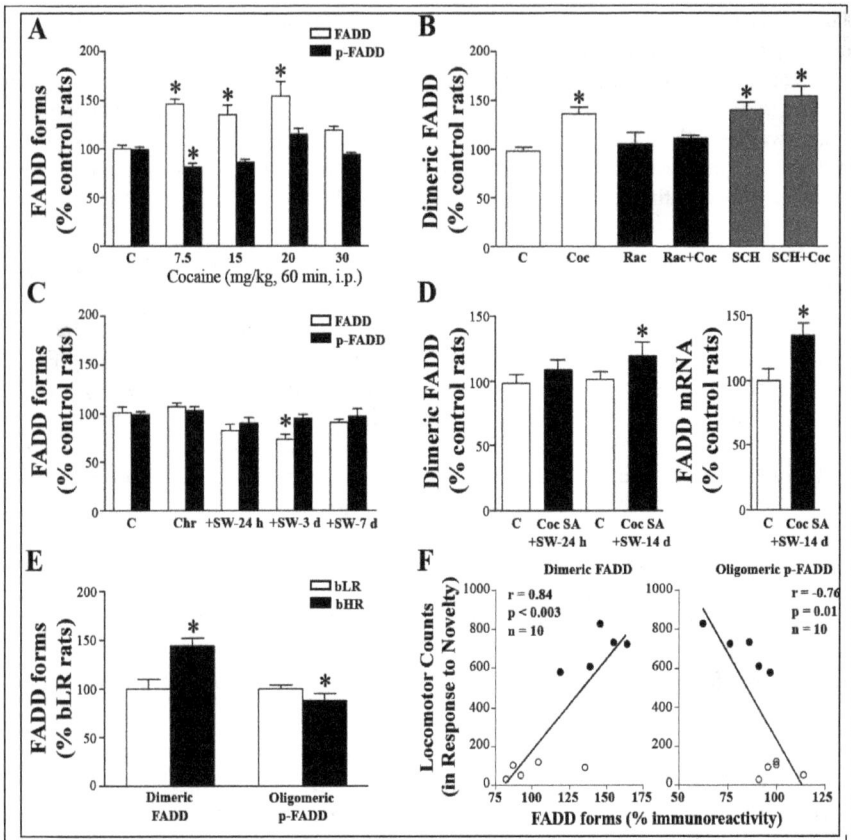

Fig. 9. (A) Acute dose-response effects of cocaine (7.5-30 mg/kg) on FADD and p-FADD in rat brain cortex. (B) FADD is modulated by acute cocaine (Coc, 7.5 mg/kg) through the activation of dopamine D_2 receptors in rat cortex. Rac: raclopride (0.5 mg/kg), SCH: SCH-23390 (0.5 mg/kg). (C) Non-contingent chronic cocaine (Chr, 15 mg/kg for 7 days) and spontaneous withdrawal (+SW) time course effects on cortical FADD and p-FADD. (D) Effects of spontaneous withdrawal (+SW) following contingent cocaine self-administration (Coc SA) on hippocampal FADD protein and mRNA. (E) Basal cortical differences in FADD and p-FADD in bred low-responder (bLR) and high-responder (bHR) rats. (F) Individual differences in locomotor response to novelty correlated (Pearson's r) with basal contents of FADD and p-FADD in rat cortex; non-parametric analysis (Spearman's ρ) also resulted in significant correlations for FADD (ρ=0.85; p<0.003; n=10) and p-FADD (ρ=-0.70; p<0.05; n=10) (open circle: bLR rats; closed circles: bHR rats). *At least $p<0.05$ *versus* control (C) or bLR rats. (Modified from García-Fuster et al., 2009, 2011; Álvaro-Bartolomé et al., 2011).

It is unlikely that cocaine-induced up-regulation of pro-apoptotic FADD in rat brain (Fig. 9A) could result in the induction of aberrant cell death. In fact, neither acute and chronic cocaine treatments nor cocaine spontaneous withdrawal altered the content of Fas receptor forms or mitochondrial cytochrome c (a potent caspase-3 activator) and AIF (a mitochondrial mediator of caspase-independent apoptosis) in rat cortex (Álvaro-Bartolomé et al., 2011). Moreover, none of these cocaine treatments altered the pattern of cleavage of nuclear PARP-1 in rat brain cortex (García-Fuster et al., 2009; Álvaro-Bartolomé et al., 2011).

A recent study has examined how a contingent extended daily access to cocaine self-administration impacts the hippocampus at the cellular and molecular levels, and how these alterations can change over the course of cocaine withdrawal (García-Fuster et al., 2011). This animal model has good validity in that it results in the escalation of drug intake (as controlled by the animal, see Ahmed and Koob, 1998) and in cognitive deficits (Briand et al., 2008) similar to those seen in human addicts. Moreover, hippocampal plasticity likely plays an important role in addiction-related behaviors. For example, suppression of hippocampal neurogenesis enhanced resistance to extinction of drug-seeking behavior (Noonan et al., 2010). The results of this study indicated that 5-hour of extended daily access to cocaine for 14 days elicits a profound increase in drug intake from the first self-administration session to the last (García-Fuster et al., 2011), providing a model to study the hippocampal adaptations associated with cocaine withdrawal after abuse of the psychostimulant. This cocaine paradigm led to alterations of hippocampal cell fate regulation (in various hippocampal subregions) during the course of withdrawal (1, 14 and 28 days) with significant changes observed at 14 days (García-Fuster et al., 2011). Notably, FADD adaptor (protein and mRNA; Fig. 9D) was increased in the hippocampus of rats with impaired cell proliferation rates (Ki-67+ mitotic progenitor cells and NeuroD+ neural progenitor cells). The increase in hippocampal FADD (14 days of cocaine withdrawal) did not parallel changes in apoptotic cell death, as measured by cleavage of nuclear PARP-1 (García-Fuster et al., 2011). These data suggest that FADD adaptor is an important hippocampal cell fate regulator during cocaine withdrawal in rats.

4.2 Relevance of FADD in novelty-seeking behaviour and cocaine abuse

Selectively breeding for divergence in locomotor reactivity to a novel environment (bred high-responder (bHR) and low-responder (bLR) lines of Sprague-Dawley rats) has been shown to display reliable differences across multiple behavioural and neurochemical dimensions (Stead et al., 2006). For example, bHR compared to bLR rats have shown an increased behavioural sensitization to cocaine (García-Fuster et al., 2010) and a greater initial propensity to self-administer cocaine (Davis et al., 2008). Interestingly, bHR and bLR rats showed significant basal differences in cortical FADD (higher content in bHR) and p-FADD (lower content in bHR) (Fig. 9E) (García-Fuster et al., 2009). However, bHR/bLR rats showed similar levels of basal nuclear PARP-1 cleavage, indicating similar rates of basal induction of cell death in the cortex (García-Fuster et al., 2009). Moreover, locomotion in a novel environment (bLR *versus* bHR) correlated with the basal content of cortical FADD (positive relation) and p-FADD (inverse relation) (Fig. 9F, n=10). Similarly to the acute, chronic and withdrawal cocaine effects observed in commercially purchased Sprague-Dawley rats (see Fig. 9A/C), the basal differences observed between bHR and bLR rats were maintained post-cocaine (i.e., increased FADD after acute cocaine with a reversal following 3 days of withdrawal) for both phenotypes (García-Fuster et al., 2009). These results suggest that FADD signalling could represent a molecular correlate for the bHR and/or bLR phenotype and therefore the initial propensity to initiate cocaine use (Belin et al., 2008).

4.3 Regulation of apoptotic pathways and associated signalling in brains of cocaine addicts: Increased degradation of nuclear PARP-1

In a recent study (Álvaro-Bartolomé et al., 2011), the hypothesis was tested that cocaine addiction in humans results in abnormal activation of canonical (extrinsic and intrinsic) apoptotic pathways leading to increased cell death in the brain (Fig. 10).

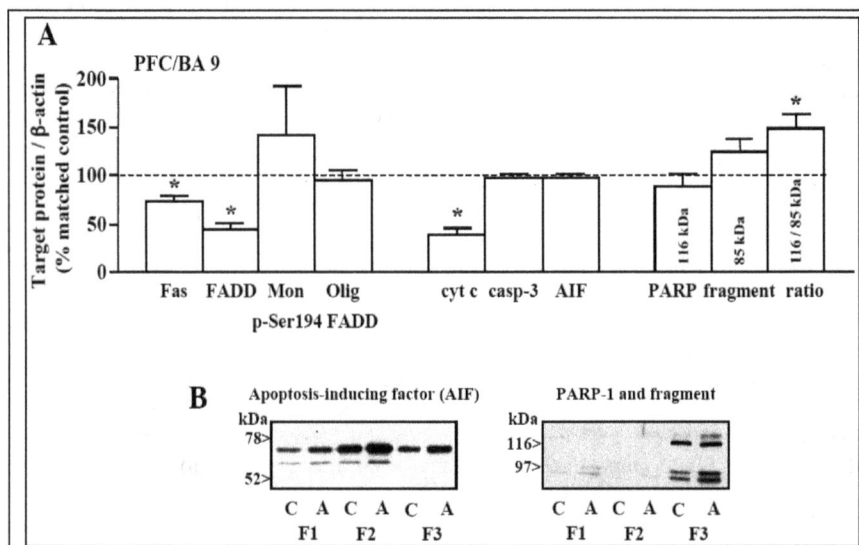

Fig. 10. (A) Contents of apoptotic proteins of the intrinsic (Fas receptor, FADD adaptor and p-FADD) and intrinsic (cytochrome c, caspase-3 and AIF) pathways, as well as the cleavage of nuclear PARP-1 in the prefrontal cortex/Brodmann's area 9 (PFC/BA9; total homogenate samples) of cocaine abusers. (B) Subcellular content of AIF and PARP-1 (F1: cytosol; F2: membranes; F3: nucleus) in the PFC/BA9 of a representative chronic cocaine addict. *At least $p<0.05$ versus matched controls. (Modified from Álvaro-Bartolomé et al., 2011).

In a small (n=10) and well-characterized cohort of "pure" cocaine abusers (including the assessment of cocaine and metabolites in blood, urine, and hair samples), Fas aggregates and FADD adaptor were down-regulated in the PFC/BA9 (Fig. 10A), which was associated with a modest increase in p-FADD/FADD ratio. Moreover, mitochondrial cytochrome c was also reduced, but not caspase-3 or AIF (Fig. 10A) (AIF, however, was increased in the nuclear fraction, Fig. 10B). Importantly, the proteolytic cleavage of nuclear PARP-1 (ratio of 85 kDa fragment to 116 kDa PARP-1) was augmented in the same brain samples of cocaine addicts (Fig. 10A), including an increase in the cortical nuclear fraction (Fig. 10B). In chronic cocaine abusers (PFC/BA9), several signalling molecules associated with cocaine/dopamine and/or apoptotic pathways (Akt1, PEA-15, JNK1/2) were found unaltered, with the exception of DARPP-32 and anti-apoptotic t-DARPP whose contents were decreased.

These findings indicate that cocaine addiction in humans is not associated with abnormal upregulation of major components of the extrinsic and intrinsic apoptotic machineries in the

PFC/BA9. On the contrary, the downregulation of Fas–FADD receptor complex and cytochrome c could reflect the induction of contraregulatory adaptations or non-apoptotic (neuroplastic) actions induced by the repeated abuse of the psychostimulant. In any case, the enhanced degradation of nuclear PARP-1 (Fig. 10B), a hallmark of apoptosis, clearly indicates the possibility of aberrant cell death in brains of chronic cocaine addicts. The molecular mechanism appears to involve the induction of oxidative stress by cocaine metabolites (norcocaine and derivatives) and the activation of the mitochondrial death effector AIF after its translocation to the nucleus (Fig. 10B) (Álvaro-Bartolomé et al., 2011), where it interact with PARP-1 and induces chromatin condensation and large-scale DNA fragmentation (Strosznajder et al., 2010). This particular (caspase-independent) cell death subroutine, involving the nuclear interaction of AIF and PARP-1, has been named *parthanatos* and has a role in multiple pathophysiological conditions (Galluzzi et al., 2011), which could include the induction of neurotoxic effects in the brain of human cocaine addicts (see Fig. 3).

5. Role of FADD adaptor in the neurobiology of the cannabinoid system

Among the many effects induced by natural and synthetic cannabinoids (Pertwee, 1997), their beneficial or deleterious actions on neuronal survival remain a controversial topic (Guzmán et al., 2002; Álvaro-Bartolomé et al., 2010). Although cannabinoids can induce pro-apoptotic activity in several cellular models (Maccarrone and Finazzi-Agró, 2003), recent evidence also demonstrates that these compounds, acting through cannabinoid CB_1 (Aguado et al., 2007) or CB_2 receptors (Viscomi et al., 2009) can also protect neurons from death. It is conceivable therefore that the neuroprotection induced by some cannabinoids *in vivo* could be the result of a favorable balance between the relative activation of anti- and pro-apoptotic signalling pathways in the brain.

5.1 Regulation of basal Fas/FADD complex by cannabinoid receptors: Pro-apoptotic CB_1 receptor tone

CB_1 receptors are highly expressed in the CNS (Howlett et al., 2002) and display a high level of constitutive activity (Gifford and Ashby, 1996). This contrasts with brain CB_2 receptors, which pharmacological activation has been questioned in conscious rats (Chin et al., 2008) and, therefore, the presence of any receptor constitutive activity is uncertain. Similarly to δ-opioid receptors (see Fig. 4; García-Fuster et al., 2007b), the remarkable constitutive activity of CB_1 receptors was also postulated to be involved in the tonic control of pro-apoptotic Fas/FADD complex. This possibility was investigated using gene-targeted mice lacking CB_1 or CB_2 receptors (Álvaro-Bartolomé et al., 2010).

In brain regions of CB_1-KO mice (cerebral cortex, corpus striatum and cerebellum), the content of Fas receptor and/or FADD was reduced (Fig. 11A), suggesting that endocannabinoids acting on CB_1 receptors stimulate the expression of pro-apoptotic Fas/FADD complex. In these mice, non-apoptotic p-FADD and p-FADD/FADD ratio are increased (Fig. 11A), indicating that CB_1 receptors tonically inhibit the phosphorylation of brain FADD, which could also favour the induction of pro-apoptotic actions. In brain regions of CB_2-KO mice, in contrast, the changes of Fas receptor, FADD and p-FADD (somehow opposite to those observed in CB_1-KO mice) did not indicate that CB_2 receptors are involved in the tonic regulation of Fas/FADD complex. The alterations of Fas/FADD in brains of CB_1 and CB_2 receptors KO mice did not appear to result in an increased cell death because the pattern of cleavage of nuclear PARP-1 was very similar to that measured in WT mice (Álvaro-Bartolomé et al., 2010).

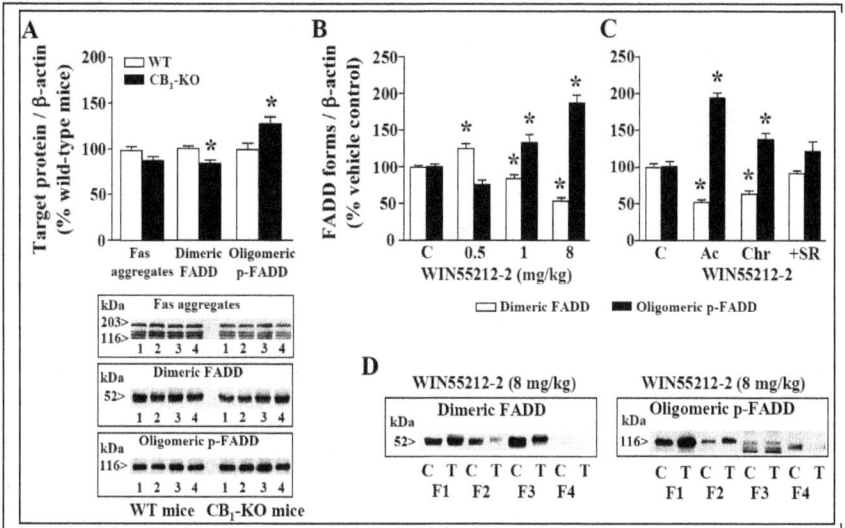

Fig. 11. (A) Fas receptor aggregates, FADD adaptor, and p-FADD in the cerebral cortex of WT mice and cannabinoid CB_1 receptor KO mice. (B) Acute (dose-response) effects of the CB_1 receptor agonist WIN55212-2 on the content of FADD and p-FADD in mouse brain cortex. (C) Acute (Ac, 8 mg/kg), chronic (Chr, 1-8 mg/kg, increasing doses for 5 days) and withdrawal effects (SR, 10 mg/kg; precipitated with the antagonist SR141716A or rimonabant) of WIN55212-2 on FADD and p-FADD content in mouse brain cortex. (D) Effects of WIN55212-2 (8 mg/kg) on the content of FADD and p-FADD at the subcellular level (F1: cytosol; F2: membranes; F3: nucleus; F4: cytoskeleton). *At least p<0.05 *versus* WT or control (C). (Modified from Álvaro-Bartolomé et al., 2010).

Therefore, CB_1 receptors appear to exert a tonic activation of Fas/FADD complex in brain (Fig. 11A) that is opposite to that induced by δ-opioid receptors (inhibitory tonic control; Fig. 4). Given the interactions between cannabinoids and opiates (Bushlin et al., 2010), and particularly between CB_1 receptors and δ-opioid receptors (Urigüen et al., 2005), the opposite tonic control of these inhibitory receptors on pro-apoptotic Fas/FADD complex could be of relevance in drug mechanisms leading to neuronal cell death or neuroprotection.

5.2 Acute, chronic and withdrawal effects of cannabinoid drugs on FADD and associated signalling in the brain

Acute treatment of mice with the CB_1 receptor agonist WIN55212-2 (0.5, 1 and 8 mg/kg) did not alter the content of Fas receptor forms in the cerebral cortex. However, a low dose of WIN55212-2 (0.5 mg/kg) increased FADD, whereas higher doses of the agonist (1 and 8 mg/kg) decreased FADD content in mouse brain cortex (Fig. 11B). WIN55212-2 also induced bell-shaped dose effects on p-FADD, but in the opposite direction (Fig. 11B). Pretreatment of mice with the antagonist rimonabant prevented the opposite effects of WIN55212-2 on FADD and p-FADD, indicating a CB_1 receptor-related mechanism. At the subcellular level, WIN55212-2 increased p-FADD in the cytosol and membranes, and to a lesser extent in the nucleus (Fig. 11D right). In contrast, WIN55212-2 decreased FADD in membranes and nucleus, and increased its content in cytosol (Fig. 11D left). WIN55212-2 also increased CK1α in cytosol, which was coincident with the marked enhancement of p-FADD in this compartment (Fig. 11D right). In marked contrast to the activation CB_1 receptors, high doses of the CB_2 receptor agonist JWH133 were not associated with significant changes of Fas receptor forms, FADD or p-FADD in mouse brain cortex (Álvaro-Bartolomé et al., 2010).

These data indicate that the activation of CB_1 receptors decreases (lower dose) or increases (higher doses) the ratio of cortical p-FADD/FADD (an index of non-apoptotic activity). Interestingly, and as observed for opiate drugs, acute WIN55212-2 treatment induced opposite changes on p-FADD and FADD (Fig. 6B), and this interconversion of FADD forms associated with the activation of CB_1 receptors could be important in the actions of cannabinoids in the brain. For example and consistent with the findings observed in the cerebral cortex of CB_1 receptor KO mice (Fig. 11A: decreased FADD and increased p-FADD), a low dose of WIN55212-2 (0.5 mg/kg) increased FADD and decreased p-FADD in mouse brain cortex (Fig. 11B). This opposite regulation of FADD forms is also consistent with the existence of a pro-apoptotic CB_1 receptor tone. However, the selective CB_1 receptor antagonist/inverse agonist rimonabant (10 mg/kg) did not alter FADD or p-FADD in brains of mice, suggesting that the receptor tonic control on this system is moderate (Álvaro-Bartolomé et al., 2010).

It is noteworthy that chronic WIN55212-2 administration (1-8 mg/kg for 5 days) also resulted in down-regulation of FADD and up-regulation of p-FADD in mouse brain cortex (Fig. 11C), which indicates a sustained attenuation of apoptotic signalling in spite of the induction of some tolerance (tachyphylaxis) upon the repeated stimulation of CB_1 receptors. Rimonabant-precipitated WIN55212-2 withdrawal did not cause a rebound of FADD or p-FADD over control values (Fig. 11C). Along this line, the acute and chronic treatments of mice with WIN55212-2, as well as rimonabant-precipitated withdrawal, did not alter the contents of mitochondrial cytochrome c, AIF, or the cleavage of nuclear PARP-1 in the cerebral cortex. These negative findings further discount the induction of cell death after the activation of CB_1 receptors in the mouse brain.

On the other hand, acute, but not chronic, treatment with WIN55212-2 markedly stimulated the activation of anti-apoptotic ERK1/2 and Akt1/PEA-15, as well as pro-apoptotic JNK1/2 and p38 MAPK in the mouse cerebral cortex. This suggests that the acute neuroprotection *in vivo* induced by some cannabinoids could be the result of a favorable balance between the relative activation of anti- and pro-apoptotic signalling pathways. In contrast to FADD and p-FADD, the lack of a sustained stimulation of anti- and pro-apoptotic cascades upon chronic WIN55212-2 treatment probably reflects the rapid induction of CB_1 receptor desensitization in the regulation of these systems (Álvaro-Bartolomé et al., 2010).

The current findings indicate that the chronic stimulation of CB_1 receptors is associated with a marked downregulation of brain FADD, a major pro-apoptotic molecule of the extrinsic cell death pathway. This may represent a relevant molecular mechanism to explain, in part, the neuroprotective effects induced by natural and synthetic cannabinoids (Guzmán et al., 2002). In addition, the chronic stimulation of CB_1 receptors is also associated with up-regulation of p-FADD, the protein form that mediates non-apoptotic actions including brain plasticity (see Fig. 3). The link between CB_1 receptors and the multifunctional FADD adaptor provides new insights into the complex neurobiology of the cannabinoid system.

6. General conclusions

The modulation of FADD adaptor by drugs of abuse is a new and relevant molecular process in the complex neurobiology of addictions. The regulation of FADD and associated signalling by opiate drugs (heroin/methadone) and the psychostimulant cocaine can lead to neurotoxicity and/or neuroplasticity in brains of human addicts. The ratio of p-Ser194 FADD (anti-apoptotic form) to FADD (pro-apoptotic form) appears to represent a novel marker of cortical plasticity.

In the prefrontal cortex of long-term opiate addicts, the observed down-regulation of FADD (i.e. attenuation of Fas signals), the up-regulation of $FLIP_L$ and Bcl-2 (greater anti-apoptotic effects), the increased Bcl-2/Bax ratio (positive balance for cell survival), the reduction of cytochrome c (lesser activation of other pro-apoptotic factors), the lack of abnormal caspase-3 activation, and the normal pattern of nuclear PARP-1 cleavage (Fig. 3) clearly indicate the absence of aberrant cell death. In contrast, p-FADD and p-FADD/FADD ratio are increased in brains of opiate addicts, which suggests the induction of neuroplastic actions. In fact, other studies in laboratory rats have shown that the behavioural response to morphine-induced psychomotor sensitization, as well as the severity of opiate abstinence syndrome (two well-known neuroplastic responses) correlated with increased p-FADD and reduced FADD in the brain, which further supports the role of p-FADD/FADD ratio as a marker of neuronal plasticity.

In the prefrontal cortex of long-term cocaine addicts, Fas/FADD receptor complex and mitochrondrial cytochrome c are down-regulated, suggesting contraregulatory adaptations or non-apoptotic actions (Fig. 3). Importantly, however, the degradation of nuclear PARP-1 is increased in the absence of caspase-3 activation. This type of caspase-independent cell death (named *parthanatos*) involves the induction of oxidative stress by cocaine metabolites (norcocaine and derivatives) and the nuclear translocation of the mitochondrial death effector AIF (Fig. 3). Therefore, cocaine addiction in humans appears to be associated with aberrant cell death in the brain. However, p-FADD/FADD ratio is also increased which also suggest the induction of neuroplastic changes in brains of cocaine addicts. In fact, other studies in laboratory rats have shown that p-FADD and FADD in the cortex represent a molecular correlate of the initial brain plasticity that might predispose to some facets of addictive-like behaviours such as locomotor response to novelty.

7. Acknowledgments

The studies performed in the Laboratory of Neuropharmacology, IUNICS, UIB, were funded by MICINN/MINECO/FEDER (SAF2004-03685, SAF2008-011311, SAF2011-29918),

Plan Nacional Sobre Drogas (2007I061) and RETICS/RTA (RD06/0001/0003) ISCIII-MICINN/MINECO/FEDER, Spain. MJGF is a 'Ramón y Cajal' Researcher (MICINN/MINECO-UIB). JAGS is a member of the Institut d'Estudis Catalans (Barcelona, Catalonia, Spain).

8. References

Aguado, T.; Romero, E.; Monory, K.; Palazuelos, J.; Sendtner, M.; Marsicano, G.; Lutz, B.; Guzmán, M. & Galve-Roperh, I. (2007) The CB1 cannabinoid receptor mediates excitotoxicity-induced neural progenitor proliferation and neurogenesis. *Journal of Biological Chemistry*, Vol.282, No.33, pp. 23892-23898.

Ahmed, S.H. & Koob, G.F. (1998) Transition from moderate to excessive drug intake: change in hedonic set point. *Science*, Vol.282, No.5387, pp. 298-300.

Alappat, E.C.; Feig, C.; Boyerinas, B.; Volkland, J.; Samuels, M.; Murmann, A.E.; Thorburn, A.; Kidd, V.J.; Slaughter, C.A.; Osborn, S.L.; Winoto, A.; Tang, W.J. & Peter, M.E. (2005) Phosphorylation of FADD at serine 194 by CKIα regulates its nonapoptotic activities. *Molecular Cell*, Vol.19, No.3, pp. 321-332.

Algeciras-Schimnich, A.; Shen, L.; Barnhart, B.C.; Murmann, A.E.; Burkhardt, J.K. & Peter, M.E. (2002) Molecular ordering of the initial signaling events of CD95. *Molecular and Cellular Biology*, Vol.22, No.1, pp. 207-220.

Álvaro-Bartolomé, M.; Esteban, S.; García-Gutiérrez, M.S.; Manzanares, J.; Valverde, O. & García-Sevilla, J.A. (2010) Regulation of Fas receptor/Fas-associated protein with death domain apoptotic complex and associated signaling systems by cannabinoid receptors in the mouse brain. *British Journal of Pharmacology*, Vol.160, No.3, pp. 643-656.

Álvaro-Bartolomé, M.; La Harpe, R.; Callado, L.F.; Meana, J.J. & García-Sevilla, J.A. (2011). Molecular adaptations of apoptotic pathways and signaling partners in the cerebral cortex of human cocaine addicts and cocaine-treated rats. *Neuroscience*, Vol.196, No.1, pp.1-15.

Badiani, A.; Belin, D.; Epstein, D.; Calu, D. & Shaham, Y. (2011) Opiate versus psychostimulant addiction: the differences do matter. *Nature Reviews Neuroscience*, Vol.12, No.11, pp. 685-700.

Belin, D.; Mar, A.C.; Dalley, J.W.; Robbins, T.W. & Everitt, B.J. (2008) High impulsivity predicts the switch to compulsive cocaine taking. *Science*, Vol.320, No.5881, pp. 1352-1355.

Belin, D. & Everitt, N.J. (2010) Drug Addiction: The neural and psychological basis of a compulsive incentive habit. In Handbook of Basal Ganglia Structure and Function (Eds. H. Steiner & K. Tseng). New York, Academic Press. Chapter 33, pp. 571-592.

Bi, F.F.; Xiao, B.; Hu, Y.Q.; Tian, F.F.; Wu, Z.G.; Ding, L. & Zhou X.F. (2008) Expression and localization of Fas-associated proteins following focal cerebral ischemia in rats. *Brain Research*, Vol.1191, pp. 30-38.

Boronat, M.A.; García-Fuster, M.J. & García-Sevilla, J.A. (2001) Chronic morphine induces up-regulation of the pro-apoptotic Fas receptor and down-regulation of the anti-apoptotic Bcl-2 oncoprotein in rat brain. *British Journal of Pharmacology*, Vol.134, No.6, pp. 1263-1270.

Briand, L.A.; Flagel, S.B.; García-Fuster, M.J.; Watson, S. J.; Akil, H.; Sarter, M.; Robinson, T.E. (2008) Persistent alterations in cognitive function and prefrontal dopamine D2 receptors following extended, but not limited, access to self-administered cocaine. *Neuropsychopharmacology*, Vol.33, No.12, pp. 2969-2980.

Bushlin, I.; Rozenfeld, R.; Devi, L.A. (2010) Cannabinoid-opioid interactions during neuropathic pain and analgesia. *Current Opinion in Pharmacology*, Vol.10, No.8, pp. 80-86.

Büttner, A. (2011) Review: The neuropathology of drug abuse. *Neuropathology and Applied Neurobiology*, Vol.37, No.2, pp. 118-134.

Chin, C.L.; Tovcimak, A.E.; Hradil, V.P.; Seifert, T.R.; Hollingsworth, P.R.; Chandran, P. et al. (2008) Differential effects of cannabinoid receptor agonists on regional brain activity using pharmacological MRI. *British Journal of Pharmacology*, Vol.153, No.2, pp. 367-379.

Costa, T. & Herz, A. (1989) Antagonists with negative intrinsic activity at delta opioid receptors coupled to GTP-binding proteins. *Proceedings of the National Academy of Sciences of the United States of America*, Vol.86, No.19, pp. 7321-7325.

Cunha-Oliveira, T.; Rego A.C. & Oliveira, C.R. (2008) Cellular and molecular mechanisms involved in the neurotoxicity of opioid and psychostimulant drugs. *Brain Research Reviews*, Vol.58, No.1, pp.192-208.

Davis, B.A.; Clinton, S.M.; Akil, H.; Becker, J.B. (2008) The effects of novelty-seeking phenotypes and sex differences on acquisition of cocaine self-administration in selectively bred high-responder and low-responder rats. *Pharmacology, Biochemistry and Behavior*, Vol.90, No.3, pp. 331-338.

Dietrich, J.B.; Mangeol, A.; Revel, M.O.; Burgun, C.; Aunis, D. & Zwiller, J. (2005) Acute or repeated cocaine administration generates reactive oxygen species and induces antioxidant enzyme activity in dopaminergic rat brain structures. *Neuropharmacology*, Vol.48, No.7, pp. 965-974.

El-Rifai, W.; Smith, M.F. Jr.; Li, G.; Beckler, A.; Carl, V.S.; Montgomery, E.; Knuutila, S.; Moskaluk, C.A.; Frierson, H.F. Jr.; Powell, S.M. (2002) Gastric cancers overexpress DARPP-32 and a novel isoform, t-DARPP. *Cancer Research*, Vol.62, No.14, pp. 4061-4064.

Ferrer-Alcón, M.; García-Fuster, M.J.; La Harpe, R. & García-Sevilla, J.A. (2004) Long-term regulation of signalling components of adenylyl cyclase and mitogen-activated protein kinase in the pre-frontal cortex of human opiate addicts. *Journal of Neurochemistry*, Vol.90, No.1, pp. 220-230.

Föger, N.; Bulfone-Paus S.; Chan, A.C. & Lee, K.H. (2009) Subcellular compartmentalization of FADD as a new level of regulation in death receptor signaling. *The FEBS Journal*, Vol.276, No.15, pp. 4256-4265.

Galluzzi, L.; Vitali, I.; Abrams, J.M.; Alnemri, E.S.; Baehrecke, E.H.; Blagosklonny, M.V.; et al. (2011) Molecular definitions of cell death subroutines: recommendations of the Nomenclature Committee on Cell Death 2012. *Cell Death & Differentiation*, in press. doi: 10.1038/cdd.2011.96.

García-Fuster, M.J.; Ferrer-Alcón, M.; Miralles, A. & García-Sevilla, J.A. (2003) Modulation of Fas receptor proteins and dynamin during opiate addiction and induction of opiate withdrawal in rat brain. *Naunyn-Schmiedeberg's Archives of Pharmacology*, Vol.368, No.5, pp. 421-431.

García-Fuster, M.J.; Ferrer-Alcón, M.; Miralles, A. & García-Sevilla, J.A. (2004) Deglycosylation of Fas receptor and chronic morphine treatment up-regulate high molecular mass Fas aggregates in the rat brain. *European Journal of Pharmacology*, Vol.496, No.1-3, pp. 63-69.

García-Fuster, M.J.; Watson, S.J. & Akil, H. (2006). Effect of cocaine on Fas-Associated protein with Death Domain (FADD) in the rat brain. *Society for Neuroscience Annual Meeting*. Poster 294.19. Atlanta, USA.

García-Fuster, M.J.; Miralles, A. & García-Sevilla, J.A. (2007a) Effects of opiate drugs on Fas-associated protein with death domain (FADD) and effector caspases in the rat brain: Regulation by the ERK1/2 MAP kinase pathway. *Neuropsychopharmacology*, Vol.32, No.2, pp. 399-411.

García-Fuster, M.J.; Ferrer-Alcón, M.; Martín, M.; Kieffer, B.L.; Maldonado, R. & García-Sevilla, J.A. (2007b) Effects of constitutive deletion of opioid receptors on the basal densities of Fas and Fas-associated protein with death domain (FADD) in the mouse brain: A δ-opioid tone inhibits FADD. *European Neuropsychopharmacology*, Vol.17, No.5, pp. 366-374.

García-Fuster, M.J.; Ramos-Miguel, A.; Miralles, A. & García-Sevilla, J.A. (2008a) Opioid receptor agonists enhance the phosphorylation state of Fas-associated death domain (FADD) protein in the rat brain: Functional interactions with casein kinase Iα, Gαi proteins, and ERK1/2 signaling. *Neuropharmacology*, Vol.55, No.5, pp. 886-99.

García-Fuster, M.J.; Ramos-Miguel, A.; Rivero, G.; La Harpe, R.; Meana, J.J. & García-Sevilla, J.A. (2008b) Regulation of the extrinsic and intrinsic apoptotic pathways in the prefrontal cortex of short- and long-term human opiate abusers. *Neuroscience*, Vol.157, No.1, pp. 105-119.

García-Fuster, M.J.; Clinton, S.M.; Watson, S.J. & Akil, H. (2009) Effect of cocaine on Fas-associated protein with death domain in the rat brain: Individual differences in a model of differential vulnerability to drug abuse. *Neuropsychopharmacology*, Vol.34, No.5, pp. 1123-1134.

García-Fuster, M.J.; Perez, J.A.; Clinton, S.M.; Watson, S.J. & Akil, H. (2010) Impact of cocaine on adult hippocampal neurogenesis in an animal model of differential propensity to drug abuse. *European Journal of Neuroscience*, Vol.31, No.1, pp. 79-89.

García-Fuster, M.J.; Flagel, S.B.; Mahmood, S.T.; Mayo, L.M.; Thompson, R.C.; Watson, S.J. & Akil, H. (2011). Decreased proliferation of adult hippocampal stem cells during cocaine withdrawal: Possible role of the cell fate regulator FADD. *Neuropsychopharmacology*, Vol.36, No.11, pp. 2303-2317.

Gifford, A.N. & Ashby, C.R. Jr. (1996) Electrically evoked acetylcholine release from hippocampal slices is inhibited by the cannabinoid receptor agonist, WIN 55212-2, and is potentiated by the cannabinoid antagonist, SR 141716A. *Journal of Pharmacology and Experimental Therapeutics*, Vol.277, No.3, pp. 431-436.

Gilman, C.P. & Mattson, M.P. (2002) Do apoptotic mechanisms regulate synaptic plasticity and growth-cone motility? *Neuromolecular Medicine*, Vol.2, No.2, pp. 197-214.

Goldstein, R.Z. & Volkow, N.D. (2011) Dysfunction of the prefrontal cortex in addiction: neuroimaging findings and clinical implications. *Nature Reviews Neuroscience*, Vol.12, No.11, pp. 652-669.

Gómez-Angelats, M. & Cidlowski, J.A. (2003) Molecular evidence for the nuclear localization of FADD. *Cell Death & Differentiation*, Vol.10, No.7, pp. 91-97.

Govitrapong, P.; Suttitum, T.; Kotchabhakdi, N. & Uneklabh, T. (1998) Alterations of immune functions in heroin addicts and heroin withdrawal subjects. *Journal of Pharmacology and Experimental Therapeutics*, Vol.286, No.2, pp. 883-889.

Guzmán, M.; Sánchez, C. & Galve-Roperh, I. (2002) Cannabinoids and cell fate. *Pharmacology and Therapeutics*, Vol.95, No.2, pp. 175-184.

Hartmann, A.; Mouatt-Prigent, A.; Faucheux, B.A.; Agid, Y. & Hirsch, E.C. (2002) FADD: A link between TNF family receptors and caspases in Parkinson's disease. *Neurology*, Vol.58, No.2, pp. 308-310.

Howlett, A.C.; Barth, F.; Bonner, T.I.; Cabral, G.; Casellas, P; Devane, W.A.; Felder, C.C.; Herkenham, M.; Mackie, K.; Martin, B.R.; Mechoulam, R. & Pertwee, R.G. (2002) International Union of Pharmacology. XXVII. Classification of cannabinoid receptors. *Pharmacological Reviews*, Vol.54, No.2, pp. 161-202.

Imtiyaz, H.Z.; Zhou, X.; Zhang, H.; Chen, D.; Hu, T. & Zhang, J. (2009) The death domain of FADD is essential for embryogenesis, lymphocyte development, and proliferation. *Journal of Biological Chemistry*, Vol.284, No.15, pp. 9917-9926.

Kreek, M.J. (1990) Immune function in heroin addicts and former heroin addicts in treatment: pre- and post-AIDS epidemic. *NIDA Research Monographs*, Vol. 96, pp.192-219.

Lambert, C.; Landau, A.M. & Desbarats, J. (2003) Fas-beyond death: a regenerative role for Fas in the nervous system. *Apoptosis*, Vol.8, No.6, pp. 551-562.

Liao, D.; Lin, H.; Law, P.Y. & Loh, H.H. (2005) Mu-opioid receptors modulate the stability of dendritic spines. *Proceedings of the National Academy of Sciences of the United States of America*, Vol.102, No.5, pp. 1725-1730.

Maccarrone, M. & Finazzi-Agró, A. (2003) The endocannabinoid system, anandamide and the regulation of mammalian cell apoptosis. *Cell Death & Differentiation*, Vol.10, No.9, pp. 946-955.

Narita, M.; Kuzumaki, N.; Miyatake, M.; Sato, F.; Wachi, H.; Seyama, Y. & Suzuki, T. (2006) Role of δ-opioid receptor function in neurogenesis and neuroprotection. *Journal of Neurochemistry*, Vol.97, No.5, pp. 1494-1505.

Neilan, C.L.; Akil, H.; Woods, J.H. & Traynor, J.R. (1999) Constitutive activity of the δ-opioid receptor expressed in C6 glioma cells: identification of non-peptide δ-inverse agonists. *British Journal of Pharmacology*, Vol.128, No.3, pp. 556-562.

Noonan, M.A.; Bulin, S.E.; Fuller, D.C. & Eisch, A.J. (2010) Reduction of adult hippocampal neurogenesis confers vulnerability in an animal model of cocaine addiction. *Journal of Neuroscience*, Vol.30, No.1, pp. 304-315.

Novikova, S.I.; He, F.; Bai, J.; Badan, I.; Lidow, I.A. & Lidow, M.S. (2005) Cocaine-induced changes in the expression of apoptosis-related genes in the fetal mouse cerebral wall. *Neurotoxicology & Teratology*, Vol.27, No.1, pp. 3-14.

Nutt, D.; King, L.A.; Saulsbury, W.; Blakemore, G. (2007) Development of a rational scale to assess the harm of drugs of potential misuse. *Lancet*, Vol. 369, No.9566, pp. 1047-1053.

Park, S.M.; Schickel, R. & Peter, M.E. (2005) Nonapoptotic functions of FADD-binding death receptors and their signaling molecules. *Current Opinion in Cell Biology*, Vol.17, No.6, pp. 610-616.

Pertwee, R.G. (1997) Pharmacology of cannabinoid CB_1 and CB_2 receptors. *Pharmacology & Therapeutics*, Vol.74, No.2, pp. 129-180.

Ramos-Miguel A.; García-Fuster, M.J.; Callado, L.F.; La Harpe, R.; Meana, J.J. & García-Sevilla, J.A. (2009) Phosphorylation of FADD (Fas-associated death domain protein) at serine 194 is increased in the prefrontal cortex of opiate abusers: Relation to mitogen activated protein kinase, phosphoprotein enriched in astrocytes of 15 kDa, and Akt signaling pathways involved in neuroplasticity. *Neuroscience*, Vol.161, No.1, pp. 23-38.

Ramos-Miguel, A.; Esteban, S. & García-Sevilla, J.A. (2010) The time course of unconditioned morphine-induced psychomotor sensitization mirrors the phosphorylation of FADD and MEK/ERK in rat striatum: Role of PEA-15 as a FADD-ERK binding partner in striatal plasticity. *European Neuropsychopharmacology*, Vol.20, No.1, pp. 49-64.

Ramos-Miguel, A.; Miralles, A. & García-Sevilla, J.A. (2011) Correlation of rat cortical Fas-associated death domain (FADD) protein phosphorylation with the severity of spontaneous morphine abstinence syndrome: Role of α_2-adrenoceptors and extracellular signal-regulated kinases. *Journal of Psychopharmacology*, Vol.25, No.12, pp. 1691-1702.

Reich, A.; Spering, C. & Schulz, J.B. (2008) Death receptor Fas (CD95) signaling in the central nervous system: tuning neuroplasticity? *Trends in Neuroscience*, Vol.31, No.9, pp. 478-486.

Sandu, C.; Morisawa, G.; Wegorzewska, I.; Huang, T.; Arechiga, A.F.; Hill, J.M.; Kim, T.; Walsh, C.M. & Werner, M.H. (2006) FADD self-association is required for stable interaction with an activated death receptor. *Cell Death & Differentiation*, Vol.13, No.12, pp. 2052-2061.

Sastry, P.S. & Rao, K.S. (2000) Apoptosis and the nervous system. *Journal of Neurochemistry*, Vol.74, No.1, pp. 1-20.

Scott, F.L.; Stec, B.; Pop, C.; Dobaczewska, M.K.; Lee, J.J.; Monosov, E.; Robinson, H.; Salvesen, G.S.; Schwarzenbacher, R. & Riedl, S.J. (2009) The Fas-FADD death domain complex structure unravels signalling by receptor clustering. *Nature*, Vol.457, No.7232, pp. 1019-1022.

Screaton, R.A.; Kiessling, S.; Sansom, O.J.; Millar, C.B.; Maddison, K.; Bird, A.; Clarke, A.R. & Frisch, S.M. (2003) Fas-associated death domain protein interacts with methyl-CpG binding domain protein 4: a potential link between genome surveillance and apoptosis. *Proceedings of the National Academy of Sciences of the United States of America*, Vol.100, No.9, pp. 5211-5216.

Sharma, K.; Wang, R.X.; Zhang, L.Y.; Yin, D.L.; Luo, X.Y.; Solomon, J.C.; Jiang, R.F.; Markos, K.; Davidson, W.; Scott, D.W. & Shi, Y.F. (2000) Death the Fas way: regulation and pathophysiology of CD95 and its ligand. *Pharmacology & Therapeutics*, Vol.88, No.3, pp. 333-347.

Stead, J.D.; Clinton, S.; Neal, C.; Schneider, J.; Jama, A.; Miller, S.; Vazquez, D.M.; Watson, S.J. & Akil, H. (2006) Selective breeding for divergence in novelty-seeking traits: heritability and enrichment in spontaneous anxiety-related behaviors. *Behavior Genetics*, Vol.36, No.5, pp. 697-712.

Strosznajder, R.P.; Czubowicz, K.; Jesko, H. & Strosznajder, J.B. (2010) Poly(ADP-ribose) metabolism in brain and its role in ischemia pathology. *Molecular Neurobiology*, Vol.41, No.2-3, pp. 187-196.

Tegeder, I. & Geisslinger, G. (2004) Opioids as modulators of cell death and survival--unraveling mechanisms and revealing new indications. *Pharmacological Reviews*, Vol.56, No.3, pp. 351-369.

Tewari, R.; Sharma, V.; Koul, N. & Sen, E. (2008) Involvement of miltefosine-mediated ERK activation in glioma cell apoptosis through Fas regulation. *Journal of Neurochemistry*, Vol.107, No.3, pp. 616-627.

Tourneur, L. & Chiocchia, G. (2010) FADD: a regulator of life and death. *Trends in Immunology*, Vol.31, No.7, pp. 260-269.

Tramullas, M.; Martínez-Cué, C. & Hurlé, M.A. (2008) Chronic administration of heroin to mice produces up-regulation of brain apoptosis-related proteins and impairs spatial learning and memory. *Neuropharmacology*, Vol.54, No.4, pp. 640-652.

Urigüen, L.; Berrendero, F.; Ledent, C.; Maldonado, R. & Manzanares, J. (2005) Kappa- and delta-opioid receptor functional activities are increased in the caudate putamen of cannabinoid CB1 receptor knockout mice. *European Journal of Neuroscience*, Vol.22, No.8, pp.2106-1210.

Viscomi, M.T.; Oddi, S.; Latini, L.; Pasquariello, N.; Florenzano, F.; Bernardi, G.; Molinari, M. & Maccarrone, M. (2009) Selective CB2 receptor agonism protects central neurons from remote axotomy-induced apoptosis through the PI3K/Akt pathway. *Journal of Neuroscience*, Vol.29, No.14, pp. 4564-4570.

Wang, L.; Yang, J.K.; Kabaleeswaran, V.; Rice, A.J.; Cruz, A.C.; Park, A.Y.; Yin, Q.; Damko, E.; Jang, S.B.; Raunser, S.; Robinson, C.V.; Siegel, R.M.; Walz, T. & Wu, H. (2010) The Fas-FADD death domain complex structure reveals the basis of DISC assembly and disease mutations. *Nature Structural & Molecular Biology*, Vol.17, No.11, pp. 1324-1329.

Xiao, Y.; He, J.H.; Gilbert, R.D. & Zhang, L. (2000). Cocaine induces apoptosis in fetal myocardial cells through a mitochondria-dependent pathway. *Journal of Pharmacology and Experimental Therapeutics*, Vol.292, No.1, pp. 8-14.

Yin, D.; Mufson, R.A.; Wang, R. & Shi Y. (1999). Fas-mediated cell death promoted by opioids. *Nature*, Vol.397, No.6716, p. 218.

Yücel, M.; Lubman, D.I.; Harrison, B.J.; Fornito, A.; Allen, N.B.; Wellard, R.M.; Roffel, K.; Clarke, K.; Wood, S.J.; Forman, S.D. & Pantelis, C. (2007) A combined spectroscopic and functional MRI investigation of the dorsal anterior cingulate region in opiate addiction. *Molecular Psychiatry*, Vol.12, No.7, pp. 691-702.

Zhang, J.; Zhang, D. & Hua, Z. (2004) FADD and its phosphorylation. *IUBMB Life*, Vol.56, No.7, pp. 395-401.

Zhang, Y.; Chen, Q. & Yu, L.C. (2008) Morphine: a protective or destructive role in neurons? *Neuroscientist*, Vol.14, No.6, pp. 561-570.

9

Role of Prefrontal Cortex Dopamine and Noradrenaline Circuitry in Addiction

Ezio Carboni*, Roberto Cadeddu and Anna Rosa Carta

Dept. of Biomedical Sciences,
University of Cagliari, Cagliari,
Italy

1. Introduction

Understanding the mechanisms of drug dependence has been the goal of a large number of neuroscientists, pharmacologists and clinicians who carried out research with the hope of individuating and proposing an efficacious therapy for this disorder (Sofuoglu, 2010; Kalivas and Volkow, 2011). Unfortunately, although huge efforts, drug dependence is still a relevant health, social and economical problem (Popova et al., 2012; Hiscock et al., 2011; Shorter and Kosten, 2011). Treatments for drug abuse are for the most part ineffective because the molecular and cellular mechanisms through which drugs of abuse alter neuronal circuitry are still unexplained and above all, because drugs of abuse determine a global alteration of cerebral functions that govern behaviour through decision formation, making therefore unfocused the identification of a pharmacological target (Volkow et al., 2011; Schultz 2011). One of the first strategies pursued in drug dependence therapy was directed to removal of pleasure associated with drug taking, but the compliance with the treatment has been always limited, although it could improve when it was supported by psychology based motivational therapy as in alcohol dependence (Krampe and Ehrenreich, 2010; Simkin and Grenoble, 2010). On the other hand it is not infrequent that heavy smokers or heavy drinkers stop suddenly dependence just because their will overcome year-long habits. Decision making is a process based on the interaction between prefrontal cortex (PFC) and subcortical regions involved in reward and motivation, therefore it is likely that failure in self-regulatory behavior, that is common in addicted subjects, could be dependent upon the alteration of interactions between the prefrontal cortex and subcortical regions (Heatherton and Wagner, 2011). In this chapter we will review the role of PFC in addiction with particular attention to dopamine and norepinephrine transmission.

2. Brief overview on the prefrontal cortex

The PFC has a prominent role in governing behavior. This function is achieved through a complex interaction of many different areas within the PFC which cooperate with subcortical areas integrating cognitive and executive functions to produce the "optimal choice". The result of this interaction can be also a deleterious one, as observed in drug

---

* Corresponding Author

addicted subjects. This interaction has been elegantly discussed by Kennerley and Walton (2011) by comparing the functional correspondence between neurophysiological and neuropsychological studies to help define the roles of different PFC areas in supporting optimal decision making. The following brief overview on PFC is not intended to be exhaustive, as far as regards discussion of cognitive and executive functions of sub areas of PFC, but it will address specific features of PFC areas in which catecholamine transmission plays relevant role in drug addiction.

Dopamine transmission in PFC is directly involved in cognitive processes (Seamans and Yang, 2004), in the regulation of emotions (Sullivan, 2004), in working memory (Khan and Muly 2011), as well as in executive functions such as motor planning, inhibitory response control and sustained attention (Fibiger and Phillips, 1988; Granon et al., 2000; Robbins, 2002). The association of PFC functions with impulse control is supported by the evidence that damage to the ventromedial PFC causes persistent motivational impulsivity associated with affective instability, reduced capability for decision making, poor executive planning and general apathy towards social life (Damasio et al., 1994). In general damage of PFC function in humans can therefore affect one or more of the above functions producing personal and social difficulties as observed in disorders such as Alzheimer's disease (Melrose et al., 2011), schizophrenia (Arnsten, 2011), and Parkinson's disease (Luft and Schwarz, 2009). Loss of PFC function can be also generated by traumas (Bechara and Van Der Linden, 2005), or can result from drug addiction (Koob and Volkow, 2010; Van den Oever et al., 2010). Moreover, PFC functional or anatomical abnormalities are frequently found in individuals with drug abuse disorders (Liu et al., 1998a and 1998b; Franklin et al., 2002) and at the same time PFC is thought to have an important role in the onset and in the progression of psychiatric disorders associated with poor decision making such as schizophrenia (Arnsten, 2004), attention deficit/hyperactivity disorder (ADHD) (Sullivan and Brake, 2003) and depression (Davidson et al., 2002). Also, clinical studies report that when traumatic brain injury damages the PFC it often facilitate the emergence of drug use disorders (Ommaya et al., 1996, Delmonico et al., 1998).

The knowledge on PFC functions in mammals has been accumulated through research on different species but anatomy differences between primates and rodents is object of discussion when comparing experimental evidence on PFC function. In particular the dorsolateral PFC of mammals is thought to be involved in working memory, in attention processes, in reasoning-based decision making and in the timing of behavioural organization (Curtis and Lee, 2010; Arnsten, 2011). The prominent role of PFC catecholamine transmission in motivation is also supported by its anatomical and functional connection with other important areas of the brain, such as the nucleus accumbens (NAcc) (Di Chiara et al., 2011), and the ventral tegmental area (Omelchenko and Sesack, 2007) (Fig. 1). Chambers et al. (2003) provided an interesting definition for the role of the PFC: - It plays a determining role in the representation, execution and inhibition of motivational drives by influencing patterns of neural ensemble firing in the NAcc and poor PFC function could increase the probability of performing inappropriate motivated drives viewed clinically as impulsive. This view may acquire increasing relevance by integrating it in a scenario in which neural transmission in the NAcc is considered a common molecular pathway for addiction (Nestler, 2005; Di Chiara et al., 2004). Furthermore, one of the primary outputs of the accumbens is the gabaergic innervation (Fig. 2) directed to the ventral pallidum that in turn innervate the mediodorsal thalamic nucleus by GABA neurons. Mediodorsal thalamus in turn sends and excitatory output to the prelimbic and infralimbic PFC (O'Donnel et al., 1997). The PFC in primates receives the projection from the medio-dorsal nucleus of the thalamus that innervates the dorsolateral, medial and orbital cortices (Vertes, 2006) but in general, the thalamic innervation of PFC is a part of a loop which includes cortical thalamic glutamatergic excitatory projection that has a role in working memory (Watanabe and Funahashi, 2012) and is involved in the reward circuit (Haber and Knutoson, 2010).

Recent reviews suggest that the medial PFC in rat is functionally equivalent to the medial PFC of primates (Brown and Bowman 2002; Wilson et al. 2010). It has also been suggested that the rat PFC is not differentiated and therefore can subserve cognitive function localized in the dorsolateral PFC of primates as discussed elegantly by Brown and Bowman, (2002). These authors recognised that behavioural deficits following PFC damage in rats could reflect impaired behavioural flexibility similar to that reported in primates (De Bruin et al., 1994; Joel et al., 2005) and although the ability of shifting attention from one complex stimulus to another can be characterized by different abstraction level among different species, mammals could share executive processing mechanisms [selective attention, working memory, updating (manipulating the contents of working memory)] and rerouting attention (Shimamura, 2000; Brown and Bowman 2002). Due to the complexity of reciprocal neurotransmitter relationship in PFC, this chapter will mainly consider the role of dopamine and norepinephine in the PFC and their relationship with the effects of drugs of abuse and therapy of addiction. This choice is based on the important role of dopaminergic transmission in the effects of drugs of abuse and on the modulation of cognitive control (van Schouwenburg et al., 2010).

3. Dopamine in the prefrontal cortex: innervation, receptors and functions

The PFC receives multiple ascending innervations (Fig. 1 and Fig. 2). Whereas Acetylcholine (Ach) and serotonin (5-HT), contact widely all the subregions of PFC, dopamine innervations are more localized (e.g., prelimbic and infralimbic cortex) although they have a discrete grade of overlapping with norepinephrine innervation (Del Campo et al., 2011). The PFC is reciprocally connected with the VTA by dopaminergic afferents and glutamatergic efferents. Dopaminergic innervation of the PFC is predominantly provided by VTA dopamine cells sublocated in the parabrachialis pigmentosus nucleus which projects to cortical deep layers that contain the highest density of dopamine D1 and D2 receptors (Oades and Halliday, 1987). The main target of these innervations are the dendritic spines of pyramidal cells that project to GABA neurons of the NAcc which in turn complete a circuit by projecting back to VTA cells (Omelchenko and Sesack, 2007). A small population of PFC neurons that project to the VTA form synaptic contact with dopamine neurons that project onto the PFC, and a second population synapse onto GABA neurons that project to the nucleus accumbens, however no synaptic contact was found between PFC neurons and dopamine neurons that project to the NAcc (Carr and Sesack, 2000b). Lastly, to emphasize the complexity of the circuits in which the PFC is involved, it is important to underline that the majority of PFC terminals within the VTA area appear to target dopamine and GABA neurons that project onto target sites different from PFC and NAcc (Carr and Sesack, 2000a). Among them, some innervate ventral pallidum (Papp et al., 2012) and others, such as the putative gabaergic cells of the rostral linear nucleus that innervate the mediodorsal thalamic nucleus may have relevance in reward mechanism (Del Fava et al., 2007). Efferent projections from VTA to hippocampus influence spatial working memory performance (Martig and Mizumori, 2011). Dopamine innervation of PFC is functionally inhibitory either by direct action on pyramidal cells or via GABA interneurons (Grobin, and Deutch, 1998) reducing glutamatergic excitatory output to NAcc and VTA. Therefore, an increase in dopamine stimulation of PFC conversely attenuates dopamine activity in striatal and limibic terminal regions (Karreman and Moghaddam, 1996) and attenuates the motor stimulatory effects of systemically administered stimulants such as amphetamine and cocaine (Karler et al., 1998).

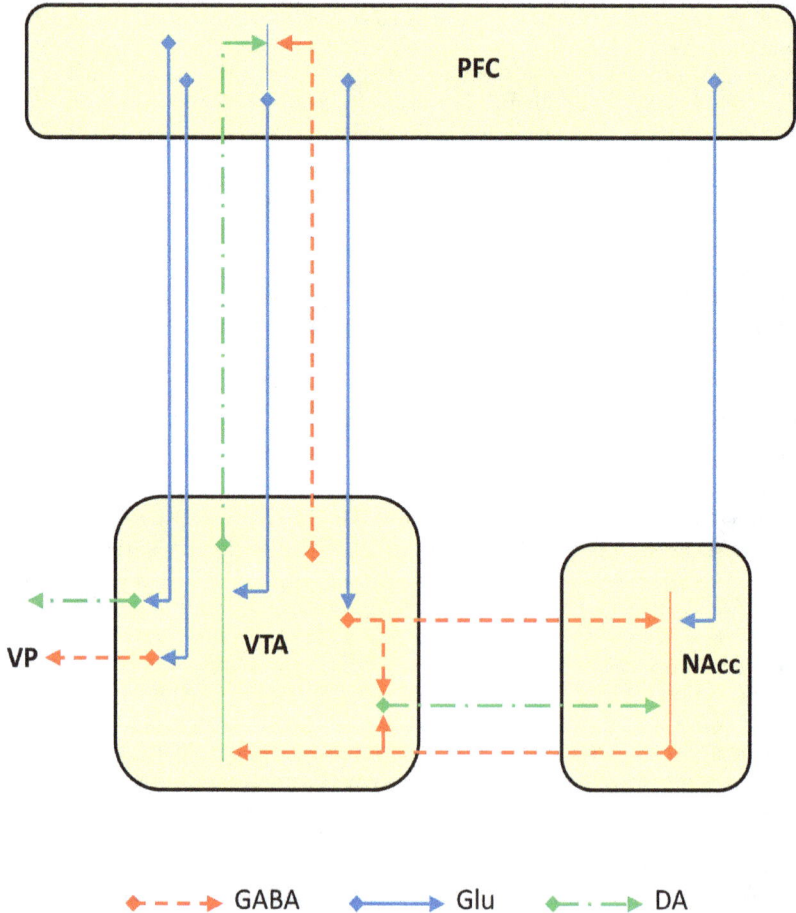

Fig. 1. Schematic representation of few major sites of interaction between prefrontal cortex (PFC) glutamate neurons, ventral tegmental area (VTA) dopamine and GABA neurons, and nucleus accumbens (NAcc) GABA neurons. Dendrites are occasionally represented for drawing clarity.

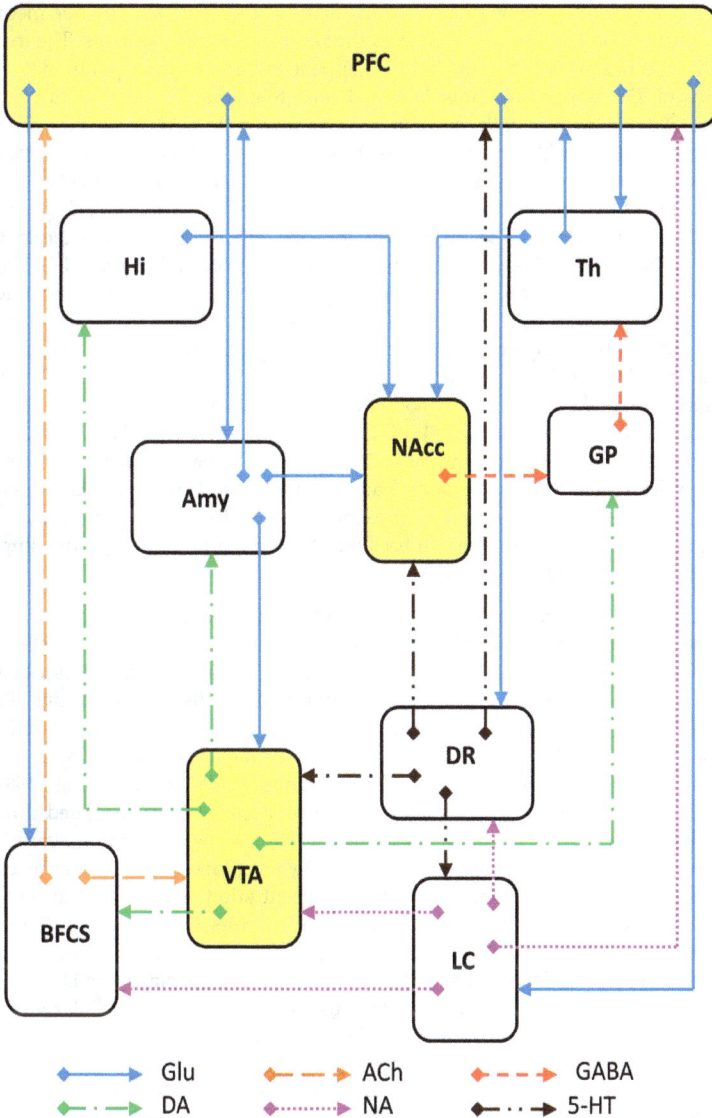

Fig. 2. Schematic representation of several major sites of interaction between prefrontal cortex (PFC) and thalamus (Th), hippocampus (Hi), amygdala (Amy), ventral tegmental area (VTA), dorsal raphe (DR), basal forebrain cholinergic system (BFCS), locus coeruleus (LC) globus pallidus (GP). Glutamate (Glu), Dopamine (DA), GABA, Acetylcholine (Ach), Norepinephrine (NA), and Serotonin (5-HT) neurons and axons are represented. The detailed connection represented in Fig. 1 have been omitted for drawing clarity.

Dopamine is a model of slow synaptic transmission; therefore it does not mediate fast synaptic transmission but instead modulates the response of other systems. The majority of D1 and D2 type receptors in the medial PFC appear to be located on pyramidal cells with the density of D2, apparently considerably lower than that of D1 (see the review by Tzschentke, 2001). Although both receptors are also present in GABAergic interneurons, the D4 subtype in particular (Ariano et al., 1997; Defagot et al., 1997a and 1997b) appears to be located on GABAergic interneurons rather than on pyramidal cells (Mrzljak et al., 1996). It is interesting to note that in the same postsynaptic pyramidal cell of the mPFC, dopaminergic terminals are localized in close opposition to each other with glutamatergic terminal originating in both the mediodorsal thalamus and the controlateral medial PFC. The former is not affected by VTA activation which instead inhibits the excitation of pyramidal cells generated by the input from recurrent collaterals of efferent glutamatergic output (Tzschentke, 2001). By acting on D1 receptors and through cAMP for the activation of cAMP sensitive protein kinase, dopamine determines an increase in the phosphorylation of DARP-32 and an inhibition of phosphatase 1 modulating mechanisms that involve ion channel and transcription factors (Greengard, 2001). D1 receptor optimal stimulation is essential to working memory process (Williams and Goldman-Rakic, 1995) and therefore either an increase or a decrease of the transmission leads to an inverted U response (Desimone, 1995). The involvement of dopamine activity through D1 receptor in cognitive function has a strong impact in schizophrenia research because of the importance of cognitive impairment in this disorder (Barch and Ceaser, 2012).

Although the result of dopamine interaction on pyramidal cells is complex and is influenced by a number of factors (e.g. dopamine concentration, receptor interaction, direct or indirect effect, depolarization status of the cells), dopamine generally, as also described in the previous paragraph, inhibits the activity of pyramidal cells in the medial PFC (see Tzschentke, 2001 for a review). The direct dopamine action on pyramidal cells (Geijo-Barrietos and Pastore, 1995; Gulledge and Jaffe, 1998) or the indirect action by a stimulation of the GABA interneurons may in turn inhibit pyramidal cells (Mercuri et al., 1985; Penit-Soria et al., 1987; Pirot et al., 1992). This latter action appears to be mediated through D2 receptors (Retaux et al., 1991; Grobin and Deutch, 1998). On the other hand, pyramidal cells respond more to NMDA stimulation through D1 receptors in the presence of a low concentration of dopamine, whereas a high concentration would instead reduce this response (Zheng et al., 1999) by acting through D2 receptors. The role of D1/5 receptor is also crucial in suppressing the sustained neuronal firing that takes place during working memory activity (Vijayraghavan et al., 2007). This property is displayed by D1/5 dopamine receptor agonists, which have been found to cause a decrease in extracellular glutamate in PFC in vivo (Abekawa et al. 2000; Harte and O'Connor 2004). Interestingly D1/5 dopamine receptor agonists are also effective in normalizing aberrant network activity induced by both hallucinogens and minimal GABAA antagonism, although clinical efficacy remains to be determined (Aghajanan, 2009). The close relationship between dopamine and glutamate is functionally expressed at NAcc level where medial PFC efferents terminate in close opposition to dopamine terminals originating in the VTA, often in the same spine of GABAergic accumbal cells (Bouyer et al, 1984; Sesack and Pickel, 1992). It is interesting to note that only about 30-40 % of the VTA projection to PFC is dopaminergic, while the rest is likely to be an inhibitory GABAergic innervation (Carr and Sesack 2000a). Of further relevance is that PFC glutamate innervations of the NAcc is part of the motivational circuit completed by accumbal GABA neurons projecting onto the ventral globus pallidus, by pallidal GABA neurons that project to the thalamus and lastly by thalamic glutamate neurons that project back to the PFC (see Chambers et al., 2003, for a review). Hence, PFC and NAcc work together to produce a behavioral output resulting from brain activity that processes input information concerning the internal status of the individual and the external environment (Dorman and Gaudiano, 1998). Considering that firing patterns in both the NAcc and PFC are influenced by glutamatergic input from the hippocampus and amygdala (Aggleton, 2011; Miller et al., 2010), it may be suggested that abnormalities in these distal structures may produce both psychiatric disorders as well as higher vulnerability to drug addiction (Chambers et al., 2001). As far as regards dopamine transmission in the PFC it is necessary to remind that dopamine could be captured by norepinephrine reuptake system (Carboni et al., 1990; Carboni et al., 2006)

4. Noradrenaline in the prefrontal cortex: Innervation, receptors and interactions

The long established observation that catecholamine depletion in PFC can be considered as destructive as tissue ablation (Brozoski et al., 1979) confirms the prominent role of catecholamine innervation in the PFC. The noradrenergic system that originates in the locus coeruleus and in other small nuclei in the medulla and the pons has the peculiar feature of projecting onto the entire neuraxis, although it originates in a relatively small group of cells. This extensive, irradiating anatomical arrangement allows the noradrenergic system to potentially influence all brain activity. In particular, noradrenaline innervations of PFC depend on neurons located in the locus coeruleus (Foote et al., 1983; Bjorklund and Lindvall, 1986) that project to dendrites of both pyramidal cells and interneurons. An interesting feature of locus coeruleus noradrenergic innervation of the cerebral cortex is that individual locus coeruleus neurons simultaneously innervate functionally and cyto-architectonically distinct cortical regions. In fact, locus coeruleus neurons arborize more extensively in the anterior-to-posterior axis of the cortex and exhibit relatively minimal medial-to-lateral collateralization (Swanson, 1976; Aoki et al., 1998). Individual locus coeruleus cells were also shown to innervate both superficial and deep layers of a cortical region (Loughlin et al., 1982). Furthermore, the PFC projects back to the locus coeruleus thereby completing a circuitry which plays a role in relevant brain activity, i.e. maintaining vigilance (reviewed by Aston Jones, 1985) or modulating the behavioural response to stress (Morilak et. al., 2005). Functionally, the noradrenergic system can be viewed as a modulatory system because it can increase the "signal to noise ratio" of responses evoked by other neurotransmitters that excite or inhibit target cells (Woodward et al., 1991). Modulatory actions of this type can be mediated through either α or β noradrenergic receptors (Waterhouse et al., 1991; Woodward et al., 1991). This modulatory type action is also supported by the fact that in the monkey PFC noradrenaline produces its effects predominantly through α2A adrenoceptors that occur in spines, localized discretely over postsynaptic membranes that are most likely PFC pyramidal cells (Aoki et al., 1998). Yet α2A receptors are most prevalent along axons, and are found also in dendritic shafts and astrocytic processes that lack evident synaptic junction. This suggests that these receptors are activated by volume transmission (Aoki et al., 1998). In particular, axonal α2A adrenoceptors have a pre-terminal location; by closing voltage dependent Ca^{++} channels, they are probably able to reduce neurotransmitter release such as serotonin as well as noradrenaline release (Frankhuyzen and Mulder, 1980; Maura et al., 1982).

Moreover, it appears that noradrenaline receptors with different affinities may mediate responses triggered by different extracellular concentrations of this transmitter. As reviewed by Arnsten (2007), moderate levels of noradrenaline released during waking act on high affinity α2A adrenoceptors coupled with Gi proteins to inhibit cAMP signalling, whereas higher levels released during stress not only activate lower affinity β1 coupled to phosphatidyl inositol signalling but also low affinity β1 adrenoceptors coupled to Gs, to increase cAMP signalling (Arnsten, 2000). In general, the role of noradrenaline in the PFC can be seen as being an inhibitory action with a long onset and protracted effect, and can be defined as being neuromodulatory. By inhibiting ongoing background discharge, noradrenaline produces an increase in the signal–to-noise ratio that helps to filter irrelevant stimuli while enhancing behaviorally significant stimuli (Bjorklund and Lindvall, 1986). According to this view NA is crucial for many PFC functions mediated by α2A post synaptic adrenoceptors, such as working memory, attention regulation, planning and behavioural inhibition as suggested by experimental research on various mammals (Arnsten, 2006 and 2009).

Catecholamine transmission in PFC is also dependent on the location of receptors in the dendritic tree of pyramidal cells and may occur through both α2A adrenoceptors increasing delay-related firing for the preferred spatial direction or through D1 receptor decreasing delay-related firing for the nonpreferred direction (Vijayraghavan et al., 2007). Catecholamine transmission is thus essential for reducing the effect of distracting stimulus, or "noise" (Miller et al., 1996) and inhibiting inappropriate behaviours (Funahashi et al., 1993 Arnsten, 2007). More recent data have indicated that both D1 and α2A adrenoceptors can either stimulate or reduce cAMP production respectively, i.e. may increase or reduce the probability of hyperpolarization-activated cyclic nucleotide gated cation channels opening (HCN) (Arnsten, 2007). Moreover, dopamine and NA can inhibit GABA interneurons in the PFC via D4 receptors for which noradrenaline has a high affinity (Wang et al., 2002).

5. Addiction and prefrontal cortex function: Similarities and differences between humans and other mammals

Addiction is the result of numerous factors and the PFC circuitry contributes to the expression of several behaviours that are associated with addiction (Goldstein and Volkow, 2011; Heatherton and Wagner, 2011, George and Koob, 2010). A large majority of addicted subjects do not seek treatment, likely because they do not even recognize their condition as a disease that requires a therapeutic intervention (Goldstein et al. 2009). This condition is probably generated by viewing the abused substance as an essential ingredient of their life, regardless of the consequences of its use. The knowledge of mPFC role in drug dependence can be improved comparing the results of studies performed in animals with those performed in humans although the complexity of addiction behaviour suggests attention in comparing directly specific components of drug dependence (i.e. chronic drug exposure, drug abstinence, drug seeking, cue or drug induced relapse and stress induced relapse). Indeed, if drug addiction in humans can be considered a disorder of self-control because the reinforcing properties of drugs of abuse prevail on the conscious awareness of the negative consequences of addiction behaviour (Heatherton and Wagner, 2011), in animals drug self-administration is supported mostly by the direct rewarding property of the drug (see O'Connor et al. 2011 for a critical evaluation). Therefore, if a man is conscious of the risk associated with drug taking either as far as regards legal or health or social consequences, the same cannot apply to monkeys or rats.

A second important difference among humans and animals deals with the beginning of drug taking. In man it is often the consequence of a complex psychological motivation in which expectations is a strong component (Berridge et al., 2009) while it is often a passive outcome in animals. Moreover, the consequences of drug taking may vary substantially depending on the age of the first experience. In fact drug taking can be started in adolescence, or at adult age and the consequences can be very different because the incomplete brain maturation at adolescence age can offer a fertile ground to the strong reinforcing properties of drugs of abuse (Casey and Jones, 2010). On the other hand, at adult age drug taking can be started to react to a stressful situation and although it may have multiple origin, it may offer again a common fertile ground because the altered status of brain circuitry. Now, if drug taking produces relevant changes in the mPFC of humans and animals, those changes are produced upon a rather different brain circuitry status and therefore the intrinsic rewarding effects in humans can be basically different from those produced in other mammals. When a drug of abuse is administered to animals, the effects observed are those produced on a brain circuitry ensemble that is in a balanced basal condition (unless specific treatments have been applied previously), therefore a great caution should be taken comparing those results to men.

6. Drugs of abuse: Acute effects on prefrontal cortex dopamine and noradrenaline transmission

Substantial evidence confirms the direct involvement of mPFC in addiction. Firing of mPFC neurons is strictly related to i.v. injections of cocaine and heroin (Chang et al., 1998), whereas 6-OH dopamine lesions of mPFC enhance cocaine self-administration (Schenk et al., 1991) and excitotoxic lesions of mPFC determine facilitation of cocaine self-administration (Weissenborn et al., 1997). In particular mPFC has a critical role in drug seeking, craving and relapse either triggered by drugs or by stress or cues associated with drug taking either in humans or in animals (Kalivas et al, 2005; Kalivas and Volkow, 2005). Moreover image studies allowed to observe a reduction in blood flow and cellular metabolism in dorsal PFC of individuals who abused psychostimulants and opioids (Daglish et al., 2001; Bolla et al., 2003; Adinoff et al., 2012). On the contrary an increase has been observed when addicts are exposed to drug-associated cues (Goldstein and Volkow, 2002; Langleben et al., 2008). Nevertheless a reduction in blood flow and cellular metabolism in ventral PFC has been observed in cocaine abusers upon exposition to cocaine related cues (Bonson et al., 2002). Taken together these data support the view that drug addiction increases the motivational value of drug-associated cues while, most likely, negatively affects the function of mPFC in reducing the value of natural reinforcers (see Van den Oever et al., 2010).

Nevertheless, although the dorsal mPFC is critically involved in reinstatement of drug seeking behaviour after abstinence (Berglind et al., 2007) pharmacological inactivation of the dorsal mPFC had no effect on cocaine seeking induced by cocaine cues (Koya et al., 2009). Psychostimulants and other drugs that block dopamine or noradrenaline carrier increase directly extracellular concentration of these catecholamine in all brain areas innervated by dopamine and noradrenaline neurons (Carboni et al., 1989; Tanda et al., 1997; Carboni et al.,

1990; Carboni et al., 2006) including the PFC. The increase in dopamine extracellular concentration can determine the inhibition of the firing of dopamine neurons through an action on D2 auto-receptors and in turn increase K^+ conductance at cell body level (Mercuri et al., 1992). The simultaneous reduction of firing and increase of transmitter extracellular concentration at terminal level produced by psychostimulants and cocaine on catecholamine transmission in the mPFC cortex and other brain areas determines a complex effect on cognition, attention and learning circuitry. Indeed either an increase or a decrease in dopamine transmission in the mPFC may lead to dysfunctions in the ability to inhibit inappropriate actions or thoughts (Arnsten and Li, 2005).

Investigations on the effects of non-psychostimulants substances of abuse on dopamine and norepinephrine transmission in the rat PFC have produced disaccording results. Devoto et al., (2002) have found that acute morphine reduced extracellular norepinephrine, and failed to modify extracellular dopamine level in the mPFC whereas the administration of naloxone, in morphine dependent rats, precipitated a typical abstinence syndrome associated with a concomitant dramatic increase of extracellular dopamine and noreadrenaline (by about 200 and 100%, respectively) in the PFC. The direct role of norepinephrine transmission in the effects of morphine was demonstrated by the alpha(2)-adrenoceptor agonist clonidine that suppressed naloxone-precipitated abstinence symptoms and brought both noradrenaline and dopamine output in PFC to less than 50 % of basal levels (Devoto et al., 2002). In contrast it has been reported that morphine enhances norepinephrine and dopamine release in the mPFC and that norepinephrine transmission is necessary for morphine rewarding effects, reinstatement and mesoaccumbens dopamine release (Ventura et al., 2005). More recently it was found that the released levels of dopamine and its major metabolites in the anterior cingulate cortex were increased by either the electrical stimulation of VTA neurons or by microinjection of a selective μ-opioid receptor agonist, (D-Ala²,N-MePhe⁴,Gly⁵-ol) enkephalin (DAMGO), into the VTA (Narita et al., 2010).

The ability of nicotine to stimulate dopamine and norepinephrine release in the mPFC has been also investigated to assess the involvement of PFC circuitry in the addiction mechanism of nicotine and to explore the potential of modulation of this transmission for cognition enhancement. At this regard Livingstone et al., (2010) reported that a selective alpha7 nicotinic acetylcholine receptors (nAChRs) agonist evoked dopamine overflow in the prefrontal cortex in vivo, and this effect was potentiated by PNU-120596, an allosteric modulator of alpha7 nACh receptor. Moreover, antagonists of NMDA and AMPA receptors blocked [³H]dopamine release from tissue prisms in vitro. On these bases the authors proposed that alpha7 nAChRs were present on glutamate terminals and could increase glutamate release that in turn coordinately could enhances dopamine release from neighboring buttons.

The effect of other drugs of abuse such ethanol and cannabinoids on dopamine and noradrenaline transmission in the PFC received less attention although the effects of these drugs on cognition and mental health are well known. It has been found that posterior VTA dopamine neurons projecting to the ventral pallidum and mPFC are stimulated by local administration of ethanol and that these stimulating effects are mediated, at least in part, by 5-HT(3)receptors (Ding et al., 2011). The presence of cannabinoid receptors in the PFC has been shown by neuroanatomical data suggesting that cortical norepinephrine release may be modulated, in part, by CB1 receptors that are presynaptically distributed on noradrenergic axon terminals (Oropeza et al., 2006). Moreover, repeated treatment with delta-9-tetrahydrocannabinol (THC), the major psychoactive constituent of marijuana, or WIN 55,212-2 (WIN), a synthetic cannabinoid receptor agonist caused a persistent and selective reduction in mPFC dopamine turnover (Verrico et al., 2003). Thereby these evidences suggest that dopamine and norepinephrine transmission in the PFC are involved in the effects of many drugs of abuse, although their precise role is far to be clarified.

7. Abstinence, dopamine and noradrenaline transmission in the PFC

Although the intrinsic meaning of abstinence, as far as regards drug addiction, is referred to a drug free condition, the status of PFC during abstinence may vary depending on the time interval elapsed from the interruption of drug use. Abrupt drug removal can produce a rather similar abstinence syndrome as both men and rats will experience a neuro-physiological adaptation to drug absence. This effect cannot be trivial considering the strong impact of drug effects on brain. Nevertheless once the acute abstinence has been overtaken, strong differences may be found between men and other mammals, in particular when abstinence is generated by a gradual quitting process in humans or extinction process in animals as in self-administration experiments. For instance, in these experiments, upon removal of the reinforcing drug, rats will soon experience the absence of drug effect. This condition will initially generate an enhanced activity at the operant administration mechanism (e.g. lever pressing, nose poke etc.) that will be followed by a reduction because operant activity becomes emptied of pleasurable consequences. This condition will activate a parsimonious process that drives rat behaviour to ignore the ineffective lever pressing with a come back to the routine cage activity. Thus, drug disappearance can be view as an uncontrollable variable and it is likely that rats will not go through the experience of choosing whether or not going back to the drug. Therefore, although it is hard to appraise in rats the role of memories associated with drug administration, we can suggest that medial PFC circuitry will respond to drug removal through adapting progressive changes, thus generating the relative abstinence condition.

On the other hand in man, abstinence is a multiple component condition in which the lack drug effects is strictly associated with an internal struggle between the desire of the reward associated with drug taking and the evaluation of the consequences of that behaviour in terms of money, social life and health involvement (e.g. smoking, cocaine use). It is therefore likely that mPFC circuitry response to abstinence in man will be unique, although it is obviously dependent on the abused drug and on plenty of other environmental factors such as recreational habits, family or economic problems or other stress related conditions. Therefore, craving for drugs is characterized in animals by an initial stereotyped search for drug, that ends relatively quickly with the reaching of a relatively stable brain circuitry equilibrium. Instead in man, mPFC brain circuitry reaches only a pseudo-equilibrium to which contribute the lack of drug effects and its desire (in common with animals), together with of the effort of self-controlling environmental stimuli that often were those that generated drug addiction. In this scenario the result of the exposition to cues associated with drug taking can trigger relapse either in animals or humans, but again involvement of mPFC circuitry can be completely different. The role of PFC in extinction has been recently investigated in humans and animals though the circuitry involved is poorly understood (See the recent review by Millan et al., 2011).

Here we will briefly discuss mPFC changes related to immediate abstinence generated from drug withdrawal. For instance interruption of nicotine exposure in humans, determines a rather fast appearance of withdrawal syndrome that is characterized by depressed mood, irritability, mild cognitive deficits accompanied by other peripheral physiological symptoms (Shiffman et al., 2004). We observed that either mecamylamine or naloxone determine the precipitation of an abstinence syndrome in rats carrying an osmotic minipump that continuously delivers nicotine (Carboni et al., 2000). This syndrome was characterized by physical abstinence signs appearing to be dissociated from dopamine extracellular concentration. Mecamylamine decreased dopamine in the NAcc while increasing it the mPFC whereas naloxone did not (Carboni et al., 2000). Interestingly withdrawal from a schedule of increasing doses of morphine or the administration of naloxone determined an increase in the extracellular concentration of dopamine mPFC (Bassareo et al., 1995). Preclinical research in animal models have also shown that early nicotine withdrawal is characterized by decreased function of presynaptic inhibitory metabotropic glutamate 2/3 receptors (Markou, 2008). At the same time it has been observed an increased expression of postsynaptic glutamate receptor subunits in limbic and frontal brain sites. This increase may explain why a protracted abstinence may be associated with increased glutamate response to stimuli associated with nicotine administration (as reviewed by Markou, 2008).

As far as regards cocaine addiction it has been reported (Kalivas et al., 2005) that enhanced D1 activity would lead to an increased inhibitory state of the PFC during withdrawal, so that only particularly strong stimuli, such as those associated with drug consumption, would be able to activate and guide behaviour. Moreover repeated cocaine administration change functional properties of the D1 receptors in the PFC through an enhancement of the activity of the G protein signalling 3 (AGS3), coupled to D1 receptors, whereas the G protein activity coupled to D2 was reduced following cocaine withdrawal (Bowers et al., 2004). These alterations in the mPFC may determine alteration of prefrontal glutamatergic innervation of the accumbens promoting the compulsive character of drug seeking in addicts by decreasing the value of natural rewards, diminishing cognitive control (choice), and enhancing glutamatergic drive in response to drug-associated stimuli.

8. Relapse, dopamine and noradrenaline transmission in the prefrontal cortex

The relapse to drug use is a major problem in drug addiction therapy. Essentially, relapse can be categorized in three major types: drug induced relapse, reinstatement of self-administration behaviour upon exposition to drug related cues and stress induced relapse (Stewart, 2003; Crombag et al., 2008; Van den Oever et al., 2010). Drug-induced relapse could be associated with similar processes in humans and animals and will determine the resumption of drug intake behaviour, whereas cue-induced relapse may engage different brain circuitry depending on the involvement of self-control mechanisms. If a rat will just start pressing a lever, a man, who probably went through a strong involving process to achieve drug taking interruption, will go through a complex decision making process (e.g. a man will evaluate the strong effect of the cue and only when self control processes will be defeated will resume drug taking; alternatively he can resume drug taking without craving, or even he can rationally decide to take the drug because he has the conviction to be able to control drug taking). Thus, it is likely that reinstatement in man involves a more complex mPFC circuitry than in other mammals. Nevertheless one of the major determinants of reinstatement to cocaine use among human addicts is acute re-exposure to the drug, which often precipitates cocaine craving and relapse (Cromabag et al., 2008; Volkow et al., 2010). As far as regards animal studies, it has been reported that the mPFC plays a major role during reinstatement, either because its direct role in cognition or because its connections with subcortical areas (Kalivas et al., 2005; Crombag et al., 2008; Van den Oever et al., 2010). Projections from the mPFC to the NAcc are stratified in a dorso-ventral pattern with the dorsal mPFC projecting predominantly to the NAcc core and the ventral mPFC projecting to the NAcc shell (Heidbreder and Groenewegen, 2003; Voorn et al., 2004). These anatomical features have been used to assume that during reinstatement the increase in extracellular glutamate in the NAcc core is associated with an increased excitatory activity of pyramidal neurons of dorsal mPFC that in turn may drive heroin (LaLumiere and Kalivas, 2008) or cocaine seeking behaviour in rats (Mac Farland et al., 2003).

On the other hand, glutamatergic projections from the ventral mPFC to the NAcc shell have been found to suppress conditioned drug seeking after extinction learning (Peters et al., 2009) whereas interruption of this neuronal link or pharmacological inactivation of the NAcc shell produce resumption of drug craving (Peters et al., 2008; Fuchs et al., 2008). At this regard it has been proposed that the mPFC regulates the expression of both fear and drug memories after extinction, through divergent projections to the amygdala and nucleus accumbens, respectively. Therefore a common neural circuit for extinction of fear and drug memories would suggest shared mechanisms and treatment strategies across both domains (Peters et al., 2009). These experimental evidences support the view of mPFC neurons controlling drug craving whereas its suppression may occur through two separate but balanced pathways by acting directly in the two NAcc sub-regions. This view has been contradicted by numerous studies (for a review see Van den Oever et al., 2010) and therefore it can be suggested that drug dependence in rats cannot be the product of a single neuronal pathway

VTA dopaminergic neurons that innervate the dorsal mPFC have been reported to be involved in the initiation of drug seeking responses (for a review see Crombag et al., 2008 and Van den Over et al., 2010). In particular dopamine administration into the dorsal mPFC has been shown to be sufficient to elicit a reinstatement of self-administration behavior (McFarland and Kalivas, 2001), whereas microinjections of the D1/D2 antagonist fluphenazine into the dorsal PFC but not into the NAcc core or ventral pallidum, prevented cocaine induced reinstatement (McFarland and Kalivas 2001). A role for dopamine transmission in reinstatement is also supported by the findings of Park and coworkers (Park et al., 2002). These authors showed that intra-mPFC administration of the dopamine antagonist flupentixol blocked cocaine reinstatement triggered by systemic cocaine administration in rats that were first trained to self-administer cocaine intravenously and later underwent through extinction by substitution of cocaine (i.v.) with saline (Park et al., 2002). These authors also showed that reinstatement of cocaine seeking behavior could be induced by intra-mPFC cocaine and could be blocked by local administration of the AMPA receptor antagonist CNQX into NAcc shell or the border with the core (Park et al., 2002). Interestingly, it has been recently reported that the infralimbic mPFC, and specifically its glutamatergic and beta-adrenergic systems, regulates the consolidation of extinction of cocaine self-administration. Therefore the transmission at level of infralimbic cortex can be manipulated to influence the retention of extinction (LaLumiere and Kalivas, 2008).

Moreover, a role for dopamine transmission in the mPFC has been also proposed in cue and in stress induced reinstatement of self-administration behavior. In fact intracranial infusion of the dopamine D1 receptor antagonist, SCH 23390 into the prelimbic cortex potently, and dose dependently, attenuated heroin-seeking in response to either cue presentations or a priming dose of heroin, confirming that dopamine D1 receptors regulate prefrontal cortex pathways necessary for the reinstatement of heroin-seeking in rats (See, 2009). In addition systemic blockade of D1 receptors prevents an increase in Fos expression in the dorsal mPFC (Ciccocioppo et al., 2001) suggesting an increase in dopamine transmission in this area during reinstatement. Moreover the role of the mPFC and in particular the involvement of dopamine transmission in stress induced reinstatement of cocaine seeking have been investigated in rats (Capriles et al., 2003). These authors have shown that inactivation of prelimbic cortex by tetrodotoxin blocked reinstatement of cocaine seeking induced by either foot shock or by cocaine priming, whereas the effects of tetrodotoxin injections in the orbitofrontal cortex (OFC) were mixed. Moreover, Capriles and coworkers found that infusion of the D1 dopamine antagonist SCH23390 into either the prelimbic or into the OFC blocked foot-shock induced reinstatement. These results suggest that the prelimbic and the orbitofrontal cortices form part of the circuitry mediating the effects of foot shock stress in reinstatement of drug seeking and that the prelimbic region may be a common pathway for cue, drug and foot-shock stress-induced reinstatement of drug seeking (Capriles et al., 2003). Nevertheless, the dichotomy in mPFC function, attributing to dorsal mPFC (prelimbic, cingulate subregions) promotion of drug seeking and to ventral mPFC (infralimbic) inhibition of drug seeking in cocaine-experienced rats (Peters et al., 2009), has been challenged by studies on heroin self-administration suggesting that heroin seeking is promoted by a minority of selectively activated ventral mPFC neurons (Bossert et al., 2011). These authors thus suggested that different brain mechanisms mediate heroin and cocaine relapse in the rat model.

9. Genetic variation, catecholamine transmission in the prefrontal cortex and predisposition to addictions

Dopamine neurons projecting to the PFC possess an interesting feature as compared with other systems. In fact they have a higher baseline rate firing and a higher rate of dopamine turnover. This feature renders them very sensitive to alteration in dopamine synthesis and metabolism either underlained by gene variation or induced by drugs of abuse (Bannon et al., 1981; Hallman, 1984; Garris et al., 1993; Garris and Wightman, 1994; Cass and Gerhardt, 1995). Improved performances in cognitive tasks requiring working memory and inhibition have been observed in subjects that carry variations in the catechol-O-methyltransferase (COMT) gene (Dumontheil et al., 2011). COMT degrades the catecholamine neurotransmitters dopamine, epinephrine, and norepinephrine. A functional polymorphism in the COMT gene (val[158]met) accounts for a four-fold variation in enzyme activity (Heinz and Smolka, 2006). The low activity met[158] allele causes approximately 75 % reduction in dopamine methylation and increased dopamine function. This has been associated with improved working memory, executive functioning, and attention control, but is also linked to a higher risk of anxiety-related behaviours. The latter, in turn, may be related to an excessive activation of the HPA axis and relative responses due to elevated noradrenaline transmission in the PFC (Heinz and Smolka, 2006). On the other hand, limbic and prefrontal activation elicited by unpleasant stimuli in subjects with more met[158] alleles might contribute to the observed lower emotional resilience against negative mood states (Smolka, et al., 2005). The increase in dopamine function is particularly relevant in areas such as the prefrontal cortex because it contains significantly less dopamine transporter (Sesack et al.,

1998; Lammel et al., 2008), and because dopamine clearance (approx. 60 %) is carried out by the COMT enzyme, unlike in other dopamine areas such as the striatum where dopamine is cleared promptly by the reuptake system (Karoum et al., 1994).

Furthermore, Adele Diamond (2007) makes an interesting observation on the difference found between males and females. COMT activity in females is in fact roughly 30 % lower, due probably to estrogen activity (Cohn and Axelrod, 1971; Boudikova et al., 1990). This gender variation may render females able to better perform cognitive tasks because of the more elevated dopamine function in the PFC whereas they perform worse under even minor stress. On the other hand there is also substantial evidence that males perform better or no worse if slightly stressed (Shors and Miesegaes, 2002; Shors and Leuner, 2003; Shansky et al., 2004). This observation fits well with the above reported characteristics of the PFC dopamine function being highly sensitive to stress (Thierry et al., 1972; Reinhard et al., 1982; Roth et al., 1988; Deutch and Roth, 1990; Arnsten and Goldman-Rakic 1998; Arnsten, 1999 and 2000). Thus, as reported by Diamond (2007), cognitive functioning in men would benefit from the expression of COMT variation with reduced activity whereas females would instead benefit from the expression of a faster-acting valine version of the COMT enzyme that would moderate excess dopamine functioning in the PFC. Altered activity of COMT, which has a primary role in the degradation of dopamine in the frontal cortex (Karoum et al., 1994), might thus also be involved in the magnification of the reinforcing properties of drugs of abuse. Considering that the increase of extracellular dopamine and norepinephrine in PFC is a peculiar effect of drugs such as amphetamine and cocaine one can wonder if subjects that carry variations in the catechol-O-methyltransferase (COMT) gene are predisposed to psychostimulant addiction. Genetic studies suggest that while occasional use of drugs of abuse is predominantly linked to environmental or familiar factors, over 60 % of the cocaine users inherited their vulnerability to heavy use and dependence (Kendler et al., 2000; Kendler and Prescott, 1998).

Nevertheless there are no convincing studies that correlate cocaine addiction with variation of genes related to dopaminergic system such as the genes DRD2, COMT, SLC6A3 (coding for the dopamine transporter DAT) and DBH (coding for the dopamine beta hydroxylase). However an interesting hypothesis (Brousse et al., 2010) suggested that individuals carrying genetic variation of the DBH gene, that has particularly been linked with the psychotic effects caused by cocaine, could be predisposed to cocaine-induced psychosis making the development of cocaine addiction less probable. This can also apply to mutations of the Val158Met of the gene COMT, TaqI A of the gene DRD2 and VNTR 9 repeat of the DAT. On the other hand Hosak et al., (2006) found that consumers of methamphetamine carrying the Met allele of the COMT gene Val158Met polymorphism showed higher novelty seeking scores. This polymorphism is associated with low COMT enzyme activity and high endogenous dopamine synaptic levels in the PFC. According to the authors this leads to a decrease in dopaminergic neurotransmission in the NAcc and a need to stimulate it through novelty seeking behaviour or psychostimulant use.

10. Prefrontal cortex dopamine transmission in adolescence and drug addiction

Adolescence (see chapter XX) is a crucial developmental period of life in which physical and psychological remarkable changes occurring after puberty, model the personality to allow the assumption of adult roles and responsibilities (Dahl, 2004a and 2004b; Steinberg, 2008). In this scenario PFC represents a crucial brain area because its function in expressing a specific behaviour. This may be the outcome of multiple interactions such as those between the hormonal triggered desires, and the representation of increasingly complex and distant social goals. The shaping of this objective in turn will be influenced by the social and family environment. Therefore the maturation of PFC occurring in adolescence may definitively shape the adult personality and at the same time, dysfunctions happening in this process may constitute a milieu necessary and often sufficient for developing psychiatric disorders such as schizophrenia and depression or for predisposing individuals to a high vulnerability to drug addiction (see Davey, et al., 2008).

The PFC has a prominent role in controlling impulsiveness (Fineberg et al., 2010) and in adolescence it is likely that this control is insufficient due to incomplete maturation of cognitive function. Accordingly, working memory, abstract thinking and complex problem solving improve during adolescence to peak at late adolescence (Feinberg, 1983; Woo et al., 1997; Williams et al., 1999). These acquired abilities are supported by distinct developmental changes occurring in the PFC during adolescence and involve changes in densities of dendritic processes and synapses, increased myelination, increased neuronal membrane synthesis and in turn, increase in white matter (Paus et al., 1999; Giedd et al., 1999a, 1999b). Among these changes, synaptic pruning has been considered a way to reduce energy use through a selective reduction of synaptic contacts that are not necessary to sustain a particular ability; in humans PFC synaptic density, after reaching a maximum at the age of 5 years, diminishes by about 35 % by late adolescence (Lewis, 1997). This synapse reduction involves mostly local PFC circuits (Woo et al., 1997) and both excitatory and inhibitory inputs are implicated (Anderson et al., 1995). During the pruning that occurs in adolescence there is a prevalent reduction of the excitatory stimulation that reaches the PFC (Rakic et al., 1994). In particular synapse elimination of presumed glutamatergic inputs occurs in PFC. Binding to NMDA receptors in rat brain peaks at 28 post natal day (PND) whereas a successive reduction leads to a 33 % reduction by the 60 PND (Insel et al., 1990).

On the contrary, dopamine functional activity in the PFC increases in adolescence, peaking to levels much higher than those seen in adulthood (for a review see Lewis et al., 1998). In rats, dopamine innervation is maximum at 35 PND in superficial layers and at 60 PND in deeper layers (Kalsbeek et al., 1988); moreover, the density of DAT, often used as an index of dopamine innervation in the PFC, is about 70 % of adult levels in weaning rats. On the other hand the increase in dopamine fiber density observed in development may be associated to a decline in synthesis and turnover; in fact synthesis peaks at PND 30 and then declines in late adolescence (Andersen, et al., 1997). Adolescence has a peculiar feature from an energetically point of view. In fact cortex energy consumption in humans peaks at 3-4 years and is maintained up to the age of 20, to progressively decline in later life (Chugani et al., 1987). In general synaptic pruning and myelination can be considered parallel processes that apparently have the role of strengthening regularly used innervations rendering them able to fire in a more concerted pattern (Lewis, 1997; Miller, 1996). At the same time infrequently used innervations are eliminated (Rutherford et al., 1998). Furthermore dopamine modulation of fast-spiking interneurons changes dramatically during adolescence (PND 45-50 in rats) with D2 agonists switching from being mildly inhibitory in prepubertal rats to strongly excitatory in young adult rats. In vivo recordings in adult rats reveal that deep-layer pyramidal neurons respond to endogenous DA release with suppression of firing while interneurons are activated (Tseng and O'Donnell, 2007; Gruber et al., 2010). Thus the increase in dopamine functional activity that peaks in adolescence together with the reduction of excitatory innervation are two delicate processes which reduce the activity of pyramidal cells. Therefore either a deficiency in excitatory reduction or a defective increased inhibitory activity may lead to an excessive pyramidal cell activity that in turn may be reflected by the onset of a psychiatric disorder or drug abuse.

Substantial evidence points to the higher risk of drug exposure in adolescence (Barron et al., 2005; Crews and Hodge, 2007; Schramm-Sapyta et al., 2009). In particular alcohol consumption during adolescence causes diffuse brain alterations and greatly increases the likelihood that an alcohol use disorder will develop later in life (Nixon and McClain, 2010). Diffusion tensor imaging studies have shown that adolescent binge drinking damages white matter tracts throughout the brain, including main hippocampus efferent fibers and those interconnecting the PFC (McQueeny et al., 2009; Jacobus et al., 2009). Adolescents respond to the effects of alcohol distinctly from adults in fact they are less sensitive to negative effects of alcohol, they do no perceive cues that may suggest reduction of intake, but are more sensitive to positive effects such as those related to social interaction, which may serve to reinforce or promote excessive intake (Spear et al., 2005). Adolescence is also critical for cannabis abuse, indeed it is widely reported that cannabis use during adolescence increases the risk of developing psychotic disorders later in life (Bossong and Niesink, 2010, Malone et al, 2010). However, although the neurobiological processes underlying this relationship are unknown, alteration of PFC circuitry is more than likely. Very recently it was found that marijuana users had decreased cortical thickness in right caudal middle frontal, bilateral insula and bilateral superior frontal cortices (Lopez-Larson, 2011). These results suggest that age of regular use may be associated with altered PFC gray matter development in adolescents. According to the authors of this study reduced insular cortical thickness may be used as a biological marker for ascertain increased risk of substance dependence (Lopez-Larson, 2011). An interesting comparison in adolescent alcohol and marijuana users has been proposed by evaluating participants who performed a verbal paired associates encoding task during functional magnetic resonance imaging (fMRI) scanning. The results of this study suggested that adolescent substance users demonstrated altered fMRI response relative to non-using controls, yet binge drinking appeared to be associated with more differences in activation than marijuana use (Schweinsburg et al., 2011). Alcohol and marijuana may have interactive effects that alter these differences, particularly in prefrontal brain regions (Schweinsburg et al., 2011).

As far as regards cocaine effects, rats with adolescent-onset cocaine self-administration experience were more impaired in an OFC-related learning task than rats with adult-onset cocaine self-administration experience (Harvey et al., 2009). Treatment with cocaine during adolescence also caused acute alterations in the expression of genes encoding cell adhesion molecules and transcription factors within the PFC. In particular, a decrease in histone methylation was observed and this effect may indicate a role for chromatin remodelling in gene expression patterns. These findings allowed the authors to suggest that exposure to cocaine during adolescence has extensive molecular and behavioural effects in the rat PFC. These consequences develop over time and endure long after drug administration has ceased (Black et al., 2006). Smoking and nicotine exposure during adolescence is a very relevant heath problem because the higher dependence developed in individuals who start smoking early (see O'Dell, 2009 for review). Early tobacco use is facilitated by the legal possibility to purchase tobacco in most of the western countries. Besides other health consequences, tobacco smoking and nicotine exposure during adolescence interfere with PFC development and leads to cognitive impairments in later life with enduring attentional disturbances (Cunotte et al., 2009). Among molecular alteration, early nicotine exposure determines reduced mGluR2 protein and function on presynaptic terminals of PFC glutamatergic synapses. Interestingly restoring mGluR2 activity in vivo by local infusion of a group II mGluR agonist in adult rats that received nicotine as adolescents rescued attentional disturbances (Counotte et al., 2011).

Among others, novelty directed behavior is highly expressed in adolescence. It may represent a strong risk for the use of addictive drugs and consequently for the developing of drug dependence. Novelty directed behavior can be observed in periadolescent rats, in fact they show a strong exploratory behavior in a novel open field. Although it is not clear the role of dopamine and norepinephrine transmission in this behavior, periadolescent rats show hypo-responsivity to dopamine agonists and hypersensitivity to antagonist action suggesting that their dopamine transmission is hyperactive as compared with adult rats (Spear and Brake, 1983). Moreover the response of adolescent animals to amphetamine (an indirect dopamine and noradrenaline agonist) supports the peculiarity of catecholamine transmission in adolescence (Mathews and McCormick, 2011). Paradoxically amphetamine reduces novelty preference when adolescent mice are paired with a novel environment while it increases novelty preference when this test is performed in normal adult mice (Adriani et al., 1998). Thus we can hypothesize that typical adolescent behaviors such as novelty seeking, impulsivity and risk taking are the result of a natural drive that emerges in adolescence possibly linked to the need of spreading individuals of a species in a territory. It may be likely that this behaviour could be maintained by an overactive excitatory transmission in the prefrontal cortex and in subcortical areas that are balanced by an increasing active inhibitory catecholamine transmission. On the other hand catecholamine innervations reaching their maximal inhibitory activity at the end of adolescence, may have a role in stabilizing those brain processes that have been developed in adolescence and will be then acquired as behaviour reference in adult life.

As far as nicotine effect in adolescents, we observed that nicotine-stimulated dopamine release was higher in the mPFC of adolescent rats as compared with adults (Carboni et al., 2010). These results suggest that the higher response observed in adolescents might be correlated to their higher sensitivity to the effects of nicotine. This trait might have a contributory role in the strong nicotine addiction that is observed in smokers who start nicotine abuse during adolescence (see the review of O'Dell, 2009). In fact, although nicotine abuse has much in common with other drugs of abuse in that it increases dopamine output in the NAcc shell (Di Chiara, 2000) or in other brain areas (Carboni et al., 2000), its ability to determine a higher increase of dopamine in the PFC of adolescents could potentially be correlated to the alteration of the brain maturation process that occurs in adolescent smokers (Carboni et al., 2010). Consequently this feature may alter the PFC's role in the ability to establish a rational evaluation of smoking even during adult age. We also observed that nicotine increased noradrenaline release in the PFC (Carboni et al., 2010) thus suggesting that this increase may have a role in the nicotine enhancement of cognition (see the review of Poorthuis et al., 2009). Furthermore local infusion of nicotine in the prelimbic mPFC can increase mPFC glutamate extracellular concentration supporting the role of nAChRs in modulating thalamocortical input to the PFC (Gioanni et al., 1999). These findings therefore suggest that such a mechanism may be relevant to the cognitive effects of nicotine and nicotinic agonists.

11. Role of stress (prenatal, adolescent and adult) on prefrontal cortex function and drug addiction

Acute stress modulates the neuronal activity of brain regions such as mPFC (Hains and Arnsten, 2008), amygdala (Goldstein et al., 1996), hippocampus (Belujon and Grace 2011) , OFC (Capriles et al., 2003), insula, and striatum (Koob, 2009) that are also areas of the brain involved in regulation of appetitive behaviors, such as feeding and drug taking (Marchant et al., 2012). These areas share common a consistent dopaminergic innervation pointing to a role of dopamine in stress-induced reinstatement of drug taking (Erblich et al., 2004; Shaham and Stewart, 1995; Shaham et al., 2003). The preclinical early work of Piazza and collaborators has shown a clear relationship between drugs of abuse, stress and glucocorticoids levels (Piazza et al., 1996), although most of their work was focused on sub-cortical areas. They have indeed shown that drugs of abuse acutely activate the hypothalamic-pituitary-adrenal (HPA) axis and that drug dependence was characterized by a dysregulation of HPA axis (Piazza and Le Moal, 1996). Moreover they showed that stressors facilitate the acquisition of cocaine and amphetamine self-administration (Piazza and Le Moal, 1998). Stress plays and important role in drug addiction either by triggering relapse in abstinent addicts, or by altering PFC function thus predisposing for drug use and abuse (Stewart, 2003; George and Koob, 2010; Van den Oever et al., 2010). Human studies suggested that the incapacity to resist to drug cues, such as the sight of drug, can also be amplified by stress (Swan et al., 1988; Breese et al., 2011; Potenza et al., 2012). Although moderate stress can have a positive value on cognition, strong or repeated stress will either be deleterious for cognitive functions or may be a determining factor in vulnerability to mental illness and drug addiction, likely through an alteration of catecholamine transmission in the PFC (Holmes and Welman 2009, George and Koob, 2010; Goldstein and Volkow, 2011). Indeed, it has recently been reported (Radley et al., 2008) that selectively ablating noradrenergic input into the rat medial PFC attenuates the effects of stress in the paraventricular hypothalamic nucleus, as well as the HPA axis secretory responses, while stress-induced Fos expression in dorsal medial PFC was enhanced and was negatively correlated with stress-induced paraventricular hypothalamic nucleus activation. These observations identify the locus coeruleus as an upstream component of a circuitry providing for dorsal medial PFC modulation of emotional stress-induced HPA activation. Since noradrenergic projection, and its innervations of the prefrontal cortex play an important role in the modulation of working memory and attention, it may be likely that noradrenaline release in the medial PFC could modulate stress response, depending on the evaluation and comparison of environmental stimuli with past experience in mounting adequate behaviourally adaptive responses to emotional stress and environmental challenge in general.

Further, the artificial activation of catecholamine transmission in the PFC, such as that produced by amphetamine administration, similarly to stress, can have beneficial or a deleterious effects on cognition depending on the dose and on basal dopamine and noradrenaline transmission. The ability of stress to alter neuronal function has been investigated in 15 smokers undergoing functional magnetic resonance imaging who were exposed to a psychosocial stressor, followed by smoking drug cues (Dagher et al., 2009). The results allowed to observe a significant change in neural activity during stress with an increased neural response to drug cues in the medial prefrontal cortex, posterior cingulate cortex, dorsomedial thalamus, medial temporal lobe, caudate nucleus, and primary and association visual areas. A stress-induced limbic deactivation that predicted subsequent neural cue-reactivity was also observed. The authors thus suggested that stress increases the incentive salience of drug cues (Dagher et al., 2009). The role of mPFC in the ability of stress to enhance the reinforcing properties of morphine has been recently investigated (Rozeske et al., 2009). The results obtained show that escapable stress activates the ventral regions of the mPFC while inescapable stress does not. On the other hand inescapable stress potentiates morphine-conditioned place preference while escapable stress does not. Moreover these effects are modulated by intra-mPFCv microinjection of the GABAA agonist muscimol 1 h before stress session (Rozeske et al., 2009).

It was early reported that the adult offspring of stressed pregnant rats exhibited higher locomotor response to novelty and to an injection of amphetamine but also a higher level of amphetamine self-administration, suggesting that prenatal stress (PNS) could determine an individual predisposition to drug self-administration (Deminiére et al., 1992). The effect of PNS was also observed to elevate active lever responding in rats either during extinction or in cocaine-primed reinstatement, but not during self-administration or in conditioned-cued reinstatement, thus suggesting that early environmental factors contribute to an individual's initial responsiveness to cocaine and propensity to relapse to cocaine-seeking (Kipping et al., 2008). We recently investigated in rats the effect of PNS on dopamine and noradrenaline transmission in the mPFC (Carboni et al., 2010) and in the NAcc shell (Silvagni et al., 2008). We observed that PNS did not change dopamine but decreased noradrenaline basal output in the PFC of both adolescents and adult rats (Carboni et al, 2010). Moreover we observed that PNS decreased amphetamine stimulated dopamine output and increased amphetamine-stimulated noradrenaline output. PNS decreased nicotine-stimulated noradrenaline (but not dopamine output) in adults, though not in adolescents (Carboni et al., 2010). These data support a contributing role of PNS in the development of psychiatric disorders and that its effect may augment drug addiction vulnerability.

12. Areas of prefrontal cortex, decision making and drug addiction.

Preclinical and human studies have provided unequivocal evidence that drug addiction involves many subregions of the PFC. Nevertheless the correspondence between these subregions among rodents and primates has been long debated (Brown and Bowman, 2002). Moreover it is claimed that PFC function is more than the sum of the functions of individual PFC sub-regions (Wilson et al., 2010). An exhaustive review of PFC dysfunction in addiction has been recently provided (Goldstein and Volkow, 2011). In this section we will briefly consider some preclinical and human studies on the involvement of the OFC in addiction because this PFC sub region has recently received much attention in drug addiction (Shoenbaum et al., 2006). The orbitofrontal area is interconnected in both rat and primates with mediodorsal talamus, the basolateral amigdala and NAcc, and has been proposed to use associative information handled by this circuitry to guide behaviour on the basis of the expected outcome of a specific action (See the review of Shoenbaum et al., 2006 for specific anatomical location and relationship with other brain areas). In particular this area is activated in humans during anticipation of expected outcomes and therefore can allow prediction of reward or punishment using this information to guide decisions (Arana et al., 2003). Rats with OFC lesions fail to behave correctly in reinforcing devaluation tasks where they have to make decisions on the basis of outcome expectancies (Gallagher et al., 1999). As far as regards addicted they may suffer of OFC circuitry alteration because, often under the control of drug-associated cues, they are unable to control drug-seeking behaviour despite they are aware of adverse consequences associated with their compulsive and impulsive behaviour and despite a stated desire to stop. The alteration of OFC have been detected by imaging studies of addicts and in particular it has been observed a reduction in OFC activation during acute withdrawal whereas an over-activation of OFC associated with high level of craving has been observed in addicts exposed to drug-related cues (see the review of Dom et al., 2005). Furthermore, in addicts are observed impairments of OFC-dependent behaviours that strongly parallel those that are observed in individuals carrying OFC damage (Grant et al., 2000).

Nevertheless in humans it is difficult to state that functional deficits at the level of OFC are due to drug exposure because it could be attributable to pre-existing condition. At this regard Volkow and collaborators proposed an interesting hypothesis (Volkow et al., 2009). They suggested an association between an impairment of the OFC and other PFC areas involved in addiction, and a decrease of striatal dopamine D2 receptors availability. This condition would render subjects more vulnerable to drug addiction (Volkow et al., 2009). Further, a study done in subjects who have a high risk for alcoholism but were not alcoholics showed higher than normal striatal D2 receptor levels and a normal metabolism in OFC, anterior cingulate cortex and dorsolateral PFC (Volkow et al., 2006). On this basis the authors proposed that normal PFC function may have protected these subjects from alcohol abuse. A further recent evolution of this hypothesis suggested that OFC and cingulate function are involved in individual positive emotionality which in turn is a defence against drug of abuse vulnerability (Volkow et al., 2011). Nevertheless these stimulating hypotheses have to be evaluated taking into account that dopoamine D2 availability does not distinguish between an increase in the released dopamine or in a decrease of receptors. On the other hand rats trained to self-administer amphetamine show a long term (one month) reduction of dendritic spine density specifically in the OFC whereas spine density was increased in the medium spiny neurons of the NAcc and in pyramidal neurons of the mPFC (Crombag et al., 2005). Moreover others have reported an increase of dendritic spine density in the medial PFC and in the NAcc after treatment with psychostimulant (Robinson and Kolb, 1999). It has been reported that chronic cocaine use causes long lasting impairment in OFC function as established by studies on reversal learning in animals, thus suggesting that this damage is expressed by the inability of using the value of predicted outcome to guide behavior (Shoenbaum et al., 2004, 2006 and 2009). The results of these experiments allowed Shoenbaum et al. (2006) to claim that "cocaine use can drive to the loss of outcome expectancies making addicts to continue to seek drugs despite the almost inevitable negative consequences of such behaviour concluding that changes in the OFC-dependent signal would by themselves contribute powerfully to a transition from normal goal-directed behaviour to compulsive habitual responding".

Moreover a dysregulation of the ventral, dorsomedial and dorsolateral striatal systems has been hypothesized to play a fundamental role in the transition from voluntary drug use to more habitual and compulsive drug use (Everitt and Robbins, 2005; Belin and Everitt, 2008). These sub cortical areas are strictly connected with PFC regions and in particular the NAcc shell receives glutamatergic inputs from the ventromedial PFC and insular cortex, the NAcc core receives glutamatergic inputs from the dorsomedial PFC, insular cortex and OFC whereas the dorsomedial and the dorsolateral striatum receive glutamatergic inputs from the OFC, the anterior cingulate cortex and the sensory and motor cortices (Reynolds and Zahm, 2005; Gabbott et al., 2005). Therefore it is objectively possible that the dysfunction in the cortical areas observed after chronic cocaine use (Shoenbaum et al., 2006 and 2009) are a consequence of a complex neural adaptative response that occurs during the transition from voluntary drug use to a more habitual and compulsive drug use. This transition has been hypothesized to be mediated at neural level through a shift from PFC to striatal control over drug seeking and drug taking (Everitt and Robbins, 2005). Nevertheless a recent review of neuroimaging studies have revealed a generalized PFC dysfunction in drug addicted individuals and although the activity of PFC regions is highly integrated and plastic, pre-existing dysfunction of specific PFC regions may confer individual vulnerability to drug addiction (Goldstein and Volkow, 2011).

13. Addiction a disorder of awareness, motivation, or self-control

Addiction may be considered the product of an imbalance between two separate, but interacting, neural systems: an immediate one that generates decision making, based on the impulsivity-related amygdala system for signalling pain or pleasure of immediate prospects and a reflective one, based on PFC circuitry for elaborating the value of signalling pain or pleasure of future prospects (Bechara, 2005). The capacity of controlling behavior is challenged by the ability of cues associated with reinforcing activities (food, sex, drugs of abuse, pleasure) of activating circuitry in which dopamine release in the NAcc has a fundamental value (Schultz, 2010). On the other hand self-control efforts involve increased activity in regions of the PFC regulating emotions and cognition (i.e. dorsolateral and ventrolateral PFC) and a reduced activity in regions associated with reward processing and craving. These brain areas include the ventral striatum, subgenual cingulate, amygdala, ventral tegmental area and OFC as observed in neuroimaging studies in cocaine users (Volkow et al., 2010) or smokers (Kober et al., 2010) when they are required to inhibit craving. In smokers a decrease in craving correlated with a decrease in ventral striatum activity and an increase in dorsolateral prefrontal cortex activity, with ventral striatal activity fully mediating the relationship between lateral prefrontal cortex and reported craving (Kober et al., 2010).

Interestingly, the activation of similar regions was seen in healthy volunteers who were requested to control response to cues associated with monetary rewards (Delgado et al., 2008). Therefore, emotional and cognitive processes that influence decision-making and which may also lead to impulsive behavior or motivational disturbances such as food abuse, drug addiction, excessive spending, risky sexual behavior, may be indicative of an abnormal functioning of PFC or subcortical ventral striatal regions as observed in neuroimaging studies (Breiter et al., 2001). A further feature of PFC role in cognition deals with the overlapping dopamine and ACh innervations in the PFC. It suggests that all the cognitive processes in which are involved these two transmitters may occur involving local mechanisms (Briand et al., 2007). In particular it is of relevance that dopamine agonists increase Ach release and social cognition in rats (Di Cara et al., 2006). Several authors suggested that dopaminergic modulation of PFC cholinergic output is mediated primarily through activation of D1 and D5 type receptors (see Briand et al., 2007 for a review).

Moreover the importance of PFC in expressing self-control is supported by the fact that failure occurs when frontal executive control is compromised such as following alcohol consumption or injury (Crews and Boettinger, 2009) as reported in patients with frontal lobe damage (Sellito et al., 2010) and in subjects who were subjected to transient disruption of functions in the lateral PFC by repetitive transcranial magnetic stimulation in lateral PFC (Figner et al., 2010). The lateral PFC is considered the area which activity allows self-control as proposed by the top-down model although two types of subcortical activities could be distinguished: one related to drug addiction that involves primarily the control of PFC over NAcc and one related to amygdala that controls the emotions. Therefore PFC could be associated with long term outcomes whereas sub-cortical activity is associated with more immediate outcomes. The prevalence of subcortical areas in managing drug taking is gained progressively during drug taking experience. At this regard Belin and Everett (2010) have proposed the incentive habit hypothesis. According to these authors drug seeking habits progressively dominate goal directed drug seeking behavior that in turn ca be highly influenced by Pavlovian incentive mechanisms. This process in humans may crucially affect the transition from drug use to drug abuse, involves a strong emotional component but the outcome of this process likely depends on the individual resilience of neuronal circuit to resist to the neurochemical insult of the drug abused. In fact drug addiction depending on the situation can involve a strong component of emotion (Burke et al., 2008; Heatherton and Wagner, 2011; Artiges et al., 2009). The similarity between the control over drug addiction and over emotion share many commonalities although reactivity to emotion may involve an immediate response while drug addiction control is the result of a complex outcome of brain elaborating activity. According to a simplified point of view addiction is the result of a hypersensitivity of the brain reward systems that escapes the control from PFC regions (Bechara, 2005; Koob et al. 2008). In fact it has been reported that during alcohol intoxication, together with a shift toward right versus left brain metabolic laterality, can be observed a shift in the predominance of activity from cortical to limbic brain regions (Volkow et al., 2008). The widespread nature of these brain changes may contribute to the marked disruption of behaviour, mood, cognition and motor activity induced by alcohol (Volkow et al., 2008) or other drugs of abuse (Goldstein and Volkow, 2011) and can cause degeneration in cortical areas deputed to controlling impulsivity in case of heavy alcohol use (Crews and Bottinger, 2009).

14. Concluding remarks

In summary it has been proposed that according to the theory of top-down control, the PFC and in particular the lateral PFC is responsible for controlling different domains of behavior (Cohen and Lieberman, 2010) regardless their content that may vary depending on the subcortical area involved. It may range from food intake, to drug addiction behaviour up to control of emotions and may explain why the effect of resource depletion are no tied to any one self-regulatory domain, as discussed by Heatherton and Wagner (2010). Among PFC areas many are definitively involved in drug addiction as well as in self-control and decision making. Nevertheless an interesting observation suggested that the PFC is involved in cognitive functions exceeding the sum of specific functions attributed to its subregions (Wilson et al., 2010). Thus if behaviour and decision making are considered as an overall result of PFC activity it is interesting to investigate the reason why self-control fails in drug addicts. Thus it could be hypothesized as mentioned before, that chronic exposure to a drug of abuse could disrupt the balance between cortical and sub-cortical activities but it is less clear why some people start taking drugs of abuse. Do they miss an unspecified activity in brain (genetic theory) or is the environment (psychological pressure and need to emulate companion behaviour to be accepted in the group), or is the sum of each factor to push to drug use. Fortunately, in the case of prevalence of the second factor drug taking may not necessarily lead to drug abuse. Considering that an optimal therapy for drug addiction is far to be proposed it remains to pursue prevention by involving young subject, and especially those at risk for drug use and abuse with involving activities in order to occupy brain activities in thoughts that are far from drug taking. Nevertheless drug therapy aimed at controlling drug taking impulse could be directed on improving the awareness of the consequences associated with pleasure directed behaviours and the capacity to take decisions directed to break the vicious circle of drug dependence.

Abbreviations

HPA, hypothalamic-pituitary-adrenal; NAcc Nucleus Accumbens; nAChRs, nicotinic acetylcholine receptors; OFC, orbitofrontal cortex; PFC, prefrontal cortex; PND, postnatal day; PNS, prenatal stress; VTA, ventral tegmental area.

Acknowledgements

This work has been supported by the Fondazione Banco di Sardegna, and by RAS Legge Regionale 7, 2007.

This work was supported by grants from Regione Autonoma della Sardegna (RAS: Legge 7 n° 2007) and from Fondazione Banco di Sardegna.

15. References

Abekawa T., Ohmori T., Ito K., Koyama T. (2000). D1 dopamine receptor activation reduces extracellular glutamate and GABA concentrations in the medial prefrontal cortex. *Brain Res.* 867, 250-254.

Adinoff B., Braud J., Devous M.D., Harris T.S. (2012). Caudolateral orbitofrontal regional cerebral blood flow is decreased in abstinent cocaine-addicted subjects in two separate cohorts. Addict Biol. In press

Adriani W., Chiarotti F., Laviola G. (1998). Elevated novelty seeking and peculiar d-amphetamine sensitization in periadolescent mice compared with adult mice. *Behav. Neurosci.*, 112, 152-1166.

Aggleton J.P. (2011). Multiple anatomical systems embedded within the primate medial temporal lobe: Implications for hippocampal function. *Neurosci Biobehav Rev.* in press.

Aghajanian GK. (2009). Modeling "psychosis" in vitro by inducing disordered neuronal network activity in cortical brain slices. *Psychopharmacology (Berl).* 206, 575-585.

Andersen S.L., Dumont N.L., Teicher M.H. (1997). Developmental differences in dopamine synthesis inhibition by (+/-)-7-OH-DPAT. *Naunyn Schmiedebergs Arch. Pharmacol.*, 356, 173-181.

Anderson S.A., Classey J.D., Condé F., Lund J.S., Lewis D.A. (1995). Synchronous development of pyramidal neuron dendritic spines and parvalbumin-immunoreactive chandelier neuron axon terminals in layer III of monkey prefrontal cortex. *Neuroscience, 67,* 7-22.

Aoki C., Venkatesan C., Go C.G., Forman R., Kurose H. (1998). Cellular and subcellular sites for noradrenergic action in the monkey dorsolateral prefrontal cortex as revealed by the immunocytochemical localization of noradrenergic receptors and axons. *Cereb. Cortex, 8,* 269-277.

Arana F.S., Parkinson J.A., Hinton E., Holland A.J., Owen A.M,. Roberts A.C. (2003). Dissociable contributions of the human amygdala and orbitofrontal cortex to incentive motivation and goal selection. *J Neurosci.* 23, 9632-9638.

Ariano M.A., Wang J., Noblett K.L., Larson E.R., Sibley D.R. (1997). Cellular distribution of the rat D4 dopamine receptor protein in the CNS using anti-receptor antisera. *Brain Res.,* 752, 26-34.

Arnsten A.F., Goldman-Rakic P.S. (1998). Noise stress impairs prefrontal cortical cognitive function in monkeys: evidence for a hyperdopaminergic mechanism. *Arch. Gen. Psychiatry,* 55, 362-368.

Arnsten A.F. (1999). Development of the cerebral cortex: XIV. Stress impairs prefrontal cortical function. *J. Am Acad. Child Adolesc. Psychiatry,* 38, 220-222.

Arnsten A.F. (2000). Through the looking glass: differential noradenergic modulation of prefrontal cortical function. *Neural Plast.,* 7, 133-146.

Arnsten A.F. (2004). Adrenergic targets for the treatment of cognitive deficits in schizophrenia. *Psychopharmacology,* 174, 25-31.

Arnsten A.F., Li B.M. (2005). Neurobiology of executive functions: catecholamine influences on prefrontal cortical functions. *Biol Psychiatry.* 57, 1377-1384.

Arnsten A.F. (2006). Fundamentals of attention-deficit/hyperactivity disorder: circuits and pathways. *J. Clin. Psychiatry,* 67, Suppl. 8, 7-12.

Arnsten A.F. (2007). Catecholamine and second messenger influences on prefrontal cortical networks of "representational knowledge": a rational bridge between genetics and the symptoms of mental illness. *Cereb. Cortex.,* 17, Suppl 1, 6-15.

Arnsten A.F. (2009). Toward a new understanding of attention-deficit hyperactivity disorder pathophysiology: an important role for prefrontal cortex dysfunction. *CNS Drugs.* 23 Suppl 1, 33-41.

Arnsten A.F. (2011). Catecholamine Influences on Dorsolateral Prefrontal Cortical Networks. Biol Psychiatry. 69, e89–e99.

Artiges E., Ricalens E., Berthoz S., Krebs M.O., Penttilä J., Trichard C., Martinot J.L. (2009) Exposure to smoking cues during an emotion recognition task can modulate limbic fMRI activation in cigarette smokers. *Addict Biol.* 14, 469-477.

Aston-Jones, G., Foote, S.L., Segal, M. (1985). Impulse conduction properties of noradrenergic locus coeruleus axons projecting to monkey cerebrocortex. *Neuroscience,* 15, 765-777.

Bannon M.J., Bunney E.B., Roth R.H. (1981). Mesocortical dopamine neurons: rapid transmitter turnover compared to other brain catecholamine systems. *Brain Res.,* 218, 376-382.

Barch DM, Ceaser A. (2012). Cognition in schizophrenia: core psychological and neural mechanisms. *Trends Cogn Sci.* 16, 27-34.

Barron S., White A., Swartzwelder H.S., Bell R.L., Rodd Z.A., Slawecki C.J., Ehlers C.L., Levin E.D., Rezvani A.H., Spear L.P. (2005). Adolescent vulnerabilities to chronic alcohol or nicotine exposure: findings from rodent models. *Alcohol Clin Exp Res.* 29, 1720-1725.

Bassareo V, Tanda G, Di Chiara G. (1995). Increase of extracellular dopamine in the medial prefrontal cortex during spontaneous and naloxone-precipitated opiate abstinence. *Psychopharmacology (Berl).* 122, 202-205.

Belujon P., Grace A.A. (2011). Hippocampus, amygdala, and stress: interacting systems that affect susceptibility to addiction. *Ann N Y Acad Sci.* 1216, 114-121.

Bechara A. (2005) Decision makin, impulse control and loss of willpower to resist drugs: a neurocognitive perspective. *Nat Neurosci* 8, 1445-1449.

Bechara A., Van Der Linden M. (2005). Decision-making and impulse control after frontal lobe injuries. *Curr Opin Neurol.* 18, 734-739.

Belin D, Everitt BJ (2008). Cocaine seeking habits depend upon dopamine-dependent serial connectivity linking the   ventral with the dorsal striatum. *Neuron*, 57, 432-441.

Belin D, Everitt BJ (2010) The Neural and Psychological Basis of a Compulsive Incentive Habit. In: Handbook of basal   ganglia structure and function, 20 (Steiner H, Tseng K, eds), pp 571-592. Elsvier, Academic Press.

Berglind W.J., See R.E., Fuchs R.A., Ghee S.M., Whitfield T.W. Jr., Miller S.W., McGinty J.F. (2007). A BDNF *infusion into the medial prefrontal cortex suppresses cocaine seeking in rats. Eur* J Neurosci. 26, 757-766.

Berridge K.C., Robinson T.E., Aldridge J.W. (2009). Dissecting components of reward: 'liking', 'wanting', and learning. *Curr Opin Pharmacol.* 9, 65-73.

Björklund, A., Lindvall, O. (1986) Catecholaminergic brain stem regulatory systems. In: Handbook of Physiology. The Nervous System IV: Intrinsic Regulatory Systems of the Brain, (pp 677-700). American Physiology Society, Washington.

Black Y.D., Maclaren F.R., Naydenov A.V., Carlezon W.A. Jr., Baxter M.G., Konradi C. (2006). Altered attention and prefrontal cortex gene expression in rats after binge-like exposure to cocaine during adolescence. *J Neurosci.* 26, 9656-965.

Bolla K.I., Eldreth D.A., London E.D., Kiehl K.A., Mouratidis M., Contoreggi C., Matochik J.A., Kurian V., Cadet J.L., Kimes A.S., Funderburk F.R., Ernst M. (2003). Orbitofrontal cortex dysfunction in abstinent cocaine abusers performing a decision-making task. *Neuroimage.* 19, 1085-1094.

Bonson K.R., Grant S.J., Contoreggi C.S., Links J.M., Metcalfe J., Weyl H.L., Kurian V., Ernst M., London E.D. (2002). Neural systems and cue-induced cocaine craving. *Neuropsychopharmacology.* 26, 376-386.

Bossert J.M., Stern A.L., Theberge F.R., Cifani C., Koya E., Hope B.T., Shaham Y. (2011). Ventral medial prefrontal cortex neuronal ensembles mediate context-induced relapse to heroin. *Nat Neurosci.* 14, 420-422.

Bossong M.G., Niesink R.J. (2010). Adolescent brain maturation, the endogenous cannabinoid system and the neurobiology of cannabis-induced schizophrenia. *Prog Neurobiol.* 92, 370-385.

Boudíková B., Szumlanski C., Maidak B., Weinshilboum R. (1990). Human liver catechol-O-methyltransferase pharmacogenetics. *Clin. Pharmacol. Ther.*, 48, 381-389.

Bouyer J.J., Joh T.H., Pickel V.M. (1984). Ultrastructural localization of tyrosine hydroxylase in rat nucleus accumbens. *J. Comp, Neurol.*, 227, 92-103.

Bowers M.S., McFarland K., Lake R.W., Peterson Y.K., Lapish C.C., Gregory M.L., Lanier S.M., Kalivas P.W. (2004). Activator of G protein signaling 3: a gatekeeper of cocaine sensitization and drug seeking. *Neuron.* 42, 269-281.

Breese GR, Sinha R, Heilig M. (2011). Chronic alcohol neuroadaptation and stress contribute to susceptibility for alcohol craving and relapse. *Pharmacol Ther.* 129, 149-171.

Breiter H.C., Aharon I., Kahneman D., Dale A., Shizgal P. (2001). Functional imaging of neural responses to expectancy and experience of monetary gains and losses. *Neuron,* 30, 619-639.

Briand L.A., Gritton H., Howe W.M., Young D.A., Sarter M. (2007). Modulators in concert for cognition: modulator interactions in the prefrontal cortex. *Prog Neurobiol.* 83, 69-91.

Brousse G., Vorspan F., Ksouda K., Bloch V., Peoc'h K., Laplanche J.L., Mouly S., Schmidt J., Llorca P.M., Lepine J.P. (2010). Could the inter-individual variability in cocaine-induced psychotic effects influence the development of cocaine addiction? Towards a new pharmacogenetic approach to addictions. *Med Hypotheses.* 75, 600-604.

Brown V.J., Bowman E.M. (2002). Rodent models of prefrontal cortical function. *Trends Neurosci.* 25, 340-343.

Brozoski T.J., Brown R.M., Rosvold H.E., Goldman P.S. (1979). Cognitive deficit caused by regional depletion of dopamine in prefrontal cortex of rhesus monkey. *Science,* 205, 929-932.

Burke K.A., Franz T.M., Miller D.N., Schoenbaum G. (2008) The role of the orbitofrontal cortex in the pursuit of happiness and more specific rewards. *Nature* 454, 340-344.

Capriles N., Rodaros D., Sorge R.E., Stewart J. (2003). A role for the prefrontal cortex in stress- and cocaine-induced reinstatement of cocaine seeking in rats. *Psychopharmacology (Berl)* 168, 66-74.

Carboni E., Imperato A., Perezzani L., Di Chiara G. (1989). Amphetamine, cocaine, phencyclidine and nomifensine increase extracellular dopamine concentrations preferentially in the nucleus accumbens of freely moving rats. *Neuroscience,* 28, 653-661.

Carboni E., Tanda G.L., Frau R., Di Chiara G. (1990). Blockade of the noradrenaline carrier increases extracellular dopamine concentrations in the prefrontal cortex: evidence that dopamine is taken up in vivo by noradrenergic terminals. *J. Neurochem.,* 55, 1067-1070.

Carboni E., Bortone L., Giua C., Di Chiara G. (2000). Dissociation of physical abstinence signs from changes in extracellular dopamine in the nucleus accumbens and in the prefrontal cortex of nicotine dependent rats. *Drug Alcohol Depend.* 58, 93-102.

Carboni E., Silvagni A., Rolando M.T., Di Chiara G. (2000). Stimulation of in vivo dopamine transmission in the bed nucleus of stria terminalis by reinforcing drugs. *J Neurosci.* 20, RC102.

Carboni E., Silvagni A., Vacca C., Di Chiara G. (2006). Cumulative effect of norepinephrine and dopamine carrier blockade on extracellular dopamine increase in the nucleus accumbens shell, bed nucleus of stria terminalis and prefrontal cortex. *J. Neurochem,* 96, 473-481.

Carboni E., Barros V.G., Ibba M., Silvagni A., Mura C., Antonelli M.C. (2010). Prenatal restraint stress: an in vivo microdialysis study on catecholamine release in the rat prefrontal cortex. *Neuroscience.* 168, 156-66.

Carr D.B., Sesack S.R. (2000a). Projections from the rat prefrontal cortex to the ventral tegmental area: target specificity in the synaptic associations with mesoaccumbens and mesocortical neurons. *J. Neurosci.,* 20, 3864-3873.

Carr D.B., Sesack, S.R. (2000b). GABA-containing neurons in the rat ventral tegmental area project to the prefrontal cortex. *Synapse,* 38, 114-23.

Casey BJ, Jones RM. (2010). Neurobiology of the adolescent brain and behavior: implications for substance use disorders. *J Am Acad Child Adolesc Psychiatry.* 49, 1189-1201;

Cass, W.A., Gerhardt, G.A. (1995). In vivo assessment of dopamine uptake in rat medial prefrontal cortex: comparison with dorsal striatum and nucleus accumbens. *J. Neurochem., 65,* 201-207.

Chambers R.A., Krystal J.H., Self D.W. (2001). A neurobiological basis for substance abuse comorbidity in schizophrenia. *Biol. Psychiatry,* 50, 71-83.

Chambers R.A., Taylor J.R., Potenza M.N. (2003). Developmental neurocircuitry of motivation in adolescence: a critical period of addiction vulnerability. *Am. J. Psychiatry, 160,* 1041-1052.

Chang J.Y., Janak P.H., Woodward D.J. (1998). Comparison of mesocorticolimbic neuronal responses during cocaine and heroin self-administration in freely moving rats. *J. Neurosci.* 18, 3098-3115.

Chugani H.T., Phelps M.E., Mazziotta J.C. (1987). Positron emission tomography study of human brain functional development. *Ann. Neurol., 22,* 487-497.

Ciccocioppo R., Sanna P.P., Weiss F. (2001). Cocaine-predictive stimulus induces drug-seeking behavior and neural activation in limbic brain regions after multiple months of abstinence: reversal by D(1) antagonists. *Proc Natl Acad Sci U S A.* 98, 1976-1981.

Cohen J.R. and Lieberman M.D. (2010). The common neural basis of exerting self-control in multiple domains. *In Self Control in Society, Mind, and Brain* (Hassin, R. et al., eds), pp. 141–162, Oxford University Press.

Cohn C.K., Axelrod J. (1971). The effect of estradiol on catechol-O-methyltransferase activity in rat liver. *Life Sci., 10,* 1351-1354.

Counotte D.S., Spijker S., Van de Burgwal L.H., Hogenboom F., Schoffelmeer A.N., De Vries T.J., Smit A.B., Pattij T. (2009). Long-lasting cognitive deficits resulting from adolescent nicotine exposure in rats. *Neuropsychopharmacology.* 34, 299-306.

Counotte D.S., Goriounova N.A., Li K.W., Loos M., van der Schors R.C., Schetters D., Schoffelmeer A.N., Smit A.B., Mansvelder H.D., Pattij T., Spijker S. (2011). Lasting synaptic changes underlie attention deficits caused by nicotine exposure during adolescence. *Nat Neurosci.* 14, 417-419.

Crews F., He J., Hodge C. (2007). Adolescent cortical development: a critical period of vulnerability for addiction. Pharmacol Biochem Behav. 86, 189-199.

Crews F.T., Boettiger C.A. (2009). Impulsivity, frontal lobes and risk for addiction. *Pharmacol Biochem Behav.* 93, 237-247.

Crombag H.S., Gorny G., Li Y., Kolb B., Robinson TE. (2005). Opposite effects of amphetamine self-administration experience on dendritic spines in the medial and orbital prefrontal cortex. *Cereb Cortex.* 15, 341-8.

Crombag H.S., Bossert J.M., Koya E., Shaham Y. (2008). Context-induced relapse to drug seeking: a review. *Philos Trans R Soc Lond B Biol Sci.* 363, 3233-3243.

Curtis C.E., Lee D. (2010). Beyond working memory: the role of persistent activity in decision making. *Trends Cogn Sci.* 14, 216-222.

Dagher A., Tannenbaum B., Hayashi T., Pruessner J.C., McBride D. (2009). An acute psychosocial stress enhances the neural response to smoking cues. *Brain Res.* 1293, 40-48.

Daglish M.R., Weinstein A., Malizia A.L., Wilson S., Melichar J.K., Britten S., Brewer C., Lingford-Hughes A., Myles J.S., Grasby P., Nutt D.J. (2001). Changes in regional cerebral blood flow elicited by craving memories in abstinent opiate-dependent subjects. *Am J Psychiatry.* 158, 1680-168.

Dahl R.E. (2004a). Adolescent brain development: a period of vulnerabilities and opportunities. Keynote address. *Ann. N. Y. Acad. Sci.,* 1021, 1-22.

Dahl R.E. (2004b). Adolescent development and the regulation of behavior and emotion: introduction to part VIII. *Ann. N. Y. Acad. Sci.,* 1021, 294-295.

Damasio H., Grabowski T., Frank R., Galaburda A.M., Damasio A.R. (1994). The return of Phineas Gage: clues about the brain from the skull of a famous patient. *Science, 264,* 1102-1105.

Davey C.G., Yücel M., Allen N.B. (2008). The emergence of depression in adolescence: development of the prefrontal cortex and the representation of reward. *Neurosci. Biobehav. Rev.,* 32, 1-19.

Davidson R.J., Pizzagalli D., Nitschke J.B., Putnam K. (2002). Depression: perspectives from affective neuroscience. *Annu. Rev. Psychol.* 53, 545-74.

De Bruin J.P., Sànchez-Santed F., Heinsbroek R.P., Donker A., Postmes P. (1994). A behavioural analysis of rats with damage to the medial prefrontal cortex using the Morris water maze: evidence for behavioural flexibility, but not for impaired spatial navigation. *Brain Res.* 652, 323-333.

Defagot M.C., Antonelli M.C. (1997a). Autoradiographic localization of the putative D4 dopamine receptor in rat brain. *Neurochem. Res.,* 22, 401-407.

Defagot M.C., Malchiodi E.L., Villar M.J., Antonelli M.C. (1997b) Distribution of D4 dopamine receptor in rat brain with sequence-specific antibodies. *Brain Res. Mol. Brain Res.,* 45, 1-12.

Del Campo N., Chamberlain S.R., Sahakian B.J., Robbins T.W. (2011). The roles of dopamine and noradrenaline in the pathophysiology and treatment of attention-deficit/hyperactivity disorder. *Biol Psychiatry.* 69, 145-57.

Del-Fava F., Hasue R.H., Ferreira J.G., Shammah-Lagnado S.J. (2007). Efferent connections of the rostral linear nucleus of the ventral tegmental area in the rat. *Neuroscience.* 145, 1059-1076.

Delgado M.R., Gillis M.M., Phelps E.A. (2008). Regulating the expectation of reward via cognitive strategies. *Nat Neurosci.* 11, 880-881.

Delmonico R.L., Hanley-Peterson P., Englander J. (1998). Group psychotherapy for persons with traumatic brain injury: management of frustration and substance abuse. *J. Head Trauma Rehabil.* 13, 10-22.

Deminière JM, Piazza PV, Guegan G, Abrous N, Maccari S, Le Moal M, Simon H. (1992) Increased locomotor response to novelty and propensity to intravenous amphetamine self-administration in adult offspring of stressed mothers. *Brain Res.* 586, 135-139.

Desimone R. (1995). Neuropsychology. Is dopamine a missing link? *Nature, 376,* 549-550.

Deutch A.Y., Roth R.H. (1990). The determinants of stress-induced activation of the prefrontal cortical dopamine system. *Prog. Brain Res.,* 85, 367-402.

Devoto P., Flore G., Pira L., Diana M., Gessa G.L. (2002). Co-release of noradrenaline and dopamine in the prefrontal cortex after acute morphine and during morphine withdrawal. *Psychopharmacology,* 160, 220-224.

Diamond A. (2007). Consequences of variations in genes that affect dopamine in prefrontal cortex. *Cereb. Cortex,* 17, Suppl 1, i161-i170.

Di Cara B., Panayi F., Gobert A., Dekeyne A., Sicard D., De Groote L., Millan M.J. (2006). Activation of dopamine D1 receptors enhances cholinergic transmission and social cognition: a parallel dialysis and behavioural study in rats. *Int J Neuropsychopharmacol.* 10, 383-399.

Di Chiara G. (2000). Role of dopamine in the behavioural actions of nicotine related to addiction. *Eur J Pharmacol.* 393, 295-314.

Di Chiara G., Bassareo V., Fenu S., De Luca M.A., Spina L., Cadoni C., Acquas E., Carboni E., Valentini V., Lecca D. (2004) Dopamine and drug addiction: the nucleus accumbens shell connection. *Neuropharmacology* 47, Suppl 1, 227-241.

Ding Z.M., Oster S.M., Hall S.R., Engleman E.A., Hauser S.R., McBride W.J., Rodd Z.A. (2011). The stimulating effects of ethanol on ventral tegmental area dopamine neurons projecting to the ventral pallidum and medial prefrontal cortex in female Wistar rats: regional difference and involvement of serotonin-3 receptors. *Psychopharmacology (Berl).* 216, 245-55.

Dom G., Sabbe B., Hulstijn W., van den Brink W. (2005). Substance use disorders and the orbitofrontal cortex: systematic review of behavioural decision-making and neuroimaging studies. *Br. J Psychiatry.* 187, 209-220.

Dorman C., Gaudiano P. (1998). Motivation in: Arbib, M.A. (Ed) The Handbook of Brain Theory and Neuronal Networks. (pp 189-226).Cambridge, Mass. MIT Press.

Dumontheil I, Roggeman C, Ziermans T, Peyrard-Janvid M, Matsson H, Kere J, Klingberg T. (2011). Influence of the COMT genotype on working memory and brain activity changes during development. *Biol Psychiatry.* 70, 222-229.

Erblich J., Lerman C., Self D.W., Diaz G.A., Bovbjerg D.H. (2004). Stress-induced cigarette craving: effects of the DRD2 TaqI RFLP and SLC6A3 VNTR polymorphisms. *Pharmacogenomics J.* 4, 102-109.

Everitt BJ, Robbins TW (2005). Neural systems of reinforcement for drug addiction: from actions to habits to compulsion.   *Nat Neurosci,* 8, 1481-1489.

Feinberg I. (1983). Schizophrenia: caused by a fault in programmed synaptic elimination during adolescence? *J. Psychiatr. Res.,* 17, 319-334.

Fibiger H.C. and Phillips A.G. (1988). Mesocorticolimbic dopamine systems and reward. *Ann. N. Y. Acad. Sci.* 537, 206-215.

Figner B., Knoch D., Johnson E.J., Krosch A.R., Lisanby S.H., Fehr E., Weber E.U. (2010). Lateral prefrontal cortex and self-control in intertemporal choice. *Nat Neurosci.* 13, 538-539.

Fineberg N.A., Potenza M.N., Chamberlain S.R., Berlin H.A., Menzies L., Bechara A., Sahakian B.J., Robbins T.W., Bullmore E.T., Hollander E. (2010). Probing compulsive and impulsive behaviors, from animal models to endophenotypes: a narrative review. Neuropsychopharmacology. 35, 591-604.

Foote S.L., Bloom F.E., Aston-Jones G. (1983). Nucleus locus coeruleus: new evidence of anatomical and physiological specificity. *Physiol. Rev.,* 63, 844-914.

Frankhuyzen A.L., Mulder A.H. (1980). Noradrenaline inhibits depolarization-induced 3H-serotonin release from slices of rat hippocampus. *Eur. J. Pharmacol.,* 63, 179-182.

Franklin T.R., Acton, P.D., Maldjian, J.A., Gray, J.D., Croft, J.R., Dackis, C.A., O'Brien, C.P., Childress, A.R. (2002). Decreased gray matter concentration in the insular, orbitofrontal, cingulate, and temporal cortices of cocaine patients. *Biol. Psychiatry,* 51, 134-142.

Fuchs R.A., Ramirez D.R., Bell G.H. (2008). Nucleus accumbens shell and core involvement in drug context-induced reinstatement of cocaine seeking in rats. *Psychopharmacology (Berl).* 200, 545-556.

Funahashi S., Inoue M., Kubota K. (1993). Delay-related activity in the primate prefrontal cortex during sequential reaching tasks with delay. *Neurosci. Res.,* 18, 171-175.

Gabbott PL, Warner TA, Jays PR, Salway P, Busby SJ (2005). Prefrontal cortex in the rat: projections to subcortical autonomic, motor, and limbic centers. *J Comp Neurol,* 492, 145-177.

Gallagher M., McMahan R.W., Schoenbaum G. (1999). Orbitofrontal cortex and representation of incentive value in associative learning. *J Neurosci.* 19, 6610-4.

Garris P.A., Collins L.B., Jones S.R., Wightman R.M. (1993). Evoked extracellular dopamine in vivo in the medial prefrontal cortex. *J. Neurochem.,* 61, 637-647.

Garris P.A., Wightman R.M. (1994). Different kinetics govern dopaminergic transmission in the amygdala, prefrontal cortex, and striatum: An in vivo voltammetric study. *J. Neurosci,* 14, 442-450.

Geijo-Barrientos E., Pastore C. (1995). The effects of dopamine on the subthreshold electrophysiological responses of rat prefrontal cortex neurons in vitro. *Eur. J. Neurosci.,* 7, 358-366.

George O., Koob G.F. (2010). Individual differences in prefrontal cortex function and the transition from drug use to drug dependence. *Neurosci Biobehav Rev.* 35, 232-247.

Giedd J.N., Jeffries, N.O., Blumenthal J., Castellanos F.X., Vaituzis A.C., Fernandez T., Hamburger S.D., Liu H., Nelson J., Bedwell J., Tran L., Lenane M., Nicolson R., Rapoport J.L. (1999a). Childhood-onset schizophrenia: progressive brain changes during adolescence. *Biol. Psychiatry,* 46, 892-898.

Giedd J.N., Blumenthal J., Jeffries N.O., Castellanos F.X., Liu H., Zijdenbos A., Paus T., Evans A.C., Rapoport J.L. (1999b). Brain development during childhood and adolescence: a longitudinal MRI study. *Nat. Neurosci.,* 2, 861-863.

Gioanni Y., Rougeot C., Clarke P.B., Lepousé C., Thierry A.M., Vidal C. (1999). Nicotinic receptors in the rat prefrontal cortex: increase in glutamate release and facilitation of mediodorsal thalamo-cortical transmission. *Eur J Neurosci.* 11, 18-30.

Goldstein L.E., Rasmusson A.M., Bunney B.S., Roth R.H. (1996). Role of the amygdala in the coordination of behavioral, neuroendocrine, and prefrontal cortical monoamine responses to psychological stress in the rat. *J Neurosci.* 16, 4787-4798.

Goldstein RZ, Craig AD, Bechara A, Garavan H, Childress AR, Paulus MP, Volkow ND (2009). The neurocircuitry of impaired insight in drug addiction. *Trends Cogn Sci.* 13, 372-380.

Goldstein R.Z., Volkow N.D. (2002). Drug addiction and its underlying neurobiological basis: neuroimaging evidence for the involvement of the frontal cortex. *Am J Psychiatry.* 159, 1642-52.

Goldstein R.Z., Volkow N.D. (2011). Dysfunction of the prefrontal cortex in addiction: neuroimaging findings and clinical implications. *Nat Rev Neurosci.* 12, 652-669.

Granon S., Passetti F., Thomas K.L., Dalley J.W., Everitt B.J., Robbins T.W. (2000). Enhanced and impaired attentional performance after infusion of D1 dopaminergic receptor agents into rat prefrontal cortex. *J. Neurosci.,* 20, 1208-1215.

Grant S., Contoreggi C., London ED. (2000). Drug abusers show impaired performance in a laboratory test of decision making. *Neuropsychologia.* 38, 1180-1187.

Greengard P. (2001). The neurobiology of slow synaptic transmission. *Science, 294,* 1024-1030.

Grobin A.C., Deutch A.Y. (1998). Dopaminergic regulation of extracellular gamma-aminobutyric acid levels in the prefrontal cortex of the rat. *J. Pharmacol. Exp. Ther.,* 285, 350-357.

Gulledge A.T., Jaffe D.B. (1998). Dopamine decreases the excitability of layer V pyramidal cells in the rat prefrontal cortex. *J. Neurosci.,* 18, 9139-9151.

Haber S.N., Knutson B. (2010). The reward circuit: linking primate anatomy and human imaging. *Neuropsychopharmacology.* 35, 4-26.

Gruber AJ, Calhoon GG, Shusterman I, Schoenbaum G, Roesch MR, O'Donnell P (2010). More is less: a disinhibited prefrontal cortex impairs cognitive flexibility. *J Neurosci.* 30, 17102-17110.

Hains A.B., Arnsten A.F. (2008). Molecular mechanisms of stress-induced prefrontal cortical impairment: implications for mental illness. *Learn Mem.* 15, 551-564.

Hallman H., Jonsson G. (1984). Neurochemical studies on central dopamine neurons--regional characterization of dopamine turnover. *Med. Biol.,* 62, 198-209.

Hamlin A.S., Clemens K.J., McNally G.P. (2008). Renewal of extinguished cocaine-seeking. *Neuroscience.* 151, 659-670.

Harte M., O'Connor W.T. (2004). Evidence for a differential medial prefrontal dopamine D1 and D2 receptor regulation of local and ventral tegmental glutamate and GABA release: a dual probe microdialysis study in the awake rat. *Brain Res.* 1017, 120-9.

Harvey R.C., Dembro K.A., Rajagopalan K., Mutebi M.M., Kantak K.M. (2009). Effects of self-administered cocaine in adolescent and adult male rats on orbitofrontal cortex-related neurocognitive functioning. *Psychopharmacology (Berl).* 206, 61-71

Heatherton T.F., Wagner D.D. (2011). Cognitive neuroscience of self-regulation failure. *Trends Cogn Sci.* 15, 132-139.

Heidbreder C.A., Groenewegen H.J. (2003). The medial prefrontal cortex in the rat: evidence for a dorso-ventral distinction based upon functional and anatomical characteristics. *Neurosci Biobehav Rev.* 27, 555-79.

Heinz A., Smolka,M.N. (2006). The effects of catechol O-methyltransferase genotype on brain activation elicited by affective stimuli and cognitive tasks. *Rev. Neurosci.,* 17, 359-367.

Hiscock R., Bauld L., Amos A., Fidler J.A., Munafò M. (2012). Socioeconomic status and smoking: a review. Ann N Y Acad Sci. 1248, 107-123.

Holmes A, Wellman CL. (2009). Stress-induced prefrontal reorganization and executive dysfunction in rodents. *Neurosci Biobehav Rev. 33,* 773-783.

Hosák L., Libiger J., Cizek J., Beránek M., Cermáková E. (2006). The COMT Val158Met polymorphism is associated with novelty seeking in Czech methamphetamine abusers: preliminary results. *Neuro Endocrinol Lett.* 27, 799-802.

Insel T.R., Miller L.P., Gelhard R.E. (1990). The ontogeny of excitatory amino acid receptors in rat forebrain--I. N-methyl-D-aspartate and quisqualate receptors. *Neuroscience,* 35, 31-43.

Jacobus J., McQueeny T., Bava S., Schweinsburg B.C., Frank L.R., Yang T.T., Tapert S.F. (2009). White matter integrity in adolescents with histories of marijuana use and binge drinking. *Neurotoxicol Teratol.* 31, 349-355.

Joel D., Doljansky J., Schiller D. (2005). 'Compulsive' lever pressing in rats is enhanced following lesions to the orbital cortex, but not to the basolateral nucleus of the amygdala or to the dorsal medial prefrontal cortex. *Eur J Neurosci.* 21, 2252-2262.

Kalivas P.W., Volkow N., Seamans J. (2005). Unmanageable motivation in addiction: a pathology in prefrontal-accumbens glutamate transmission. *Neuron.* 45, 647-650.

Kalivas P.W., Volkow N.D. (2005). The neural basis of addiction: a pathology of motivation and choice. *Am J Psychiatry.* 162, 1403-1413.

Kalivas P.W., Volkow N.D. (2011). New medications for drug addiction hiding in glutamatergic neuroplasticity. *Mol Psychiatry.* 16, 974-86.

Kalsbeek A., Voorn P., Buijs R.M., Pool C.W., Uylings H.B. (1988). Development of the dopaminergic innervation in the prefrontal cortex of the rat. *J. Comp. Neurol.*, 269, 58-72.

Karler R., Calder L.D., Thai D.K., Bedingfield J.B. (1998). The role of dopamine and GABA in the frontal cortex of mice in modulating a motor-stimulant effect of amphetamine and cocaine. *Pharmacol. Biochem. Behav.*, 60, 237-244.

Karoum F., Chrapusta S.J., Egan M.F. (1994). 3-Methoxytyramine is the major metabolite of released dopamine in the rat frontal cortex: reassessment of the effects of antipsychotics on the dynamics of dopamine release and metabolism in the frontal cortex, nucleus accumbens, and striatum by a simple two pool model. *J. Neurochem.*, 63, 972-979.

Karreman M., Moghaddam B. (1996). The prefrontal cortex regulates the basal release of dopamine in the limbic striatum: an effect mediated by ventral tegmental area. *J. Neurochem.*, 66, 589-598.

Kendler K.S., Prescott C.A. (1998). Cocaine use, abuse and dependence in a population-based sample of female twins. *Br J Psychiatry.* 173, 345-350.

Kendler K.S., Karkowski L.M., Neale M.C., Prescott C.A. (2000). Illicit psychoactive substance use, heavy use, abuse, and dependence in a US population-based sample of male twins. *Arch Gen Psychiatry.* 57, 261-269.

Kennerley SW, Walton ME. (2011). Decision making and reward in frontal cortex: *Behav Neurosci.* 125, 297-317.

Khan ZU, Muly EC. (2011). Molecular mechanisms of working memory. *Behav Brain Res.* 219, 329-341.

Kippin T.E., Szumlinski K.K., Kapasova Z. Rezner B., See R.E. (2008). Prenatal stress enhances responsiveness to cocaine. *Neuropsychopharmacology.* 33, 769-782.

Kober H., Mende-Siedlecki P., Kross E.F., Weber J., Mischel W., Hart C.L., Ochsner K.N. (2010). Prefrontal-striatal pathway underlies cognitive regulation of craving. *Proc Natl Acad Sci U S A.* 107, 14811-14816.

Koob G.F. (2008). A role for brain stress systems in addiction. *Neuron.* 59(1), 11-34.

Koob G.F., Volkow N.D. (2010). Neurocircuitry of addiction. *Neuropsychopharmacology.* 35, 217-238.

Koya E., Uejima J.L., Wihbey K.A., Bossert J.M., Hope B.T., Shaham Y. (2009). Role of ventral medial prefrontal cortex in incubation of cocaine craving. *Neuropharmacology.* 56 (S 1), 177-185.

Krampe H., Ehrenreich H. (2010). Supervised disulfiram as adjunct to psychotherapy in alcoholism treatment. *Curr Pharm Des.* 16, 2076-2090.

LaLumiere R.T., Kalivas P.W. (2008). Glutamate release in the nucleus accumbens core is necessary for heroin seeking. *J Neurosci.* 28, 3170-3177.

Lammel S., Hetzel A., Häckel O., Jones I., Liss B., Roeper J. (2008). Unique properties of mesoprefrontal neurons within a dual mesocorticolimbic dopamine system. *Neuron*, 57, 760-773.

Langleben D.D., Ruparel K., Elman I., Busch-Winokur S., Pratiwadi R., Loughead J., O'Brien C.P., Childress A.R. (2008). Acute effect of methadone maintenance dose on brain FMRI response to heroin-related cues. *Am J Psychiatry*. 165, 390-394.

Lewis D.A. (1997). Development of the prefrontal cortex during adolescence: insights into vulnerable neural circuits in schizophrenia. *Neuropsychopharmacology, 16*, 385-398.

Lewis D.A., Sesack S.R., Levey A.I., Rosenberg D.R. (1998). Dopamine axons in primate prefrontal cortex: specificity of distribution, synaptic targets, and development. *Adv. Pharmacol., 42*, 703-706.

Liu X., Vaupel D.B., Grant S., London E.D. (1998a). Effect of cocaine-related environmental stimuli on the spontaneous electroencephalogram in polydrug abusers. *Neuropsychopharmacology, 19*, 10-17.

Liu X., Matochik J.A., Cadet J.L., London E.D. (1998b). Smaller volume of prefrontal lobe in polysubstance abusers: a magnetic resonance imaging study. *Neuropsychopharmacology, 18*, 243-252.

Livingstone P.D., Dickinson J.A., Srinivasan J., Kew J.N., Wonnacott S. (2010). Glutamate-dopamine crosstalk in the rat prefrontal cortex is modulated by Alpha7 nicotinic receptors and potentiated by PNU-120596. *J Mol Neurosci.* 40, 172-176.

Lopez-Larson M.P., Bogorodzki P., Rogowska J., McGlade E., King J.B., Terry J., Yurgelun-Todd D. (2011). Altered prefrontal and insular cortical thickness in adolescent marijuana users. *Behav Brain Res.* 220, 164-172.

Loughlin S.E., Foote S.L., Fallon J.H. (1982). Locus coeruleus projections to cortex: topography, morphology and collateralization. *Brain Res. Bull., 9*, 287-294.

Luft A.R., Schwarz S. (2009). Dopaminergic signals in primary motor cortex. *Int J Dev Neurosci.* 27, 415-421.

Malone D.T., Hill M.N., Rubino T. (2010). Adolescent cannabis use and psychosis: epidemiology and neurodevelopmental models. *Br J Pharmacol.* 160, 511-522.

Marchant N.J., Millan E.Z., McNally G.P. (2012). The hypothalamus and the neurobiology of drug seeking. *Cell Mol Life Sci.* 69, 581-597.

Markou A. (2008). Review. Neurobiology of nicotine dependence. *Philos Trans R Soc Lond B Biol Sci.* 363, 3159-3168.

Markram H., Toledo-Rodriguez M., Wang Y., Gupta A., Silberberg G., Wu C.(2004). Interneurons of the neocortical inhibitory system. *Nat Rev Neurosci.* 5, 793-807.

Martig A.K., Mizumori S.J. (2011). Ventral tegmental area disruption selectively affects CA1/CA2 but not CA3 place fields during a differential reward working memory task. *Hippocampus.* 21, 172-184.

Mathews IZ, McCormick CM. (2011). Role of medial prefrontal cortex dopamine in age differences in response to amphetamine in rats: Locomotor activity after intra-mPFC injections of dopaminergic ligands. *Dev Neurobiol.* In press

Maura G., Gemignani A., Raiteri M. (1982). Noradrenaline inhibits central serotonin release through alpha 2-adrenoceptors located on serotonergic nerve terminals. *Naunyn Schmiedebergs Arch. Pharmacol., 320*, 272-274.

McFarland K., Kalivas P.W. (2001). The circuitry mediating cocaine-induced reinstatement of drug-seeking behavior. *J Neurosci.* 21, 8655-8663.

McFarland K., Lapish C.C., Kalivas P.W. (2003). Prefrontal glutamate release into the core of the nucleus accumbens mediates cocaine-induced reinstatement of drug-seeking behavior. *J Neurosci.* 23, 3531-3537.

McQueeny T., Schweinsburg B.C., Schweinsburg A.D., Jacobus J., Bava S., Frank L.R., Tapert S.F. (2009). Altered white matter integrity in adolescent binge drinkers. Alcohol *Clin Exp Res.* 33, 1278-1285.

Melrose R.J., Ettenhofer M.L., Harwood D., Achamallah N., Campa O., Mandelkern M., Sultzer DL. (2011). Cerebral metabolism, cognition, and functional abilities in Alzheimer disease. *J Geriatr Psychiatry Neurol.* 24, 127-34.

Mercuri N., Bernardi G., Calabresi P., Cotugno A., Levi G., Stanzione P. (1985). Dopamine decreases cell excitability in rat striatal neurons by pre- and postsynaptic mechanisms. *Brain Res.,* 358, 110-121.

Mercuri N.B., Calabresi P., Bernardi G. (1992). The electrophysiological actions of dopamine and dopaminergic drugs on neurons of the substantia nigra pars compacta and ventral tegmental area. *Life Sci.* 51, 711-718.

Millan E.Z., Marchant N.J., McNally G.P. (2011). Extinction of drug seeking. *Behav Brain Res.* 217, 454-462.

Miller E.K., Erickson C.A., Desimone R. (1996). Neural mechanisms of visual working memory in prefrontal cortex of the macaque. *J. Neurosci.,* 16, 5154-5167.

Miller E.J., Saint Marie L.R., Breier M.R., Swerdlow N.R. (2010). Pathways from the ventral hippocampus and caudal amygdala to forebrain regions that regulate sensorimotor gating in the rat. *Neuroscience.* 165, 601-611.

Morilak D.A., Barrera G., Echevarria D.J., Garcia A.S., Hernandez A., Ma S., Petre C.O. (2005). Role of brain norepinephrine in the behavioral response to stress. *Prog Neuropsychopharmacol Biol. Psychiatry,* 29, 1214-1224.

Mrzljak L., Bergson C., Pappy M., Huff R., Levenson R., Goldman-Rakic PS. (1996) Localization of dopamine D4 receptors in GABAergic neurons of the primate brain. *Nature,* 381, 245-248.

Narita M., Matsushima Y., Niikura K., Narita M., Takagi S., Nakahara K., Kurahashi K., Abe M., Saeki M., Asato M., Imai S., Ikeda K., Kuzumaki N., Suzuki T. (2010). Implication of dopaminergic projection from the ventral tegmental area to the anterior cingulate cortex in μ-opioid-induced place preference. *Addict Biol.* 15, 434-47.

Nestler E.J. (2005) Is there a common molecular pathway for addiction? *Nature Neurosci* 8, 1445-1449.

Nixon K., McClain J.A. (2010). Adolescence as a critical window for developing an alcohol use disorder: current findings in neuroscience. *Curr Opin Psychiatry.* 23, 227-232.

Oades R.D., Halliday G.M. (1987). Ventral tegmental (A10) system: neurobiology. 1. Anatomy and connectivity. *Brain Res.* 434, 117-165.

O'Connor EC, Chapman K, Butler P, Mead AN. (2010). The predictive validity of the rat self-administration model for abuse liability. *Neurosci Biobehav Rev.* 35, 912-938.

O'Dell LE. (2009). A psychobiological framework of the substrates that mediate nicotine use during adolescence. *Neuropharmacology.* 56 Suppl 1, 263-78.

O'Donnell P. (2010). Adolescent maturation of cortical dopamine. *Neurotox Res.* 18, 306-312.

O'Donnell P, Lavín A, Enquist LW, Grace AA, Card JP. (1997). Interconnected parallel circuits between rat nucleus accumbens and thalamus revealed by retrograde transynaptic transport of pseudorabies virus. *J Neurosci.* 17, 2143-2167.

Omelchenko N., Sesack S.R. (2007). Glutamate synaptic inputs to ventral tegmental area neurons in the rat derive primarily from subcortical sources. *Neuroscience,* 146, 1259-1274.

Ommaya A.K., Salazar A.M., Dannenberg A.L., Ommaya A.K., Chervinsky A.B., Schwab K. (1996). Outcome after traumatic brain injury in the U.S. military medical system. *J. Trauma.* 41, 972-975.

Oropeza VC, Mackie K, Van Bockstaele EJ. (2006). Cannabinoid receptors are localized to noradrenergic axon terminals in the rat frontal cortex. *Brain Res.* 1127,36-44.

Papp E., Borhegyi Z., Tomioka R., Rockland K.S., Mody I., Freund T.F. (2012). Glutamatergic input from specific sources influences the nucleus accumbens-ventral pallidum information flow. *Brain Struct Funct.* 217, 37-48.

Park W.K., Bari A.A., Jey A.R., Anderson S.M., Spealman R.D., Rowlett J.K., Pierce R.C. (2002). Cocaine administered into the medial prefrontal cortex reinstates cocaine-seeking behavior by increasing AMPA receptor-mediated glutamate transmission in the nucleus accumbens. *J Neurosci.* 22, 2916-2925.

Paus T., Zijdenbos A., Worsley K., Collins D.L., Blumenthal J., Giedd J.N., Rapoport J.L., Evans A.C. (1999). Structural maturation of neural pathways in children and adolescents: in vivo study. *Science,* 283, 1908-1911.

Penit-Soria J., Audinat E., Crepel F. (1987). Excitation of rat prefrontal cortical neurons by dopamine: an in vitro electrophysiological study. *Brain Res.,* 425, 263-274.

Peters J., LaLumiere R.T., Kalivas P.W. (2008). Infralimbic prefrontal cortex is responsible for inhibiting cocaine seeking in extinguished rats. *J Neurosci. 28 (23),* 6046-53.

Peters J., Kalivas P.W., Quirk G.J. (2009). Extinction circuits for fear and addiction overlap in prefrontal cortex. *Learn Mem.* 16, 279-288.

Piazza PV, Rougé-Pont F, Deroche V, Maccari S, Simon H, Le Moal M. (1996). Glucocorticoids have state-dependent stimulant effects on the mesencephalic dopaminergic transmission. Proc Natl Acad Sci U S A. 93, 8716-8720.

Piazza PV, Le Moal ML. (1998). Pathophysiological basis of vulnerability to drug abuse: role of an interaction between stress, glucocorticoids, and dopaminergic neurons. Annu Rev Pharmacol Toxicol. 36, 359-378.

Pirot S., Godbout R., Mantz J., Tassin J.P., Glowinski J., Thierry A.M. (1992). Inhibitory effects of ventral tegmental area stimulation on the activity of prefrontal cortical neurons: evidence for the involvement of both dopaminergic and GABAergic components. *Neuroscience,* 49, 857-865.

Poorthuis R.B., Goriounova N.A., Couey J.J., Mansvelder H.D. (2009). Nicotinic actions on neuronal networks for cognition: general principles and long-term consequences. *Biochem Pharmacol.* 78, 668-676.

Popova S., Mohapatra S., Patra J., Duhig A., Rehm J. (2011). A literature review of cost-enefit analyses for the treatment of alcohol dependence. *Int J Environ Res Public Health.* 8, 3351-3364.

Potenza MN, Hong KI, Lacadie CM, Fulbright RK, Tuit KL, Sinha R. Neural correlates of stress-induced and cue-induced drug craving: influences of sex and cocaine dependence. *Am J Psychiatry.* 169, 406-414.

Radley J.J., Williams B., Sawchenko P.E. (2008). Noradrenergic innervation of the dorsal medial prefrontal cortex modulates hypothalamo-pituitary-adrenal responses to acute emotional stress. *J. Neurosci.,* 28, 5806-5816.

Rakic P., Bourgeois J.P., Goldman-Rakic P.S. (1994). Synaptic development of the cerebral cortex: implications for learning, memory, and mental illness. *Prog. Brain Res.*, 102, 227-243.

Reinhard J.F. Jr, Bannon M.J., Roth R.H. (1982). Acceleration by stress of dopamine synthesis and metabolism in prefrontal cortex: antagonism by diazepam. *Naunyn Schmiedebergs Arch. Pharmacol.*, 318, 374-377.

Rétaux S., Besson M.J., Penit-Soria J. (1991). Opposing effects of dopamine D2 receptor stimulation on the spontaneous and the electrically evoked release of [3H]GABA on rat prefrontal cortex slices. *Neuroscience*, 42, 61-71.

Reynolds SM, Zahm DS (2005). Specificity in the projections of prefrontal and insular cortex to ventral striatopallidum and the extended amygdala. *J Neurosci*. 14, 25, 11757-11767.

Robbins T.W. (2002). The 5-choice serial reaction time task: behavioural pharmacology and functional neurochemistry. *Psychopharmacology*, 163, 362-380.

Robinson T.E., Kolb B. (1999). Alterations in the morphology of dendrites and dendritic spines in the nucleus accumbens and prefrontal cortex following repeated treatment with amphetamine or cocaine. *Eur J Neurosci*. 11, 1598-1604.

Roth R.H., Tam S.Y., Ida Y., Yang J.X., Deutch A.Y. (1988). Stress and the mesocorticolimbic dopamine systems. *Ann. N. Y. Acad. Sci.*, 537, 138-147.

Rozeske R.R., Der-Avakian A., Bland S.T., Beckley J.T., Watkins L.R., Maier S.F. (2009). The medial prefrontal cortex regulates the differential expression of morphine-conditioned place preference following a single exposure to controllable or uncontrollable stress. *Neuropsychopharmacology*. 34, 834-843.

Rutherford L.C., Nelson S.B., Turrigiano G.G. (1998). BDNF has opposite effects on the quantal amplitude of pyramidal neuron and interneuron excitatory synapses. *Neuron*, 21, 521-530.

Schenk S., Horger B.A., Peltier R., Shelton K. (1991). Supersensitivity to the reinforcing effects of cocaine following 6-hydroxydopamine lesions to the medial prefrontal cortex in rats. *Brain Res*. 543, 227-235.

Schoenbaum G., Saddoris M.P., Ramus S.J., Shaham Y., Setlow B. (2004). Cocaine-experienced rats exhibit learning deficits in a task sensitive to orbitofrontal cortex lesions. *Eur J Neurosci*. 19, 1997-2002.

Schoenbaum G., Roesch M.R., Stalnaker T.A. (2006). Orbitofrontal cortex, decision-making and drug addiction. *Trends Neurosci*. 29, 116-124.

Schoenbaum G., Roesch M.R., Stalnaker T.A., Takahashi Y.K. (2009). A new perspective on the role of the orbitofrontal cortex in adaptive behaviour. Nat *Rev Neurosci*. 10, 885-892.

Schramm-Sapyta N.L., Walker Q.D., Caster J.M., Levin E.D., Kuhn C.M. (2009). Are adolescents more vulnerable to drug addiction than adults? Evidence from animal models. *Psychopharmacology (Berl)*. 206, 1-21.

Schultz W. (2010). Multiple functions of dopamine neurons. *F1000 Biol Rep*. 2, pii: 2.

Schultz W. (2011). Potential vulnerabilities of neuronal reward, risk, and decision mechanisms to addictive drugs. *Neuron*. 69, 603-617.

Schulz S. (2011). MDMA & cannabis: a mini-review of cognitive, behavioral, and neurobiological effects of co-consumption. Curr Drug Abuse Rev. 4, 81-86.

Schweinsburg A.D., Schweinsburg B.C,. Nagel B.J., Eyler L.T., Tapert S.F. (2011). Neural correlates of verbal learning in adolescent alcohol and marijuana users. *Addiction.* 106, 564-573

Seamans J.K.and Yang C.R. (2004). The principal features and mechanisms of dopamine modulation in the prefrontal cortex. *Prog. Neurobiol.* 74, 1-58.

See R.E. (2009). Dopamine D1 receptor antagonism in the prelimbic cortex blocks the reinstatement of heroin-seeking in an animal model of relapse. *Int J Neuropsychopharmacol.* 12, 431-436.

Sellitto M., Ciaramelli E., di Pellegrino G. (2010). Myopic discounting of future rewards after medial orbitofrontal damage in humans. *J Neurosci.* 30, 16429-16436.

Sesack S.R., Pickel V.M. (1992). Prefrontal cortical efferents in the rat synapse on unlabeled neuronal targets of catecholamine terminals in the nucleus accumbens septi and on dopamine neurons in the ventral tegmental area. *J. Comp. Neurol.,* 8, 145-160.

Sesack S.R., Hawrylak V.A., Guido M.A., Levey A.I. (1998). Cellular and subcellular localization of the dopamine transporter in rat cortex. *Adv. Pharmacol.,* 42, 171-174.

Shaham Y., Stewart J. (1995). Stress reinstates heroin-seeking in drug-free animals: an effect mimicking heroin, not withdrawal. *Psychopharmacology (Berl).* 119, 334-341.

Shaham Y., Shalev U., Lu L., De Wit H., Stewart J. (2003). The reinstatement model of drug relapse: history, methodology and major findings. *Psychopharmacology (Berl).* 168, 3-20.

Shansky R.M., Glavis-Bloom C., Lerman D., McRae P., Benson C., Miller K., Cosand L., Horvath T.L., Arnsten A.F. (2004). Estrogen mediates sex differences in stress-induced prefrontal cortex dysfunction. *Mol. Psychiatry,* 9, 531-538.

Shiffman S., Waters A., Hickcox M. (2004). The nicotine dependence syndrome scale: a multidimensional measure of nicotine dependence. *Nicotine Tob Res.* 6, 327-348.

Shimamura A.P. (2000). Toward a cognitive neuroscience of metacognition. *Conscious Cogn.* 9(2 Pt 1), 313-323.

Shors T.J., Miesegaes G. (2002). Testosterone in utero and at birth dictates how stressful experience will affect learning in adulthood. *Proc. Natl. Acad. Sci. U S A,* 99, 13955-13960.

Shors T.J., Leuner B. (2003). Estrogen-mediated effects on depression and memory formation in females. *J. Affect. Disord.,* 74, 85-96.

Shorter D., Kosten T.R. (2011). Novel pharmacotherapeutic treatments for cocaine addiction. *BMC Med.* 9, 119.

Silvagni A, Barros VG, Mura C, Antonelli MC, Carboni E (2008). Prenatal restraint stress differentially modifies basal and stimulated dopamine and noradrenaline release in the nucleus accumbens shell: an 'in vivo' microdialysis study in adolescent and young adult rats. *Eur J Neurosci.* 28, 744-758.

Simkin D.R., Grenoble S. (2010). Pharmacotherapies for adolescent substance use disorders. *Child Adolesc Psychiatr Clin N Am.* 19, 591-608.

Smolka M.N., Schumann G., Wrase J., Grüsser S.M., Flor H., Mann K., Braus D.F., Goldman D., Büchel C., Heinz A. (2005). Catechol-O-methyltransferase val158met genotype affects processing of emotional stimuli in the amygdala and prefrontal cortex. *J. Neurosci.,* 25, 836-842.

Sofuoglu M. (2010). Cognitive enhancement as a pharmacotherapy target for stimulant addiction. *Addiction.* 105, 38-48.

Spear L.P., Brake S.C. (1983). Periadolescence: age-dependent behavior and psychopharmacological responsivity in rats. *Dev. Psychobiol.,* 16, 83-109.

Spear L.P., Varlinskaya E.I. (2005). Adolescence. Alcohol sensitivity, tolerance, and intake. *Recent Dev Alcohol.* 17, 143-59.

Steinberg L. (2008). A Neurobehavioral Perspective on Adolescent Risk-Taking. *Dev. Rev.,* 28, 78-106.

Stewart J. (2003). Stress and relapse to drug seeking: studies in laboratory animals shed light on mechanisms and sources of long-term vulnerability. *Am J Addict.* 12, 1-17.

Sullivan R.M., Brake, W.G. (2003). What the rodent prefrontal cortex can teach us about attention-deficit/hyperactivity disorder: the critical role of early developmental events on prefrontal function. *Behav. Brain Res.* 146, 43-55.

Sullivan R.M. (2004) Hemispheric asymmetry in stress processing in rat prefrontal cortex and the role of mesocortical dopamine. *Stress,* 7,131-143.

Sun W., Rebec G.V. (2005). The role of prefrontal cortex D1-like and D2-like receptors in cocaine-seeking behavior in rats. *Psychopharmacology (Berl).* 177, 315-323.

Swanson L.W. (1976). The locus coeruleus: a cytoarchitectonic, Golgi and immunohistochemical study in the albino rat. *Brain Res.,* 110, 39–56.

Swan G.E., Denk C.E., Parker S.D., Carmelli D., Furze C.T., Rosenman R.H. (1988). Risk factors for late relapse in male and female ex-smokers. *Addict Behav.* 13, 253-266.

Tanda G., Pontieri F.E., Frau R., Di Chiara G. (1997). Contribution of blockade of the noradrenaline carrier to the increase of extracellular dopamine in the rat prefrontal cortex by amphetamine and cocaine. *Eur. J. Neurosci.,* 9, 2077-2085.

Thierry A.M. (1972). Effect of stress on various characteristics of norepinephrine metabolism in central noradrenergic neurons. *Adv. Exp. Med. Biol.,* 33, 501-508.

Tseng KY, O'Donnell P (2007). D2 dopamine receptors recruit a GABA component for their attenuation of excitatory synaptic transmission in the adult rat prefrontal cortex. *Synapse.* 61, 843-850.

Tzschentke T.M. (2001). Pharmacology and behavioral pharmacology of the mesocortical dopamine system. *Prog. Neurobiol.,* 63, 241-320.

Van den Oever M.C., Spijker S., Smit A.B., De Vries T.J. (2010). Prefrontal cortex plasticity mechanisms in drug seeking and relapse. *Neurosci Biobehav Rev.* 35, 276-284.

Van Schouwenburg M., Aarts E., Cools R. (2010). Dopaminergic modulation of cognitive control: distinct roles for the prefrontal cortex and the basal ganglia. *Curr Pharm Des.* 16, 2026-2032.

Ventura R., Alcaro A., Puglisi-Allegra S. (2005). Prefrontal cortical norepinephrine release is critical for morphine-induced reward, reinstatement and dopamine release in the nucleus accumbens. *Cereb Cortex.* 15, 1877-1886

Verrico C.D., Jentsch J.D., Roth R.H. (2003). Persistent and anatomically selective reduction in prefrontal cortical dopamine metabolism after repeated, intermittent cannabinoid administration to rats. *Synapse.* 49, 61-66.

Vertes R.P. (2006). Interactions among the medial prefrontal cortex, hippocampus and midline thalamus in emotional and cognitive processing in the rat. *Neuroscience.* 142, 1-20.

Vijayraghavan S., Wang M., Birnbaum S.G., Williams G.V., Arnsten A.F. (2007). Inverted-U dopamine D1 receptor actions on prefrontal neurons engaged in working memory. *Nat. Neurosci.,* 10, 376-384.

Volkow ND, Wang GJ, Begleiter H, Porjesz B, Fowler JS, Telang F, Wong C, Ma Y,Logan J, Goldstein R, Alexoff D, Thanos PK. (2006). High levels of dopamine D2 receptors in unaffected members of alcoholic families: possible protective factors. *Arch Gen Psychiatry.* 63, 999-1008.

Volkow N.D., Ma Y., Zhu W., Fowler J.S., Li J., Rao M., Mueller K., Pradhan K., Wong C., Wang GJ. (2008). Moderate doses of alcohol disrupt the functional organization of the human brain. *Psychiatry Res.* 162, 205-213.

Volkow ND, Fowler JS, Wang GJ, Baler R, Telang F. (2009). Imaging dopamine's role in drug abuse and addiction. *Neuropharmacology.* 56 Suppl 1, 3-8.

Volkow N.D., Fowler J.S., Wang G.J., Telang F., Logan J., Jayne M., Ma Y., Pradhan K., Wong C., Swanson J.M. (2010). Cognitive control of drug craving inhibits brain reward regions in cocaine abusers. *Neuroimage.* 49, 2536-2543.

Volkow N.D., Wang G.J., Fowler J.S., Tomasi D., Telang F. (2011). Addiction: beyond dopamine reward circuitry. *Proc Natl Acad Sci U S A.* 108, 15037-15042.

Voorn P., Vanderschuren L.J., Groenewegen H.J., Robbins T.W., Pennartz C.M. (2004). Putting a spin on the dorsal-ventral divide of the striatum. *Trends Neurosci.* 27, 468-474.

Wang X., Zhong P., Yan Z. (2002). Dopamine D4 receptors modulate GABAergic signaling in pyramidal neurons of prefrontal cortex. *J. Neurosci.,* 22, 9185-9193.

Watanabe Y., Funahashi S. (2012). Thalamic mediodorsal nucleus and working memory. *Neurosci Biobehav Rev.* 36, 134-42.

Waterhouse B.D., Sessler F.M., Liu W., Lin C.S. (1991). Second messenger-mediated actions of norepinephrine on target neurons in central circuits: a new perspective on intracellular mechanisms and functional consequences. *Prog. Brain Res.,* 88, 351-362.

Weissenborn R., Robbins T.W., Everitt B.J. (1997). Effects of medial prefrontal or anterior cingulate cortex lesions on responding for cocaine under fixed-ratio and second-order schedules of reinforcement in rats. *Psychopharmacology (Berl)* 134, 242-57.

Williams B.R., Ponesse J.S., Schachar R.J., Logan G.D., Tannock R. (1999). Development of inhibitory control across the life span. *Dev. Psychol.,* 35, 205-213.

Williams G.V., Goldman-Rakic P.S. (1995). Modulation of memory fields by dopamine D1 receptors in prefrontal cortex. *Nature, 376,* 572-575.

Wilson S.J., Sayette M.A., Fiez J.A. (2004) Prefrontal responses to drug cues: a neurocognitive analysis. *Nat Neurosci.* 7, 211-214.

Wilson CR, Gaffan D, Browning PG, Baxter MG (2010). Functional localization within the prefrontal cortex: missing the forest for the trees? *Trends Neurosci.* 33, 533-540.

Woo T.U., Pucak M.L., Kye C.H., Matus C.V., Lewis D.A. (1997). Peripubertal refinement of the intrinsic and associational circuitry in monkey prefrontal cortex. *Neuroscience, 80,* 1149-1158.

Woodward D.J., Moises H.C., Waterhouse B.D., Yeh H.H., Cheun J.E. (1991). Modulatory actions of norepinephrine on neural circuits. *Adv. Exp. Med. Biol.,* 287, 193-208.

Zheng P., Zhang X.X., Bunney B.S., Shi W.X. (1999). Opposite modulation of cortical N-methyl-D-aspartate receptor-mediated responses by low and high concentrations of dopamine. Neuroscience, 91, 527-535.

Permissions

The contributors of this book come from diverse backgrounds, making this book a truly international effort. This book will bring forth new frontiers with its revolutionizing research information and detailed analysis of the nascent developments around the world.

We would like to thank David Belin, PhD, for lending his expertise to make the book truly unique. He has played a crucial role in the development of this book. Without his invaluable contribution this book wouldn't have been possible. He has made vital efforts to compile up to date information on the varied aspects of this subject to make this book a valuable addition to the collection of many professionals and students.

This book was conceptualized with the vision of imparting up-to-date information and advanced data in this field. To ensure the same, a matchless editorial board was set up. Every individual on the board went through rigorous rounds of assessment to prove their worth. After which they invested a large part of their time researching and compiling the most relevant data for our readers. Conferences and sessions were held from time to time between the editorial board and the contributing authors to present the data in the most comprehensible form. The editorial team has worked tirelessly to provide valuable and valid information to help people across the globe.

Every chapter published in this book has been scrutinized by our experts. Their significance has been extensively debated. The topics covered herein carry significant findings which will fuel the growth of the discipline. They may even be implemented as practical applications or may be referred to as a beginning point for another development. Chapters in this book were first published by InTech; hereby published with permission under the Creative Commons Attribution License or equivalent.

The editorial board has been involved in producing this book since its inception. They have spent rigorous hours researching and exploring the diverse topics which have resulted in the successful publishing of this book. They have passed on their knowledge of decades through this book. To expedite this challenging task, the publisher supported the team at every step. A small team of assistant editors was also appointed to further simplify the editing procedure and attain best results for the readers.

Our editorial team has been hand-picked from every corner of the world. Their multi-ethnicity adds dynamic inputs to the discussions which result in innovative outcomes. These outcomes are then further discussed with the researchers and contributors who give their valuable feedback and opinion regarding the same. The feedback is then collaborated with the researches and they are edited in a comprehensive manner to aid the understanding of the subject.

Apart from the editorial board, the designing team has also invested a significant amount of their time in understanding the subject and creating the most relevant covers. They scrutinized every image to scout for the most suitable representation of the subject and create an appropriate cover for the book.

The publishing team has been involved in this book since its early stages. They were actively engaged in every process, be it collecting the data, connecting with the contributors or procuring relevant information. The team has been an ardent support to the editorial, designing and production team. Their endless efforts to recruit the best for this project, has resulted in the accomplishment of this book. They are a veteran in the field of academics and their pool of knowledge is as vast as their experience in printing. Their expertise and guidance has proved useful at every step. Their uncompromising quality standards have made this book an exceptional effort. Their encouragement from time to time has been an inspiration for everyone.

The publisher and the editorial board hope that this book will prove to be a valuable piece of knowledge for researchers, students, practitioners and scholars across the globe.

List of Contributors

Aude Belin-Rauscent and David Belin
INSERM U 1084, LNEC, Université de Poitiers, INSERM AVENIR Team "Psychology of Compulsive Disorders", Poitiers, France

M.L. Laorden, M. V. Milanés and P. Almela
Department of Pharmacology, University of Murcia, Murcia, Spain

Karen M. von Deneen
Xidian University, China

Yijun Liu
University of Florida, USA

José Vicente Negrete-Díaz and Gonzalo Flores
Universidad Autonoma de Puebla, Puebla, Mexico

Antonio Rodríguez-Moreno
Universidad Pablo de Olavide, Sevilla, Spain

Talvinder S. Sihra
University College London, London, UK

Edgar Antonio Reyes-Montaño and Edwin Alfredo Reyes-Guzmán
Protein Research Group (Grupo de Investigación en Proteínas, GRIP), Universidad Nacional de Colombia, Sede Bogotá, Colombia

Sonia Luz Albarracín Cordero, Bernd Robert Stab II and Felipe Guillen
Pontificia Universidad Javeriana, Colombia

Edgar Antonio Reyes Montano
Universidad Nacional de Colombia, Colombia

Alfredo Ramos-Miguel, María Álvaro-Bartolomé, M. Julia García-Fuster and Jesús A. García-Sevilla
University of the Balearic Islands, Spain

Ezio Carboni, Roberto Cadeddu and Anna Rosa Carta
Dept. of Biomedical Sciences, University of Cagliari, Cagliari, Italy